Core Topics in Vascular Anaesthesia

Core Topics in Vascular Anaesthesia

Edited by

Carl Moores
Consultant Anaesthetist, Royal Infirmary of Edinburgh

Alastair F. Nimmo
Consultant Anaesthetist, Royal Infirmary of Edinburgh

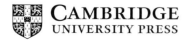

CAMBRIDGE UNIVERSITY PRESS
Cambridge, New York, Melbourne, Madrid, Cape Town,
Singapore, São Paulo, Delhi, Mexico City

Cambridge University Press
The Edinburgh Building, Cambridge CB2 8RU, UK

Published in the United States of America by
Cambridge University Press, New York

www.cambridge.org
Information on this title: www.cambridge.org/9781107001817

First published 2012

Printed in the United Kingdom at the University Press, Cambridge

A catalogue record for this publication is available from the British Library

Library of Congress Cataloging-in-Publication Data

Core topics in vascular anaesthesia / [edited by] Carl Moores,
Alastair F. Nimmo.
    p. ; cm.
  Includes bibliographical references and index.
  ISBN 978-1-107-00181-7 (Hardback)
  I. Moores, Carl. II. Nimmo, Alastair F. [DNLM: 1. Anesthesia.
2. Vascular Surgical Procedures. WG 170]
  617.96–dc23

                                                                2011052384

ISBN 978-1-107-00181-7 Hardback

Contents

List of contributors   vi
Preface   vii

1   **Arterial disease and its management**   1
Rod T. A. Chalmers

2   **Preoperative risk assessment of vascular surgery patients**   10
John Carlisle and Michael Swart

3   **Co-existing disease in vascular surgery patients**   22
John Carlisle

4   **Reducing perioperative cardiac risk**   32
Craig Beattie and Bruce Biccard

5   **Anaesthesia in the vascular surgery patient**   48
Carl Moores

6   **Monitoring in the vascular surgery patient**   52
Suzy O'Neill and Chris P. Snowden

7   **Intravenous fluid therapy**   62
Michael F. M. James and Ivan A. Joubert

8   **Haemostasis and thrombosis**   71
Gary A. Morrison and Alastair F. Nimmo

9   **Transfusion and blood conservation**   92
Alastair F. Nimmo and Danny McGee

10   **Anaesthesia for elective abdominal aortic aneurysm surgery**   101
Richard Telford

11   **Anaesthesia for thoracoabdominal aortic aneurysm surgery**   108
Carl Moores and Alastair F. Nimmo

12   **Anaesthesia for endovascular aortic repair surgery**   119
Maged Argalious

13   **Anaesthesia for emergency abdominal aortic surgery**   137
Alastair F. Nimmo

14   **Anaesthesia for aorto-iliac occlusive disease and lower limb revascularisation procedures**   146
Alastair J. Thomson

15   **Anaesthesia for lower limb amputation and the management of post-amputation pain**   161
Charles Morton and John A. Wilson

16   **Anaesthesia for carotid artery disease**   170
Mark D. Stoneham

17   **Anaesthesia for vascular surgery to the upper limb**   182
Carl Moores

18   **Surgery for vascular access in renal dialysis**   188
Carl Moores

Index   194
The colour plates are situated between pages 120 and 121.

Contributors

Maged Argalious
Associate Professor of Anesthesiology, Cleveland Clinic Lerner College of Medicine, Cleveland, OH, USA

Craig Beattie
Consultant Anaesthetist, Royal Infirmary of Edinburgh, Edinburgh, UK

Bruce Biccard
Department of Anaesthetics, Nelson R. Mandela School of Medicine, University of Kwazulu–Natal, Republic of South Africa

John Carlisle
Consultant Anaesthetist, Torbay Hospital, Torquay, UK

Rod T. A. Chalmers
Consultant Vascular Surgeon, Royal Infirmary of Edinburgh, Edinburgh, UK

Michael F. M. James
Professor of Anaesthesia, University of Cape Town and Groote Schuur Hospital, Western Cape, Republic of South Africa

Ivan A. Joubert
Head of Clinical Unit (Critical Care, Department of Anaesthesia), University of Cape Town and Groote Schuur Hospital, Western Cape, Republic of South Africa

Danny McGee
Specialist Practitioner in Blood Transfusion, Better Blood Transfusion, Scottish National Blood Transfusion Service, Edinburgh, UK

Carl Moores
Consultant Anaesthetist, Royal Infirmary of Edinburgh, Edinburgh, UK

Gary A. Morrison
Consultant Anaesthetist, Royal Infirmary of Edinburgh, Edinburgh, UK

Charles Morton
Consultant Anaesthetist, Royal Infirmary of Edinburgh, Edinburgh, UK

Alastair F. Nimmo
Consultant Anaesthetist, Royal Infirmary of Edinburgh, Edinburgh, UK

Suzy O'Neill
Consultant Anaesthetist, Freeman Hospital, Newcastle upon Tyne, UK

Chris P. Snowden
Consultant Anaesthetist, Freeman Hospital. Newcastle upon Tyne, UK

Mark D. Stoneham
Consultant Anaesthetist, Nuffield Department of Anaesthesia, Oxford, UK

Michael Swart
Consultant Anaesthetist, Torbay Hospital, Torquay, UK

Richard Telford
Consultant Anaesthetist, Royal Devon and Exeter Hospital, Exeter, UK

Alastair J. Thomson
Consultant Anaesthetist, Royal Infirmary of Edinburgh, Edinburgh, UK

John A. Wilson
Consultant Anaesthetist, Royal Infirmary of Edinburgh, Edinburgh, UK

Preface

Vascular surgery and anaesthesia have undergone great changes during the past decade so that this book is very different from previous books describing the anaesthetic and perioperative management of vascular surgical patients. Endovascular repair has been widely adopted for the elective repair of abdominal aortic aneurysms and is increasingly being used in the treatment of ruptured aneurysms. Advanced fenestrated and branched stent grafts have been introduced for the treatment of suprarenal and thoracoabdominal aneurysms, and 'hybrid' repair – the combination of endovascular and open surgery – now offers another alternative to the treatment of complex aneurysms. However, all of these procedures are accompanied by their own risks for the patient and challenges for the surgeon and anaesthetist. The number of elderly patients with comorbidities presenting for vascular surgery and their expectations of what medical care can provide have increased and many patients continue to require open surgery. This book provides extensive coverage of the current perioperative management of both endovascular and open vascular surgical procedures including aneurysm surgery, carotid surgery and revascularisation and amputation for limb ischaemia.

Patient assessment before surgery, and monitoring during surgery, have advanced greatly in recent years. Cardiopulmonary exercise testing (CPET) has become widely used, often as part of anaesthetist-led pre-assessment clinics which aim to help the surgeon and patient decide whether the benefits of intervention outweigh the risks. The chapter on preoperative risk assessment gives a clear description of the role of CPET in patients being considered for surgery. Advances in intraoperative monitoring that are discussed include the use of transoesophageal echocardiography and minimally invasive cardiac output monitoring.

Our understanding of normal haemostasis and how it is disturbed during surgery has also advanced greatly, while new anticoagulant drugs have been introduced and the risks of blood transfusion have become more widely appreciated. The causes, diagnosis and treatment of coagulation abnormalities in vascular surgery patients are described including the value of point-of-care testing of haemostasis. Modern transfusion practice and blood conservation are discussed as is the controversial area of intravenous fluid therapy during surgery.

Much has been published in recent years on reducing the risk of perioperative cardiac complications and on the benefits and risks of drug therapy including beta-blockers, coronary artery stents and coronary artery bypass grafts before vascular surgery. However, this also remains an area of controversy. The chapter on reducing perioperative cardiac risk provides a clear review of the literature and recommendations for practice.

The contributing authors are acknowledged experts in their fields and we would like to thank them for the time and effort that they have put into producing contributions that are not only informative but also interesting and stimulating. And, finally, we would like to thank our publishers for their support and patience.

Arterial disease and its management

Rod T. A. Chalmers

Introduction

In this chapter, an overview of the arterial pathologies that present commonly to the vascular surgeon will be given. Included will be a summary of pathophysiology and epidemiology of these conditions as well as their clinical assessment and the imaging modalities used in contemporary practice. Finally, available treatment options, both open surgery and endovascular, will be summarised.

Atherosclerosis

Atherosclerosis is a disease of large and medium-sized arteries and results in the build-up of cholesterol, lipid, calcium, smooth muscle cells and other cell debris in the tunica intima of the involved vessel. The cause of this accumulation is complex and multifactorial, but the common theme is an injury to the vascular endothelium that sets off a cascade of events leading to plaque formation. There are different types of injury at work simultaneously including chemical (e.g. noxious agents present in cigarette smoke, hyperglycaemia, hyperlipidaemia) and physical issues (e.g. the presence of untreated hypertension, a predisposition for plaque development at points of high shear stress in the arterial tree such as at the carotid bifurcation). A section of carotid endothelium, excised during a carotid endarterectomy, is shown in Figure 1.1. The specimen contains an ulcerated atheromatous plaque. The earliest manifestation of atherosclerosis is the 'fatty streak' and as the name suggests this is the visible accumulation of lipids and inflammatory cells in the tunica intima below the endothelium. In the Western world, most people in their 20s will have evidence of fatty streak formation. With lesion progression,

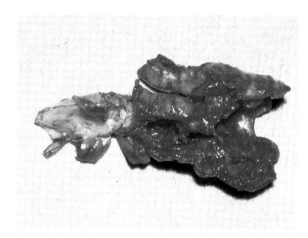

Figure 1.1 Specimen from carotid endarterectomy showing acute ulceration of active carotid plaque.

lipid and smooth muscle cell proliferation results in a fibrous plaque, which encroaches on the vessel lumen. On the luminal aspect the endothelium becomes increasingly attenuated as a so-called fibrous cap. Eventually this cap gives way and plaque rupture occurs. It is at this juncture that acute vessel occlusion can occur or distal atheroembolisation and these events correlate with significant clinical sequelae (for example, acute myocardial infarction, limb ischaemia, carotid territory transient ischaemic attack or stroke).

Although it is clearly a systemic disorder, vascular surgeons encounter atherosclerotic occlusive disease in certain specific locations. Most common is lower limb disease giving rise to intermittent claudication and if more severe, limb-threatening critical ischaemia. Carotid artery disease is a common cause of stroke and is a frequent manifestation of the disease.

Core Topics in Vascular Anaesthesia, ed. Carl Moores and Alastair F. Nimmo. Published by Cambridge University Press.
© Cambridge University Press 2012.

Peripheral arterial disease

Epidemiology

The Edinburgh Artery Study demonstrated that symptomatic peripheral arterial disease (intermittent claudication) is present in 2–7% of 50–74-year-olds [1]. Asymptomatic disease, detected by ankle–brachial pressure measurements is commoner, affecting about a quarter of the population over 50 years of age. The major risk factors for the development of peripheral arterial disease (PAD) include cigarette smoking, hypertension, diabetes mellitus and hypercholesterolaemia.

The recently published REACH registry data confirm the serious prognosis for patients with a diagnosis of lower limb arterial disease [2]. Over the first 12 months of the study, 21% of patients with PAD either died from cardiovascular disease, suffered a non-fatal myocardial infarction or stroke or were admitted to hospital because of another vascular event. Patients who in addition to PAD also had symptoms of coronary artery disease and/or cerebrovascular disease had a substantially higher incidence of these events.

Clinical presentation

Clearly the mode of presentation will be dictated by the vascular bed involved.

Lower limb ischaemia presents as either non-limb-threatening intermittent claudication or critical ischaemia with the presence of opiate-dependent rest pain and/or tissue loss or gangrene. Clinically, the level of occlusion(s) can be estimated by the presence or absence of pulses at groin, popliteal or ankle level. The measurement of ankle–brachial pressure indices is helpful but beware patients with heavily calcified vessels (e.g. diabetics) in whom the ankle vessels are incompressible and pressure measurements not particularly helpful.

Cerebrovascular events (transient ischaemic attack or stroke) can frequently be caused by embolisation from active plaques affecting the proximal internal carotid arteries. The decision about management is made based upon the degree of carotid stenosis present and the time from event to presentation. Drop attacks due to subclavian steal typically arise when patients have been using the upper limb above head level. Absent ipsilateral upper limb pulses will be the clinical clue to the diagnosis.

Mesenteric ischaemia is often a diagnosis made too late when irreversible bowel ischaemia has

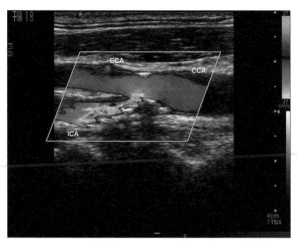

Figure 1.2 Duplex ultrasound demonstrates the presence of plaque at the carotid bifurcation. See plate section for colour version.

developed. When chronic, the symptoms of weight loss, post-prandial abdominal pain and diarrhoea and fear of food should point to the diagnosis. Co-existing atherosclerotic disease (lower limb ischaemia, ischaemic heart disease) should heighten clinical suspicion.

Aggressive surgical or endovascular intervention for renovascular disease presenting as either deteriorating renal function or drug-resistant hypertension has become far less common than was previously the case. Evidence gathered over the years indicates that most interventions do not confer any advantage over drug therapy, the ASTRAL trial being the most recent evidence base for this approach [3].

Investigation of arterial disease

Nowadays, the vast majority of patients can be investigated non-invasively. Duplex ultrasound gives very clear images of much of the arterial tree. As well as a grey-scale image, colour flow and spectral waveform analysis allow accurate delineation of the extent and degree of arterial stenosis and occlusion. Figure 1.2 is a duplex ultrasound of a carotid bifurcation with colour flow imaging which shows narrowing and turbulent flow in the internal carotid artery. In some situations, such as aorto-iliac disease not easy to visualise with duplex or mesenteric arterial disease, alternative imaging modalities are necessary. Magnetic resonance angiography (MRA) has become a very valuable tool in this setting. There is no need for ionising radiation or iodinated contrast and often it complements information obtained from duplex ultrasound. One has to remember that MRA is not safe for patients with significantly deranged renal function as there is a well-documented potential risk of disseminated systemic fibrosis [4]. Computerised tomographic angiography (CTA) can be helpful in such patients, but heavy calcification can compromise the quality of images obtained.

It is relatively rare in contemporary practice to use intra-arterial angiography as a tool to investigate occlusive disease. Rather this technique comes to the fore during (endovascular) intervention.

Treatment

Lower limb ischaemia

At initial presentation, patients with intermittent claudication will be carefully assessed clinically. All risk factors should be corrected, especially smoking. It is not uncommon to diagnose diabetes mellitus in this patient group and this should be managed appropriately. Hypercholesterolaemia and hyperlipidaemia should be identified and appropriate treatment with statin therapy commenced. There is strong evidence for administering statins to these patients irrespective of their lipid profile [5].

Depending on the social circumstances (e.g. symptoms threatening employment) most surgeons manage newly diagnosed claudicants conservatively in the first instance with risk factor control and exercise. There is considerable evidence for the beneficial outcome of this approach [6].

However, as angioplasty and stenting are readily available, particularly when risk factors have been controlled, intervention is not unreasonable. Certainly iliac artery disease giving rise to disabling buttock and thigh claudication responds very well to angioplasty and stenting with durable results [7]. Compared to the available surgical options (e.g. aortofemoral and iliofemoral bypass) with the attendant risks and complications, percutaneous intervention is a good option.

Infrainguinal disease is not so straightforward. Although the results of balloon angioplasty for short stenoses and occlusions are reasonable, more often than not there will be disease of considerable lengths of the superficial femoral artery. Although these lesions can usually be reopened percutaneously, either transluminally or more often subintimally, the medium and long-term patency rates are not great and failure necessitates reintervention or even conversion to surgery.

It is relatively uncommon to proceed with surgery for intermittent claudication in modern practice. This is largely a result of the available endovascular options and the not inconsiderable risk of surgery in these patients. However, there are a few exceptions. Younger patients with extensive aorto-iliac disease get the most durable long-term result from direct aortobifemoral bypass. Careful assessment for occult coronary disease is important prior to surgery. Unilateral iliac occlusions can be treated with low risk either by iliofemoral or femorofemoral bypass.

The approach to surgical intervention for infrainguinal occlusive disease has changed considerably. In the 1980s it was common practice to insert prosthetic above-knee grafts in such patients. Time has taught us that often these grafts fail due to disease progression and patients re-present with critical ischaemia. Good-quality long saphenous vein should be the bypass conduit of choice in this setting [8].

The situation in critical ischaemia is different. Investigations will confirm the location and extent of disease. Often disease is present at multiple levels and so this needs to be taken into account. The underlying principle is that good inflow is a must. Often if this is achieved (percutaneously or surgically) and the profunda femoris artery is patent, adequate revascularisation will result.

For infrainguinal disease many surgeons will adopt an angioplasty-first approach as these patients have a poor prognosis (40–50% mortality at 2 years). The BASIL trial indicated that this was reasonable for patients with a short life expectancy but for patients with greater than 2 years' life expectancy who had good-quality saphenous vein, surgical bypass was the better option [9].

Carotid artery disease

Since the early 1990s, clinical practice has been guided by the results of the North American and European Symptomatic Carotid Surgery Trials (NASCET and ECST) [10,11]. For patients with high-grade symptomatic carotid artery stenosis, carotid endarterectomy (CEA) provides significant protection from stroke compared to best medical therapy (BMT). The subsequent asymptomatic carotid surgery trials, albeit the North American trial was stopped early because of the steering committee's feeling that surgery was significantly superior to BMT, also showed a benefit but far less impressive than for symptomatic patients [12,13], In the UK, most vascular surgeons are fairly selective about offering CEA to asymptomatic patients. The group with greatest benefit appears to be men under the age of 68 years with bilateral high-grade carotid stenoses.

There is increasing evidence to suggest that the benefit of intervention is greatest in the first few days after the index event. There is now an ongoing effort to educate the public and non-vascular medical practitioners to recognise the emergent nature of transient ischaemic attack (TIA) and the need for immediate assessment of these patients. Many hospitals have developed TIA clinics that operate in a similar fashion to acute chest pain clinics. Pathways have been developed for urgent referral to vascular services for CEA within 2 weeks of the index event [14].

There are a lot of data in the Cochrane Database now regarding the conduct of CEA. Conventional endarterectomy with routine patching are recommended. The GALA trial failed to demonstrate a significant advantage in terms of operative stroke, death or complication for the use of regional over general anaesthesia and so it is recommended that the operating team use the approach that yields the best results in their hands. The use of shunts is another controversial subject. Under regional anaesthesia this use can be selective with most surgeons shunting about 10% of patients. Operators using general anaesthesia use either routine shunting or selective shunting based upon intraoperative monitoring (transcranial Doppler, oximetry, EEG, etc.).

Carotid angioplasty and stenting (CAS) is now fairly widespread in clinical practice in Europe and the USA. In both of these regions, the majority of patients treated are asymptomatic. Many randomised trials of variable quality have been performed over the years. Suffice it to say that the jury is still out, especially for the use of this technology in acutely symptomatic patients. The most recently published trial data indicated a significantly higher stroke rate for CAS vs. CEA in symptomatic patients [15].

Subclavian/innominate artery disease

Patients with occlusive disease of these vessels present in a variety of ways depending on the extent of disease. Subclavian artery origin disease is often asymptomatic but can give rise to subclavian steal. Investigations will demonstrate reversal of flow in the vertebral artery affected.

Traditional surgical options are carotid to subclavian bypass or subclavian transposition. The majority of symptomatic patients can be treated by balloon angioplasty and stenting.

Similarly innominate stenosis can be managed by endovascular means but there is a not insignificant stroke risk. Also these lesions tend to be heavily calcified and often cannot be reopened by balloon techniques. Occasionally direct surgical bypass from the ascending aorta is necessary. This is a major procedure with considerable operative risk and requires sternotomy. Such operations are seen pretty rarely.

Mesenteric arterial disease

The options for patients with chronic mesenteric ischaemia are either surgical bypass or balloon angioplasty and/or stenting. Surgery is probably the more durable reconstruction but is associated with risk of mortality and morbidity. The traditional procedures are either bypass to the superior mesenteric artery (SMA) directly from the infrarenal aorta, retrograde bypass from the right iliac system (if the aorta is heavily diseased) or bypass from the supracoeliac aorta often combined with coeliac revascularisation. The key is adequate revascularisation of the SMA [16].

There is a growing pool of data on the results of endovascular mesenteric revascularisation. Results are best for short proximal lesions usually combining angioplasty and stenting [17].

Aortic aneurysm disease
Pathology

The development of aneurysmal disease of the aorta is a complex, multifactorial pathology.

There are probably a number of different mechanisms at play including enzymatic degradation of the aortic wall (increased collagenase, metalloproteinase and elastase activity has been demonstrated), inflammatory cell infiltration (macrophages and lymphocytes) giving rise to increased cytokine activity and enzyme secretion, biomechanical factors including wall shear stress in combination with biochemical events and a likely genetic predisposition in combination with these other factors.

Histologically, aneurysm tissue demonstrates loss of elastin and collagen in the tunica media together with decreased numbers of smooth muscle cells, inflammatory cell infiltration and neovascularisation.

About 90% of aortic aneurysms involve the infrarenal aorta, the remaining 10% variably involving

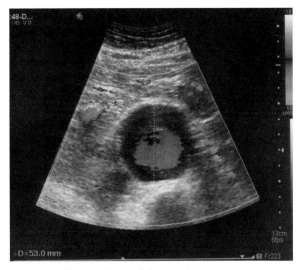

Figure 1.3 Ultrasound scan of abdominal aortic aneurysm.
See plate section for colour version.

the thoracic and thoracoabdominal aorta. The male : female ratio for infrarenal abdominal aortic aneurysm (AAA) is at least 5 : 1. whereas that for thoracic and thoracoabdominal aneurysms is about 1.5 : 1. There is a strong familial tendency with male siblings being ten times more likely to have an aneurysm. The disease affects patients in their 60s and 70s although younger patients can be affected if they have an underlying connective tissue disease such as Marfan syndrome.

Clinical presentation

The majority of patients are asymptomatic. Diagnosis is often made during routine abdominal palpation or more commonly as a coincidental finding when investigations are performed for other reasons (e.g. investigation of the urinary tract). Figure 1.3 shows an abdominal ultrasound scan demonstrating an aortic aneurysm.

As population screening is unfortunately not yet undertaken in most countries, today still a considerable proportion of patients with AAA present acutely with aortic rupture.

Management

Asymptomatic patients with AAA maximum diameter less than 5.5 cm are typically managed in surveillance programmes with serial ultrasound measurement of maximum anteroposterior aneurysm diameter [18]. For AAA between 3 and 4 cm, scans are repeated annually; for lesions between 4 and 5 cm 6-monthly and between 5 and 5.5 cm 3-monthly.

When AAA diameter exceeds 5.5 cm, intervention should be contemplated. At this size annual rupture risk is probably between 3% and 7%, rising to about 10% at 6 cm and exceeding 20% above 7 cm.

The assessment of fitness for intervention is covered elsewhere in this book.

Assuming patients are deemed fit for intervention, the options for treatment are either open surgical repair (OR) or endovascular repair (EVAR). The EVAR I trial demonstrated a significantly lower operative mortality for EVAR vs. OR in patients fit for OR (1.75 vs. 4.7%) [19]. Over follow-up, the survival curves for the two groups remained parallel for about 4 years after which they crossed and when the trial was closed at 8 years, EVAR patients seemed to have fared rather less well in terms of aneurysm-related mortality. All late-ruptured AAA were seen in the EVAR group [20]. The Achilles heel of EVAR is the need for lifelong monitoring of the grafts and reintervention on a proportion of patients. The late results of the trial are a slight cause for concern when considering this modality for relatively young, fit patients.

The decision about the feasibility of EVAR is dictated by various anatomical issues. A proximal landing zone for the stent graft that is adequate to seal the infrarenal aorta above the aneurysm sac is necessary. This should be 15–20 mm in length, be of relatively uniform, undiseased diameter aorta and not be excessively angulated. Distally iliac involvement may dictate where the iliac limbs are deployed and this may lead to the need to sacrifice one of the internal iliac arteries. In order that the sheath containing the stent-graft can be passed safely retrograde from the femoral arteries into the aorta, it is necessary that the (external) iliac artery has a minimum diameter of 7 mm. In Figure 1.4 an endovascular stent can be seen in place following a stent-graft repair of an infrarenal aortic aneurysm.

As stent-graft technology progresses the boundaries can be pushed out to treat shorter, more angulated aneurysm necks and as the devices are mounted on lower-profile delivery devices, so smaller iliac access will not be a barrier to successful EVAR.

When it was first developed, it was envisaged that EVAR would be especially useful in treating patients with large AAA unfit for open surgery. The EVAR II trial compared the outcome for patients thought unfit

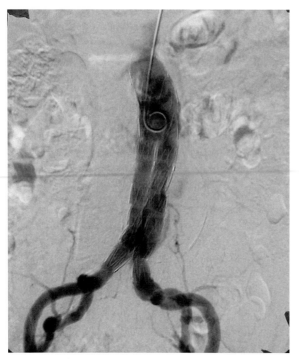

Figure 1.4 Completion angiogram at completion of endovascular stent-graft repair of aortic aneurysm.

for open repair who were randomised to EVAR or medical therapy [21]. A number of criticisms were levelled at the trial methodology. The definition of 'unfit for open repair' was not particularly well defined and so a spectrum of level of fitness was probably randomised. There was a not inconsiderable number of patients who crossed over during the trial from the medical treatment group to EVAR. Even so, at 4 years almost 70% of patients in each group had died from non-aneurysm-related causes. Thus the rather surprising and disappointing conclusion from the EVAR II trial was that patients with AAA who are unfit for open surgery should not be offered EVAR or open repair.

Suprarenal and thoracoabdominal aneurysm repair

The situation for aneurysms involving the suprarenal, thoracoabdominal and thoracic aorta is more complicated. Open surgery requires a more complex strategy as these procedures involve a degree of visceral ischaemia reperfusion. For extensive thoracoabdominal aortic aneurysms (TAAA) this includes potential ischaemic injury to the spinal cord and resulting paraplegia.

Early exponents of thoracoabdominal aneurysm repair had no choice but to adopt the so-called 'clamp

and go' technique. This involved clamping the aorta above and below the aneurysm (e.g. the proximal descending thoracic aorta and common iliac arteries), opening the entire aneurysm sac and performing proximal aortic and visceral branch anastomoses as quickly as possible. This was extremely stressful for patient and surgeon alike! Not surprisingly the complications, especially spinal cord and renal, increased significantly in direct relation to the duration of clamping. Nowadays, these operations are best performed in centres with extensive experience as the literature confirms a direct correlation between volume and outcome [22].

In addition, surgeons performing TAAA surgery make use of a number of intraoperative adjuncts to help reduce the incidence of spinal cord and abdominal organ dysfunction. The operations are done using a sequential clamp technique. In conjunction with left heart bypass and a centrifugal pump the abdominal organs and spinal cord can be perfused retrograde via a left femoral artery cannula during the procedure. Body temperature can be lowered as required (e.g. to 31–32 °C). When the visceral arteries are being anastomosed their perfusion can be maintained using selective cannulation [23]. The spinal cord is protected in a number of ways including drainage of cerebrospinal fluid, reimplantation of intercostal arteries during the operation and the maintenance of mean arterial pressure above 80 mm Hg during the first few days postoperatively. Some centres also monitor motor evoked potentials during the operation and this helps direct the best intercostals arteries to reimplant [24]. All of these techniques have greatly improved the results of this surgery. In centres of excellence repair of appropriately selected patients with extensive TAAAs is associated with operative mortality of 5–10%, paraplegia rates of 2–4% and dialysis-dependent renal failure rates of under 5%.

Thoracic endovascular aneurysm repair (TEVAR)

Endovascular stent-graft technology has revolutionised the management of thoracic aortic pathology. Isolated aneurysms of the descending thoracic aorta should all be treated using this technology nowadays. Instead of thoracotomy, heart bypass etc. grafts can be deployed via a small groin incision and femoral arteriotomy. Depending on the length of aorta to be covered cerebrospinal fluid drainage may be required and if it is necessary to cover the left subclavian artery proximally, carotid–subclavian bypass is recommended to reduce paraplegia and stroke risk. Otherwise these procedures are very straightforward and recovery time is a matter of 2 or 3 days. The procedure can be performed under regional anaesthesia. For thoracic aneurysms involving the aortic arch and thoracoabdominal lesions involving the visceral segment a number of options for endovascular treatment are available [25]. It is often possible to perform extra-anatomic grafts relocating the inflow to the carotid and left subclavian arteries thereby creating an adequate proximal landing zone for stent-graft deployment. Indeed, on occasions it is possible to ligate the origin of the innominate artery, take a graft from the proximal ascending aorta to the innominate bifurcation and perform right carotid to left carotid and left carotid to subclavian grafts creating a proximal landing zone in the ascending aorta. This means that aortic arch aneurysms can be treated by endovascular means without aortic cross-clamp. Although this approach requires a sternotomy, compared to the open surgical option which is hypothermic arrest with all of its associated complications, patients tolerate this procedure well.

Similarly, within the abdomen, retrograde revascularisation of the coeliac axis, superior mesenteric and renal arteries can be achieved with multiple grafts from the iliac arteries [26]. This allows stent-grafts to be deployed within aneurysmal disease of the thoracoabdoinal aorta including the abdominal visceral segment.

More recently, stent-graft technology has progressed further such that fenestrated and multibranched stent-grafts have been developed to allow an entirely endovascular approach to the repair of these complex aneurysms [27]. This technology is in its relative infancy and thus far is limited to highly selected patients in a few pioneering centres. Extensive coverage of the thoracoabdominal aorta during TEVAR is associated with higher paraplegia rates than one sees in open surgery.

Aortic dissection

This refers to an acute tear in the tunica intima of the aorta that leads to blood flowing in a second channel located in the tunica media and extending proximally or distally to a variable extent. The term dissection is somewhat historical (and probably a post-mortem finding in days gone by). Nowadays, largely based upon the sophisticated imaging that we have available the term acute aortic syndrome is a useful term and

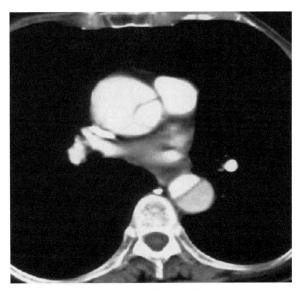

Figure 1.5 Computed tomography scan of an acute type A aortic dissection.

covers the initiating event. The site of the intimal tear can be located in the ascending or descending aorta and its location dictates the clinical sequelae.

About 60% of acute aortic dissections have an entry tear in the proximal ascending aorta and extend distally into the descending aorta to a variable extent (DeBakey type I). DeBakey type II dissections are restricted to the ascending aorta only. These two subgroups constitute the so-called Stanford type A dissections. Dissections that commence at or just beyond the left subclavian artery and propagate distally are known as DeBakey type III or Stanford type B dissections and account for about one-third of cases.

Men are affected twice as often as women. Pre-existing, poorly controlled hypertension is present in almost 80% of patients. Age at presentation is most often 50–70 years of age. Ten per cent of patients will suffer from a connective tissue disorder, most often Marfan syndrome.

Acute Stanford type A dissections are a cardiac surgical emergency. A CT scan of such a dissection is shown in Figure 1.5. If the aorta has not ruptured freely but there has been a contained rupture often with retrograde propagation involving the coronary ostia and aortic valve with or without haemopericardium, emergency surgical replacement of the ascending aorta with reimplantation of the coronaries and aortic valve resuspension or replacement if necessary is the treatment of choice. At this procedure the false lumen is closed distally just proximal to the innominate artery origin, but the remainder of the aorta is left, unless there is evidence of distal visceral or lower limb ischaemia. In a proportion of patients the false lumen remains perfused distally as there are often multiple entry tears and in this situation late aneurysmal change can develop.

Stanford type B dissections can present as acute aortic rupture. As for type A lesions, this is most likely to occur in the first 24 hours after acute dissection, decreasing in incidence with the passage of time. Conventional treatment of uncomplicated type B dissections is conservative with aggressive control of systemic blood pressure. Intervention in the acute phase has traditionally been reserved for contained leak and distal vascular compromise. About 20% of patients who survive the acute event will develop late aneurysmal change in the dissected segment of aorta due to expansion of the thin-walled, perfused false lumen. It is for this reason that some enthusiasts advocate early endovascular intervention for all type B dissections [28]. In theory, by placing a thoracic stent-graft over the entry tear within a short time of the acute event one prevents ongoing perfusion of the false lumen, and encourages flow to be directed through the true lumen thereby allowing the aorta to remodel and avoid aneurysmal change developing later. By the same token, others have argued that up to 80% of uncomplicated type B dissections do not develop late aneurysmal change and so the majority of these interventions are pointless. Most clinicians would look for evidence of early dilatation of the proximal descending aorta on CT scan soon after the acute event. In such circumstances, TEVAR is a very appealing option. Endovascular treatment of chronic type B dissections is notoriously less easy to achieve because of difficulty with adequate length of proximal landing zones and because chronic dissection flaps tend to be very rigid and difficult to seal with stent-grafts.

References

1. Fowkes FGR, Housley E, Cawood EHH, et al. Edinburgh Artery Study: prevalence of asymptomatic and symptomatic peripheral arterial disease in the general population. *Int J Epidemiol* 1991;**20**:384–92.

2. Alberts MJ, Bhatt DL, Mas JL, et al. Three-year follow-up and event rates in the International Reduction of Atherothrombosis for Continued Health. *Registry Eur Heart J* 2009; **30**:2318–26.

3. Wheatley K, Ives N, Gray R, et al. Revascularisation versus medical therapy for renal artery stenosis. *N Engl. J Med* 2009;**361**:1953–62.

4. Martin DR. Nephrogenic systemic fibrosis and gadolinium-enhanced magnetic resonance imaging: does a US Food and Drug Administration alert influence practice patterns in chronic kidney disease? *Am J Kidney Dis* 2010;**56**:427–30.

5. Ward S, Lloyd Jones M, Pandor A, et al. 2007. A systematic review and economic evaluation of statins for the prevention of coronary events. *Health Tech Assess* 2007;**11**:1–160.

6. Lee HL, Mehta T, Ray B, et al. A non-randomised clinical trial of the clinical and cost effectiveness of a supervised exercise programme for claudication. *Eur J Vasc Endovasc Surg* 2007; **33**:202–7.

7. Koizuma A, Kamakura H, Kanai H, et al. Ten year patency and factors causing restenosis after endovascular treatment of iliac artery lesions. *Circ J* 2009;**73**:860–6.

8. Norgren L, Hiatt WR, Dormandy JA, et al. Inter-society consensus for the management of peripheral arterial disease (TASC II). *J Vasc Surg* 2007;**45**:S5–67.

9. Bradbury AW, Adam DJ, Bell J, et al. Bypass versus angioplasty in severe ischaemia of the leg (BASIL) trial: a intention-to-treat analysis of amputation-free survival in patients randomised to a bypass surgery-first or balloon angioplasty-first revascularisation strategy. *J Vasc Surg* 2010;**51** (5 Suppl):5–17.

10. North American Symptomatic Carotid Endarterectomy Trial Collaborators. Beneficial effect of carotid endarterectomy in symptomatic patients with high-grade stenosis. *N Engl J Med* 1991;**325**:445–53.

11. European Carotid Trialists Group. MRC European Carotid Surgery Trial: interim results for symptomatic patients with severe (70–99%) or mild (0–29%) carotid stenosis. *Lancet* 1991;**337**: 1235–43.

12. Executive Committee for the Asymptomatic Carotid Atherosclerosis Study. Endarterectomy for asymptomatic Carotid artery stenosis. *JAMA* 1995;**273**:1421–8.

13. Halliday A, Mansfield AO, Merro J, et al. Prevention of disabling and fatal strokes by successful CEA in patients without recent neurological symptoms: randomised controlled trial. *Lancet* 2004;**363**:1491–502.

14. Scottish Intercollegiate Guidelines Network. *Management of Patients with Stroke or TIA: A National Clinical Guideline.* Edinburgh: SIGN, 2008.

15. Ederle J, Dobson J, Featherstone RL, *et al.* Carotid artery stenting compared to endarterectomy in patients with symptomatic carotid stenosis (International Carotid Stenting Trial): an interim analysis of a randomised controlled trial. *Lancet* 2010; **375**:985–97.

16. Oderich GS, Gloviczki P, Bower TC. Open surgical treatment of chronic mesenteric ischaemia in the endovascular era: when is it necessary and what is the preferred technique? *Semin Vasc Surg* 2010;**23**:36–46.

17. Sharafadden MJ, Olson CH, Sun S, *et al.* Endovascular treatment of celiac and mesenteric artery stenosis: applications and results. *J Vasc Surg* 2003;**38**:692–8.

18. UK Small Aneurysm Study Participants. Mortality results for randomised trial of early elective surgery or ultrasonic surveillance for small abdominal aortic aneurysms. *Lancet* 1999;**352**:1649–55.

19. EVAR Trial Participants. Endovascular aneurysm repair versus open repair in patients with abdominal aortic aneurysm (EVAR I trial): randomised controlled trial. *Lancet* 2005; **365**:2179–86.

20. Powell JT, Brown LC. Long-term results of the UK EVAR trials: the sting in the tail. *Eur J Vasc Endovasc Surg* 2010;**40**:44–7.

21. EVAR Trial Participants. Endovascular aneurysm repair and outcome in patients unfit for open repair of abdominal aortic aneurysm (EVAR II trial): randomised controlled trial. *Lancet* 2005;**365**:2187–92.

22. Cowan JA, Dimick JB, Henke PK, *et al.* Surgical treatment of intact thoraco-abdominal aortic aneurysms in the United States: hospital and surgeon volume-related outcomes. *J Vasc Surg* 2003;**37**:1169–74.

23. Estrera AL, Miller CC, Chen EP, *et al.* Descending thoracic aortic aneurysm: a 12-year experience using distal aortic perfusion and CSF drainage. *Ann Thorac Surg* 2005;**80**:1290–6.

24. Jacobs MJ, Mess W, Mochter B. The value of motor-evoked potentials in reducing paraplegia during thoraco-abdominal aneurysm repair. *J Vasc Surg* 2006;**43**:239–46.

25. Koullas GJ, Wheatley GH. State of the art hybrid procedures for the aortic arch: a meta-analysis. *Ann Thorac Surg* 2010;**90**:68–97.

26. Biasi L, Ai T, Loosemore T, *et al.* Hybrid repair of complex thoraco-abdominal aneurysms using applied endovascular strategies with visceral and renal revascularisation. *J Thorac Cardiovasc Surg* 2009;**138**:1331–8.

27. Greenburg RK, Steinburgh WC, Makaroum M, *et al.* 2009. Intermediate results of a US multicenter trial of fenestrated endograft repair for juxtarenal abdominal aortic aneurysms. *J Vasc Surg* 2009;**50**:730–7.

28. Tang DG, Dake MD. 2009. TEVAR for acute uncomplicated aortic dissection: immediate repair versus medical therapy. *Semin Vasc Surg* 2009;**22**:145–51.

Preoperative risk assessment of vascular surgery patients

John Carlisle and Michael Swart

Vascular surgery is a potent unnatural selector of the fittest. The more likely it is that a patient will die after scheduled surgery the more reason he or she should consult a senior anaesthetist preoperatively. This consultation should be scheduled soon after identification of pathology that could be treated surgically. This includes small abdominal aortic aneurysms (AAAs) detected by chance or through screening. Patients should have as much time as possible to consider their options and shift risk of harm to risk of benefit.

This chapter reviews preoperative survival assessment for vascular surgical patients. Further details are in chapters specific to particular operations. Throughout this chapter the word 'risk' is synonymous with 'chance'. We concentrate on assessment and preparation of patients with AAAs: screening will make this operation more common, postoperative mortality is high and it is uncertain what proportion of patients benefit and what proportion are harmed.

Benefit versus harm in surgery
Health objectives

The aim of surgery can be palliation of existing symptoms (peripheral arterial bypass surgery for pain). It can also be used to prevent future symptoms (carotid endarterectomy for stroke). Surgery can benefit patients by making life better and possibly longer. Surgery can worsen quality of life and reduce its duration. Preoperative preparation is a cooperative venture between patient, surgeon and anaesthetist intended to quantify the risks of benefit and harm, coupled with attempts to shift their balance in the patient's favour.

Evidence that vascular surgery works

The effect of an intervention is best disentangled from confounding factors by testing in randomised controlled trials (RCTs). Surgery should be justified by improved survival and quality of life. However, RCTs do not support vascular surgery except carotid endarterectomy (CEA) in symptomatic patients.

- RCT evidence does not justify bypass surgery for chronic leg ischaemia (no RCTs).
- RCT evidence does not prefer surgery to exercise for chronic leg ischaemia (one RCT).
- RCT evidence does not justify endovascular stenting for chronic leg ischaemia (two RCTs).
- RCT evidence does not justify elective repair of AAAs between 4 cm and 5.5 cm diameter (two RCTs).
- RCT evidence does not justify elective repair of AAAs larger than 5.5 cm diameter (one RCT).
- RCT evidence for endarterectomy of asymptomatic stenotic carotid arteries is equivocal (three RCTs).
- RCT evidence does not justify elective thoracic endovascular aortic repair for stable type B aortic dissections (one RCT).
- 1 in 20 symptomatic patients with >50% angiographic stenotic carotid arteries benefit within 4 years of endarterectomy, whereas 19/20 do not (outcome death from recurrent stroke or transient ischaemic attack) (two RCTs).

Other vascular surgeries continue on the assumption that other sources of evidence, such as observational data, have sufficiently evaded inherent biases that the impression we have of net benefit is correct. For instance people die from ruptured AAAs, mortality after emergency AAA surgery is higher than after elective AAA surgery, larger AAAs have a higher incidence of rupture. Of course many people with AAAs die from other causes. Interpretation of all

Core Topics in Vascular Anaesthesia, ed. Carl Moores and Alastair F. Nimmo. Published by Cambridge University Press.
© Cambridge University Press 2012.

Table 2.1 The number of vascular operations and observed postoperative 30-day mortality in the Netherlands 1991–2005: expected deaths matched for fe/male proportions and reported comorbidities, adjusted to median year of observation (1997)

Procedure	Number	Observed deaths	Expected deaths	O/E ratio
Carotid endarterectomy	20 937	256	79	3.2
Peripheral arterial bypass	104 471	3863	441	8.8
Open AAA repair	78 826	8067	331	24.4

observational evidence is made more difficult by uncertainty and a shortage of long term outcome data.

Lethal surgery

All elective vascular operations are immediately more dangerous than doing nothing. The risk of death or stroke 1 month after CEA is 2.5 times the rate of doing nothing (*Cochrane Systematic Review* of RCT data) [1]. An observational Netherlands study of 3.7 million scheduled surgeries supports the conclusion that all surgeries initially kill, proportionate to surgical severity interacting with the population's fragility (Table 2.1) [2].

The patient must decide whether or not to bear this certain risk of early harm. The chance of later benefit is uncertain and might not exist. Whether and when a survival benefit materialises is unknown for most surgeries. Patients need a thorough assessment and estimation of risk. As we detail below, the risk of dying depends upon one's Darwinian fitness to survive the selective pressure of surgery.

Choice of procedure

It seems perverse to favour one type of surgery when it might be better to do nothing. Stent technology does not benefit patients in the medium term or long term. Survival and stroke rate is no better after stenting than after open surgery for carotid stenosis (one RCT). Survival is no better after EVAR than after open AAA surgery (two RCTs) (Figure 2.1) [3,4].

Risk stratification of harm and benefit
Changing short-term to long-term assessment

Anaesthetists have stratified risk for perioperative harm, often with the important purpose of allocating resources, such as invasive intraoperative monitoring and critical care surveillance. However anaesthetists

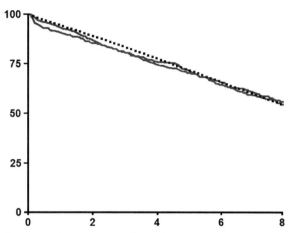

Figure 2.1 Survival 8 years after random allocation to open (blue line) or endovascular (red line) AAA repair: EVAR I study. The superimposed black dotted line is expected survival for a 77-year-old population, matched for fe/male proportions and median year of recruitment to EVAR I. Reproduced with permission from reference [3]. See plate section for colour version.

now have a much broader responsibility, through work in scheduled preoperative assessment and preparation clinics. This enhanced role makes a short-term narrow perioperative view of risk assessment inadequate. The emphasis has shifted from assessing the likelihood of postoperative coronary thrombosis and heart failure to an epidemiological estimation of long-term survival. This estimation uses survival factors common to all populations, allowing patients to understand the temporary postoperative rise in mortality within a logical framework of risk.

Darwinian postoperative survival curves

An epidemiological approach gives clinicians a tool to examine published survival trajectories. Surgical injury reduces survival by interacting with the background population survival profile. This initial deterioration is followed by improved survival, as seen following open AAA repair in Figure 2.1. This secondary, relative, survival improvement, sometimes to a rate better than expected, has usually been attributed to a survival benefit from surgery. However surgery is the most lethal man-made factor to which the population is voluntarily exposed. Patients surviving surgery do so through 'unnatural selection'. Survivors are selected through fitness to survive physiological disruption. Therefore the postoperative population is necessarily less numerous and quite different to the preoperative population. The magnitude of the differences between preoperative and postoperative populations, in number and composition, are proportionate to the selective pressure of the surgery. The stronger the perioperative selective pressure the stronger one has to be to survive it. The survival trajectory of the population winnowed by surgery is apparently improved by this selective demise of the unfit. In the EVAR I study endovascular repair was a weaker selective pressure than open surgery, post-operative mortality at 1 month being 1.8% and 4.3% respectively. The more numerous postoperative endovascular population was less fit to withstand subsequent survival pressures (than the open repair population). The survival trajectories consequently converged. This is because the less numerous survivors of open repair had to be fit.

An 'average 77-year-old survival curve' is superimposed on Figure 2.1. The survival trajectories for both the endovascular and open repair populations deviate and then join this survival curve. Mortality in the superimposed line is for the general UK population aged 77 years, matched for sex distribution and mortality in 2001 (median year of recruitment into the EVAR I study). To reiterate, scheduled surgery predominantly kills those less fit to survive ('fitness' in the general Darwinian sense, rather than aerobic capacity). This attrition continues well beyond 1 postoperative month. The mortality burden is indicated by the difference in areas under the curve.

Quality and quantity

Quality of life worsens with age, for instance as measured on the CASP-19 scale. The number of 'quality-adjusted life years' might differ even if the area of survival is the same for different populations, as in the UK small aneurysm study (Figure 2.2) [5]. The study did not report most of the variables that affect survival (see below): only the mean age and male/female ratio were reported, with probable ischaemia on ECGs substituting for the diagnosis of myocardial infarction (MI). The black diagonal line represents

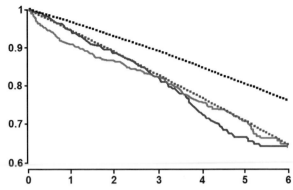

Figure 2.2 Survival 6 years after random allocation to open AAA repair (red line) or surveillance until AAA >5.4 cm diameter (blue line): UK small aneurysms study. The black dotted line is expected survival for the recruited population, matched for fe/male proportions and reported morbidities (equivalent to a 70-year-old population). The observed survival matches to a 75-year-old population (purple dotted line). Reproduced with permission from reference [5]. See plate section for colour version.

the expected survival of a population with the risk profile reported in the UK small aneurysm study and is equivalent to a 70-year-old population (adjusted to 1993, the median recruitment year). However the observed survival curve (purple line) is equivalent to a 75-year-old population. Observed mortality is 1.6 times expected. This disparity might be due to undeclared risk factors, including aerobic fitness (see below). The purple survival curve is matched from 0 to 3 years by participants allocated to surveillance and from 3 to 6 years by participants allocated to early surgery. Early surgery preferentially killed unfit participants, leaving this group depopulated but potentially fitter. Three years after allocation the survival curves for each group cross. This is due to an improved survival curve for fitter but less numerous survivors of early surgery and accumulating postoperative deaths in the surveillance cohort. Repair of AAAs was triggered in surveillance participants when aneurysms exceeded a 5.5 cm diameter. This interpretation is consistent with the statistically significant association of death with baseline aneurysm size in the surveillance group. Larger aneurysms were more likely to breach the 5.5 cm diameter threshold during follow-up, triggering both AAA repair and death. This association was not seen in the early surgery group: participants with smaller aneurysms were as likely to have surgery and die as participants with larger aneurysms. Loss of life due to surgery is probably illustrated by the two lenticular areas between the crossing survival curves, shaped like the blades of a propeller. The quality of life lost in the first area would be greater than in the second, suggesting that the net effect of surgery was to make life worse in the early surgical group than the surveillance group.

Universal survival variables

Survival curves and estimates of mortality risk can be calculated as long as one knows:

(1) mean age;

(2) proportion male (or female);

(3) proportion diagnosed with a MI;

(4) proportion diagnosed with a stroke;

(5) proportion diagnosed with heart failure;

(6) proportion diagnosed with renal failure;

(7) proportion diagnosed with peripheral arterial disease (PAD);

(8) measured aerobic fitness.

Similarly individual survival probabilities can be estimated using these variables. A reasonable though less precise estimate can be made without measuring aerobic fitness directly (see 'Cardiopulmonary exercise testing' below). However aerobic fitness differentiates to what degree a cardiovascular label (MI, stroke, heart failure and PAD) has been accompanied by cardiorespiratory incompetence. When mortality is relatively high, as it is following vascular surgery, imprecision might translate into misinformation, undermining informed decision-making and consent and disrupting attempts to manage perioperative risk.

Inadequate reporting of survival variables in vascular surgery

The separate proportions of participants with controlled heart failure, stroke, peripheral arterial disease or renal failure are not reported in the EVAR I study. A composite proportion of patients (0.423) had 'Cardiac disease': either 'cardiac valve disease', 'clinically significant arrhythmia', angina, cardiac revascularisation, MI or 'uncontrolled heart failure'. The mortality risk associated with each of these labels is different. It ranges from possibly no independent effect (valve disease, arrhythmia and cardiac revascularisation), through intermediate effect (angina increases risk 1.2 times), MI (risk increased 1.5 times, as it is for PAD, heart failure, stroke, renal failure), up to a high risk associated with 'uncontrolled' heart failure. We plotted the dotted line in Figure 2.1 using

reported mean age, sex proportions and assuming the average effect of the composite 'Cardiac disease' was to increase risk 1.5 times for the 42% of participants with one of these factors. This calculation increases expected mortality from a population aged 74 years (mean age of EVAR I participants) to the mortality associated with a 77-year-old population. The 77-year-old survival curve matches later parts of the observed survival reasonably well. The reported mortality 1 month after open surgery in EVAR I was 9.5 times the expected background mortality for a 77-year-old population in 2001. For comparison the death rate 1 month after early AAA repair in the UK small aneurysm study (5.8%) was 12 times that for the surveillance cohort in the same study. This is less than the 24-fold increase in risk associated with AAA repair in Table 2.1. The Netherlands paper reported comorbidities separately and completely, except that angina was combined with MI and transient ischaemic attack (TIA) with stroke (both angina and TIA are associated with a 1.2 times increase in mortality, MI and stroke with a 1.5 times increase). Up to 8% of surgical codes were wrong in the Netherlands database: if 8% of operations reported as scheduled AAA repair were miscoded emergent ruptured AAA repairs, then the Netherlands O/E ratio might be closer to 16 (assuming a 50% mortality following ruptured AAA repair). The observed mortality rate 1 month after AAA repair in the Netherlands (10.2%) was more than double that after open repair in EVAR I (4.3%). This disparity might be due to the background differences in population survival (people in 1998 more likely to die than in 2001), possibly a higher-risk Dutch population (no exclusion criteria, 82% with PAD, 5% renal failure, but 5 years younger), the effect of being in an RCT (the EVAR studies) and the preceding discussion concerning incorrect coding and incomplete reporting.

There was no measure of aerobic fitness in either the UK small aneurysm study, the EVAR I or II studies, or the Netherlands paper. We discuss this later: it probably explains much of the discrepancy in survival between EVAR II participants and EVAR I participants.

Chronological age, physiological age, survival age

Expected EVAR II survival does not fit the observed survival (Figure 2.3) [6]. The observed survival was equivalent to that of a 91-year-old population (red dotted curve), whereas the information provided in

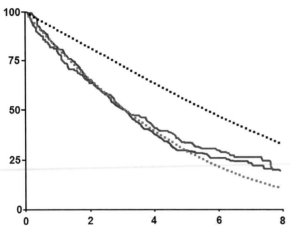

Figure 2.3 Survival 8 years after random allocation to endovascular AAA repair (red line) or no surgery (blue line): EVAR II study. The black dotted line is expected survival for the recruited population, matched for fe/male proportions and reported morbidities (equivalent to an 83-year-old population). The observed survival matches to a 91-year-old population (red dotted line). Reproduced with permission from reference [6]. See plate section for colour version.

EVAR II generated a curve expected for an 83-year-old population (black dotted curve). The observed mortality rate in EVAR II was four times that observed in EVAR I. One would have expected the EVAR II mortality rate to be 1.55 times the EVAR I rate. This calculation is based upon: mean age 3 years older in EVAR II; 29% more participants with 'Cardiac disease' in EVAR II (71% versus 42%); more women in EVAR II (14% versus 9%); 8.4% renal failure in EVAR II. Therefore there is a 2.6 relative disparity in mortality rates between EVAR I and II (4/1.55). This missing risk is composed of differences in: unreported rates of stroke, PAD and controlled heart failure; renal failure with [creatinine] between 150 μmol/l and 200 μmol/l; composition of risk factors amalgamated within the composite 'Cardiac disease'; and aerobic fitness.

Physically fit people live longer than physically unfit people. 'Fit' now refers to aerobic fitness rather than general Darwinian fitness to survive. Aerobic fitness improves survival for men and women, people of different ages and people with different comorbidities. Measurement of aerobic fitness provides unique information that when combined with the mortality rate for a given age and sex, adjusted for comorbidities, allows one to estimate general survival and how much surgery will temporarily decrease survival. One can then provide both a cross-sectional mortality risk, for instance 1 in 1000 risk of dying in the next month,

and a longitudinal risk, for instance a 50% chance of surviving 19 years.

Quantifying the survival effects of aerobic fitness

Fitness has been correlated with survival for more than 100 000 people in at least 19 studies [7]. Mortality rate is 13% less (relative risk 0.87) in people who can achieve one additional metabolic equivalent (1 MET), and 15% more in people who achieve one MET less (relative risk, RR 1.15). The fitter one is the lower one's mortality risk: if you achieve two METs more than an otherwise similar individual your mortality risk is 76% their risk (0.87 × 0.87) and their risk is 32% more than yours (1.15 × 1.15). And so on. An increase of one MET is defined as an increase in oxygen consumption of 3.5 ml/kg per minute. In an 80-kg man this amounts to 280 mls, which in turn would be elicited by an additional 28 W power: oxygen consumption and power are fixed in a 10-ml/W relationship. Fitness falls with age and is less in women. Expected peak METs average:

- 18.4 − (0.16 × age) for men [8];
- 14.7 − (0.13 × age) for women. [9].

Average mortality at a particular age can be adjusted to account for atypical fitness.

Differences in fitness, combined with incomplete reporting of comorbidity, might account for disparities in expected and observed survival curves, both within and between studies such as EVAR I and EVAR II.

Cardiopulmonary exercise testing
Peak oxygen consumption

Patients' records contain seven of the eight survival factors listed previously. Aerobic capacity, the eighth factor, cannot be accurately assessed by history. Cardiopulmonary exercise testing (CPET) measures aerobic capacity. Such testing completes estimation of general survival, including monthly mortality and median life expectancy, and the temporary mortality increase that follows surgery. Cardiopulmonary exercise testing is a unique preoperative test. Background survival cannot be reliably inferred for healthy and unhealthy people by any other investigation or combination of investigations, such as exercise ECG, resting and dobutamine stress echocardiography, dipyridamole thallium scanning and B-type natriuretic peptide concentration.

The CPET process analyses inhaled and exhaled gas flow, and O_2 and CO_2 content, during exercise that gets incrementally harder, by braking on a cycle ergometer and by speed and incline on a treadmill. Dividing the measured peak oxygen consumption ($\dot{v}O_2$ in ml/min) by 3.5 and then by mass (kg) gives peak METs. Expected monthly mortality for an individual can be extrapolated from observed general population mortality, at a given age for men or women, by adjusting for the difference between observed and expected peak METs. Comorbidities also must be adjusted for (see worked example below).

The advantage peak $\dot{v}O_2$ has over other CPET-generated variables is the weight of evidence supporting its prognostic value across numerous populations. Other CPET variables, usually measured during exercise rather than at peak power, can improve survival estimation when combined with peak $\dot{v}O_2$. However it is unclear whether their value in populations with heart failure or chronic obstructive pulmonary disease (COPD) can be extrapolated to the general population. In our preoperative CPET consultation we default to survival calculation using peak $\dot{v}O_2$. We then look for other variables with particularly abnormal values. The problem then is to determine the magnitude by which one should adjust the survival based upon peak $\dot{v}O_2$ because there are no described algorithms for doing so.

The anaerobic threshold

The anaerobic threshold (AT) is an attractive variable. It is theoretically associated with metabolic derangement, progressive acidosis, morbidity and mortality. It probably occurs when aerobic mitochondrial ATP production is supplemented by inefficient cytoplasmic anaerobic ATP production. Anaerobic ATP production rapidly evolves acid, subsequently excreted as CO_2 by the lungs, causing an increase in the measured ratio of CO_2 excreted to O_2 absorbed. The AT usually occurs when exertion is tolerable. The cyclist cannot purposefully affect onset of anaerobic ATP production. In contrast the peak $\dot{v}O_2$ in most patients represents their volitional limit rather than reflecting a physiological maximum. Therefore peak $\dot{v}O_2$ might be different in two CPETs performed on the same day with the same person.

Caveats weigh against using the AT as the primary CPET variable. Firstly, there is no algorithm equivalent to that for peak $\dot{v}O_2$ to adjust survival estimation in the general population. Secondly, determination of the AT is subjective. Two experienced assessors using the same rules for determining AT might disagree on average by between 0.5 ml/kg/ and 1.0 ml/kg per minute for a CPET that elicits a peak $\dot{v}O_2$ of 20 ml/kg per minute. By contrast the peak $\dot{v}O_2$ will have the same value for both assessors. Therefore although the physiological AT might not vary between two tests conducted over a short time its measurement will. Thirdly, there may not be an identifiable AT, common in patients with COPD, severe heart failure and peripheral vascular disease. Fourthly, the inexperienced might incorrectly identify an early spurious AT when a hyperventilating cyclist excretes CO_2 (bicarbonate) stores. Fifthly, hyperventilation before exercise depletes CO_2 stores. Consequently the apparent AT is delayed or obscured as anaerobic acid replenishes CO_2 (bicarbonate) stores and is not excreted. Finally, the AT scale is about half the peak $\dot{v}O_2$ scale so it has half the potential to describe a range of fitness, and by inference risk.

Ventilatory equivalents

How much one has to breathe to achieve gaseous exchange correlate with survival better than peak $\dot{v}O_2$ in some populations. These variables for CO_2 and O_2 exchange are called 'ventilatory equivalents' and are minute ventilation divided by CO_2 excretion ($\dot{v}_E/\dot{v}CO_2$) and O_2 absorption ($\dot{v}_E/\dot{v}O_2$) respectively. They can be calculated in a number of different ways, giving slightly different results, but are nevertheless resistant to observer bias unlike the AT. The scale for peak $\dot{v}O_2$ ranges from 5 to 95 ml/kg per minute (moribund to cross-country skier), that for the ventilatory equivalents 15 to 70 (ml/kg per minute cross-country skier to severe pulmonary hypertension).

- Mean values for $\dot{v}_E/\dot{v}CO_2$ (slope) are:
  - 21.04 + (age $\times$ 0.1) for men;
  - 22.04 + (age $\times$ 0.1) for women.
- Mean values for $\dot{v}_E/\dot{v}CO_2$ (at AT) are:
  - 21.09 + (age $\times$ 0.123) for men;
  - 22.09 + (age $\times$ 0.123) for women.

However these norms are derived from relatively few people – just over 300 individuals for male values –

so accuracy is uncertain, particularly for patients older than 60 years (only 34 men contributed to these values) [10].

The portion of the ventilatory equivalent scale achieved by most of our patients (25 to 45) is greater than for peak $\dot{v}O_2$ (10 to 20), so their potential to discriminate prognosis might be better. The problem interpreting peak $\dot{v}O_2$ (ml/kg per minute) in the underweight and overweight (see below) is avoided with ventilatory equivalents that have no unit of measure. However, as for the AT and other secondary CPET variables, there is no algorithm that converts observed–expected values into changes in survival for a general population. Authors reporting the additive prognostic value of $\dot{v}_E/\dot{v}CO_2$ to peak $\dot{v}O_2$ have disappointingly evaded doing so in a clear way. Authors presented survival hazard ratios (HRs) above and below a $\dot{v}_E/\dot{v}CO_2$ threshold – different in different papers – without reporting the HR associated with a unit increase in $\dot{v}_E/\dot{v}CO_2$. To be useful authors would need to present these HRs after the association of peak $\dot{v}O_2$ has been removed from the equation. Authors would need to then check whether a unitary change in $\dot{v}_E/\dot{v}CO_2$ was associated with the same HR throughout the range of peak $\dot{v}O_2$.

We are guilty of publishing such a paper [11]. We analysed the association of perioperative variables with survival, after scheduled open AAA repair for non-occlusive disease in 130 patients. The four CPET variables that we analysed (peak $\dot{v}O_2$, $\dot{v}_E/\dot{v}CO_2$, $\dot{v}_E/\dot{v}O_2$, AT) were all strongly associated with postoperative survival (median duration of follow-up 3 years). Although we reported the HR associated with a unit increase in $\dot{v}_E/\dot{v}CO_2$ we failed to report how ventilatory equivalents would alter a survival estimation based upon the peak $\dot{v}O_2$. On review it is apparent that 130 patients cannot reliably discriminate the contribution of ventilatory equivalents to survival estimation, independent of peak $\dot{v}O_2$. However we suggest multiplying the peak $\dot{v}O_2$ mortality estimate by about 6% (RR 1.06) for each unit $\dot{v}_E/\dot{v}CO_2$ is above expected (see normal values above) and reduce the estimate by between 5% and 6% (RR 0.943) for each unit $\dot{v}_E/\dot{v}CO_2$ is below expected.

Diagnostic patterns of other variables

We asserted that the $\dot{v}O_2$ to power relationship is fixed at about 10 ml/W. This is not always true. Pump failure, typically due to myocardial ischaemia, causes

$\dot{v}O_2/$ W ratios less than 8.5. During a CPET of a patient with known or unknown ischaemic heart disease a normal $\dot{v}O_2/$ W slope at low power is followed by an often abrupt reduction in slope. The worse the ischaemia the earlier this transition, which often coincides with the AT and a rapidly increasing heart rate. Cardiac contractility fails to increase beyond this point. This is illustrated by dividing $\dot{v}O_2$ by heart rate, a product called the 'oxygen pulse'. When plotted against time or $\dot{v}O_2$ the oxygen pulse plateaus at the transition point. These patterns can occur without pathological ECG changes: contractile deterioration precedes ECG changes in any test and also in the progression of ischaemic disease over months or years in the individual. In patients with moderate to severe heart failure the oxygen pulse may briefly rise in recovery as cardiac afterload is suddenly reduced when pedalling stops. Patients on beta-blockers may have an O_2 pulse that exceeds expected but their peak $\dot{v}O_2$ and AT will usually be less than expected, with abnormal $\dot{v}O_2/$ W if there is myocardial ischaemia.

A cause of raised ventilatory equivalents with a similarly dire prognosis to heart failure is pulmonary vascular disease, either acquired through interstitial lung disease or intrapulmonary thromboses. In heart failure arterial saturations are generally maintained, in pulmonary vascular disease significant desaturation below 85% can occur in the first half of the CPET. Occasionally desaturation is abrupt, coupled with increased end-tidal O_2 and decreased end-tidal CO_2 partial pressures. This may signal opening of a potentially patent foramen ovale with rising pulmonary vascular resistance and changes in right atrial blood flow. Blood pressure increases during CPET, with systolic blood pressures exceeding 220 mm Hg. Failure to increase blood pressure, or a fall in blood pressure, signals pump failure.

Spirometric variables, including forced vital capacity (FVC), forced expiratory volume in 1 minute (FEV_1), flow-volume loops, inspiratory capacity (IC) and maximum voluntary ventilation (MVV) are measured before CPET. Of these, IC and MVV are mechanical limits to tidal volume and minute volume respectively. Minute ventilation increases during CPET, initially through tidal volume then breathing rate. Most patients with COPD are not limited by their mechanical airway disease, with breathing reserve exceeding 10% when they stop. Restrictive lung disease causes respiratory rates above 40 breaths per minute (bpm) or 60 bpm with severe disease.

The overweight and underweight

Survival in most healthy and unhealthy populations is best at a body mass index (BMI) of about 25, i.e. overweight [12]. It is unclear whether increases in mortality above and below this BMI apply to all ranges of fitness or to what extent fitness obviates the risk associated with deviations from a BMI of 25. There is some evidence that survival in people with moderate or good fitness increases at BMIs above 25. Unmodified peak $\dot{v}O_2$ (and AT), expressed as ml/kg per minute, overestimate mortality in the obese. One can either change the unit, for instance adjust for body surface area rather than height squared, or one can adjust the predicted value for peak $\dot{v}O_2$. In an extremely useful textbook Wasserman *et al.* present modified equations to calculate predicted peak $\dot{v}O_2$ for the underweight and overweight [10]. The more weight deviates from predicted the more likely it is that a modified expected peak $\dot{v}O_2$ will represent 'true' survival risks. You could check risk predictions with and without weight corrections.

An alternative method is to use the resting metabolic rate (RMR) and to modify the expected peak $\dot{v}O_2$, by the ratio of the personalised RMR to the average RMR. The obese have a lower RMR per kilogram so this technique reduces the expected peak $\dot{v}O_2$. Dispose of the idea that 1 MET is an average RMR. The mean (SD) RMR is 2.56 (0.40) ml O_2/kg per minute. An RMR of 3.5 ml O_2/kg per minute is above the 98th centile. The RMR (ml O_2/kg per minute) is calculated:

- $3.6145 - (0.0367 \times BMI) - (0.0038 \times age) + (0.179)$ for women;
- $3.6145 - (0.0367 \times BMI) - (0.0038 \times age) + (0.358)$ for men [13].

The expected peak MET equation (see above) for men was derived from a population mean age 59, mean BMI 28. So their mean RMR was 2.72 ml O_2/kg per minute. The appropriate adjustment of observed peak $\dot{v}O_2$ should be in proportion to the difference between an individual's RMR and the reference RMR of 2.72 ml O_2/kg per minute. For example, a 65-year-old man with a BMI of 38 would have a RMR of 2.33 ml O_2/kg per minute. The correction factor for the observed peak $\dot{v}O_2$ in this man would therefore be 2.72/2.33 = 1.17. The unadjusted expected peak MET would be 8, or a peak $\dot{v}O_2$ of 28. The adjusted expected peak MET would be 8/1.17 = 6.84 and the expected peak $\dot{v}O_2$ 23.9 ml/kg per minute. If one used the unadjusted MET value mortality would be overestimated by $1.15^{1.16} = 1.18$ or 18%.

The expected peak MET equation for women was derived from a population mean age 52, mean BMI 27. So their mean RMR was 2.61 ml O_2/kg per minute. A 65-year-old woman with a BMI of 38 would have a RMR of 2.15 ml O_2/kg per minute. The correction factor for peak $\dot{v}O_2$ would be 2.61/2.15 = 1.21. The unadjusted expected peak MET would be 6.25. The adjusted expected peak MET would be 5.17. If one used the unadjusted MET value mortality would be overestimated by $1.15^{1.08} = 1.16$ or 16%.

No gas analysis

Peak power (watts) generated at the end of incremental cycling could be used in lieu of direct $\dot{v}O_2$ measurement, for instance if gas analysis was unavailable, or if cycling outside the hospital, perhaps in a gym, was used to screen patients. However, a word of warning: bicycles in gymnasiums will not be calibrated as precisely as those used in CPET, so the displayed power is likely to be inaccurate. An estimate of the increase in $\dot{v}O_2$ during exercise is given by multiplying peak power achieved by 10 ml/W. Peak $\dot{v}O_2$ is then calculated by adding this to the estimated $\dot{v}O_2$ during unloaded pedalling that precedes incremental braking. Two METs is a reasonable estimate of $\dot{v}O_2$ at the end of unloaded pedalling. So the MET value estimated at the end of exercise will be: 2 METs + [(2.86 × peak power in watts)/mass in kg]. One might be wise to view this as an overestimate if used as a screen to 'pass' patients as sufficiently fit not to merit formal CPET.

Assessing perioperative risk: a worked example

Use Excel templates with the various equations pre-loaded. All you need do is enter patient details to generate modified risk estimates. You can get these by emailing john.carlisle@nhs.net.

Mr Smith is 67 years old with a 6.2 cm diameter AAA. He had an MI 7 years ago. He has not had any other major cardiovascular events. Creatinine concentrations fluctuate between 105 and 120 μmol/l. You have not measured his aerobic capacity. He is 169 cm tall and weighs 83 kg.

(1) If this man did not have a AAA what would his monthly mortality and median life expectancy be?

The average monthly mortality risk for a 67-year-old man is 1 in 680, survival 679/680, median life expectancy (MLE) 16 years. His MI increases monthly mortality to 1.5/680, or 1/450, survival 449/450, MLE 13 years.

His renal impairment increases his mortality risk, best determined by converting [creatinine] 120 µmol/l to an estimated glomerular filtration rate (eGFR). One popular formula to calculate eGFR is the 'Modification of Diet in Renal Disease' (MDRD):

- eGFR $= 32788 \times$ [creatinine (µmol/l)]$^{-1.154} \times$ age$^{-0.203}$ for men;
- eGFR $= 32788 \times$ [creatinine (µmol/l)]$^{-1.154} \times$ age$^{-0.203} \times 0.742$ for women.

The median [creatinine] for men is about 95 µmol/l and 75 µmol/l for women. Mortality risk increases with decreasing eGFR for any age. Relative mortality increases by 0.85% (RR 1.0085) for each 1-ml fall in eGFR. Normal eGFR is 73 ml for a 67-year-old man. Mr Smith's eGFR is 56 ml. His mortality risk should be adjusted by $1.0085^{(73-56)} =$ RR 1.15.

His monthly mortality risk is therefore 1.15/450 or 1/390, survival 389/390. The MLE associated with this monthly mortality risk is about 12 years.

(2) His CPET results are: peak $\dot{v}O_2$ 15.9 ml/kg per minute, $\dot{v}_E/\dot{v}CO_2$ 37 at AT. What are his adjusted risks?

We need to adjust for BMI, which is $83/1.69^2 = 29$. His RMR is 2.65 ml O_2/kg per minute. Expected peak METs for age and sex (7.68) should be divided by 2.72/2.65 to give 7.48 METs, a peak $\dot{v}O_2$ of 26 ml. He achieved 4.54 METs, 2.94 METs less than expected. This corresponds to a relative risk of $1.15^{2.94}$ or 1.51. His adjusted monthly mortality risk is 1.51/390 or 1/260. Finally we could adjust this risk for his $\dot{v}_E/\dot{v}CO_2$ of 37. Expected $\dot{v}_E/\dot{v}CO_2$ was 29, 8 less than observed. So we adjust his risk by $1.06^8 =$ RR 1.6.

- His estimated monthly mortality risk is 1/163, MLE about 7.5 years, figures consistent with the average 81-year-old man. This compares with the average figures for a 67-year-old man of 1/680, MLE 13 years.

(3) What would his mortality risk be the month after surgery:

    (a) Open AAA repair?
    (b) EVAR?

Open AAA repair temporarily increases mortality risk by 12 times, so his risk of dying in the first postoperative month will be 1/14 or 7%. The proportionate increase in risk after EVAR is 1.8/4.3 (from EVAR I), so his risk after EVAR will increase to 1/32 or 3%.

(4) Given the absurd scenario that he didn't have a AAA, how would these surgeries alter his MLE?

    [Remember that we are talking to Mr Smith before surgery and here we are trying to calculate how long after surgery he will have a 50:50 chance of being alive.]

His background risk is consistent with an 81-year-old man. UK life tables illustrate cumulative mortality, starting with a hypothetical population of 100 000 newborns. By 81 years there will be 48 365 men left from 100 000 male neonates and after a further 7.5 years about half will be left. Open AAA surgery will deplete 48 365 men aged 81 years by 7% in the first postoperative month to 44 979, the population of 82-year-old men, reducing the MLE by about 1 year to 6.5 years.

However, it is likely that despite our best efforts to assess risk with precision, 1000 men like Mr Smith (same age, MI and CPET results) will still be heterogeneous in their Darwinian fitness to survive. As we've seen for EVAR I and II studies, initial differences in mortality do not translate into different survival rates at a later time, for instance median life expectancy. However the potential 'living time', represented by the area under the survival curve, would be less for Mr Smith should he have surgery, whether or not his MLE is changed.

Cardiac risk scoring systems

A problem with cardiac risk scoring systems is they are cardiac risk scoring systems. Two-thirds of deaths (31/43) in the population used to derive the Revised Cardiac Risk Index (RCRI) were ignored, being 'non-cardiac' [14]. The RCRI is used by the 'American College of Cardiology/American Heart Association (ACC/AHA) guideline on perioperative cardiovascular evaluation and care for noncardiac surgery'. This guideline recommends what perioperative interventions to use, when and in whom, such as beta-blockade and coronary artery bypass graft (CABG)15.

Revised Cardiac Risk Index (RCRI)

- Revised the original Goldman score published 22 years previously.
- Only estimates postoperative risks, not preoperative.
- Derived from a population >49 years, with planned admissions >1 day.
- Only estimates 'major' surgical risk.
- Outcomes were four 'major cardiac complications': MI; complete heart block; ventricular fibrillation or primary cardiac arrest; pulmonary oedema.
- Observation stopped 5 days postoperatively.

The RCRI validated the association of four perioperative factors with the four outcomes:

(1) Ischaemic heart disease: previous MI (includes ECG Q waves), positive ECG exercise test, angina, glyceryl trinitrate (GTN) use.
(2) Heart failure: history, nocturnal dyspnoea, third heart sound gallop, bilateral crackles or chest X-ray oedema.
(3) Cerebrovascular disease: TIA or stroke.
(4) High-risk elective surgery: AAA repair, intrathoracic surgery, intraperitoneal surgery.

Rates of 'cardiac complications' were associated with the number of risk factors:

- No risk factor: 1/200 risk;
- 1 risk factor: 1/100 risk;
- 2 risk factors: 1/20 risk;
- >2 risk factors: 1/10 risk.

Two other variables associated with major cardiac complications in the derivation cohort (2893 participants) were not associated with major cardiac complications in the validation cohort (1422 participants).

- Renal impairment: [creatinine] > 177 μmol/l.
- Insulin-dependent diabetes.

It is unclear whether one should use these two risk factors to estimate the postoperative risk of a major cardiac complication. Most researchers have used the six derivation variables, not the four validated variables.

Customized Probability Model (CPM)

This is more useful than the RCRI for vascular patients [16]. This risk score estimates total mortality within 30 days of surgery (153/2310). This model details the

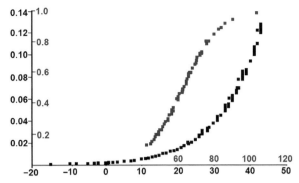

Figure 2.4 Charted postoperative mortality risk (vertical axis) according to score calculated by the Customized Probability Model (CPM). Scores −20 to +50, and associated mortality risks coloured black. Scores >50 and associated mortality risks in red. Reproduced with permission from reference [16].

odds associated with different types of vascular surgeries: carotid endarterectomy (referent odds ratio 1); infrainguinal bypass (OR 4); scheduled open AAA repair (OR between 8 and 13); thoracoabdominal (OR 22); ruptured AAA (OR between 62 and 72). As with the RCRI, diabetes was not a validated risk factor.

The score ranges from −25 to 110, the corresponding mortality estimates ranging from 0.15% to 100% (see Figure 2.4). The model summates scores for severity of surgery, comorbidity and medications:

- Acute AAA rupture +43; scheduled AAA or thoracoabdominal +26; infrainguinal bypass +15; CEA 0.
- [creatinine] >177 μmol/l +16; heart failure +14; ischaemic heart disease +13; stroke or TIA +10; hypertension +7; COPD +7.
- Beta-blockade −15; statin use −10.

The CPM predictim of Mr Smith's 30-day postoperative mortality is: 9% on clinical history; 15% if he had untreated hypertension, 4% if treated by beta-blockade, 1.5% with statin as well.

Exercise ECG, dobutamine stress echocardiography, dipyridamole thallium scanning

In symptomatic medical patients these cardiac tests assess the likelihood of coronary artery stenoses and associated risks of major adverse cardiac events (MACE – variable definitions) and cardiac death. In preoperative patients these tests have brought the unwelcome risks of coronary investigation and intervention (see chapter 4).

Of these three, dobutamine stress echocardiography (DSE) may be the best preoperative test [17, 18]. Dr Poldermans and colleagues have developed preoperative DSE as a risk assessment tool, contributing to the CPM risk factor 'ischaemia' (above). Dobutamine-induced ischaemia is defined as a biphasic response in akinetic or severely hypokinetic echocardiographic segments or an increase in wall motion score >0.

These tests are not integrated into survival estimation, either general or perioperative. They are reserved for assessing risk – again focussed upon coronary arterial disease – in patients already at high risk, for instance vascular surgical patients with poor functional capacity and at least three RCRI factors. Attempts to integrate these dynamic tests with survival epidemiology are fraught with difficulty. The first problem is that studies did not incorporate some factors into their risk models, such as renal failure, PAD, stroke or TIA or aerobic fitness. Outcomes were usually non-fatal MI and cardiac death: overall mortality was not used to generate multivariate hazard ratios that could be combined with epidemiological variables. It is therefore unclear whether these stress tests add additional information to the risk sequence described earlier in the chapter. One will double-count risk if DSE findings are not completely independent of other factors.

For the record, induced new or worsening wall motion abnormalities increase long-term non-fatal MI and cardiac death $\times 2$ to $\times 3$, whilst a unit increase in wall motion score index (WMSI) at rest increases subsequent long-term mortality $\times 2$ (men) and $\times 4$ (women). The WMSI is calculated by dividing the sum of segment scores (each scored out of 5) by the number of segments scored (range 0 to 5).

Resting echocardiography is incapable of assessing dynamic cardiac function: 50% heart failure patients have normal ejection fractions. Neither it nor coronary angiography has a place in routine preoperative risk assessment.

Biomarkers: C-reactive protein, B-type natriuretic peptide

Biomarkers share a problem with dynamic cardiac tests – how can one integrate these results with the general model of risk described above? Do these tests add prognostic information not contained by age, sex, physical fitness and histories of five morbidities? We don't know.

Attempts to integrate the results of biomarker studies into a general mortality model are hampered by:

- incomplete or no adjustment of normal ranges for known risk factors;
- incomplete or no adjustment of the concentration–mortality relationship for other risk factors;
- different units for reporting hazard ratios (log-transformed, standard deviation);
- reporting dichotomous rather than continuous concentration–mortality relationship;
- treatment of mortality as time-independent;
- odds ratios inflating apparent concentration–outcome relationship;
- follow-up unreliable;
- composite outcomes;
- mortality not reported.

There may be a continuous concentration–mortality relationship for biomarkers such as B-type natriuretic peptide (BNP) and its N-terminal propeptide (NT-proBNP). However this relationship is ill-defined, mainly due to the novelty of biomarker research. Such a relationship probably fails in healthy populations, in contrast to lower mortality in the fit compared to the unfit. So at the moment we are unable to describe how to use biomarkers in the assessment of risk in the general population or of perioperative risk in vascular surgical patients [19, 20].

Summary

Patients who survive surgery are fitter than patients who do not. The extent of this unnatural selection is determined by the surgical injury and the fitness of the population. Fitness to survive is determined by seven historical variables – age, sex and five morbidities – and measurement of physical fitness. Other historical and test variables can be incorporated in the future as they are shown to discriminate general survival or postoperative survival. The effect of surgery on survival can be gauged by comparing predicted population survival, estimated through the eight fitness-to-survive variables, with observed postoperative survival.

Preoperative risk estimation can be used:

- to inform decision-making with the patient and other clinicians;
- to identify groups and individuals in whom surgery is likely to inflict high morbidity and mortality;

- to invest stratified interventions before, during and after surgery, based upon thresholds of estimated postoperative mortalities.
- to adjust performance analyses for individual clinicians, teams and hospitals;

- to speculate on new interventions that might reduce risk;
- to model whether new variables add to the precision of prognostication.

References

1. Cina C, Clase C, Haynes RB. (2008). Carotid endarterectomy for symptomatic carotid stenoses. *Cochrane Database Syst Rev*, 2008; CD001081. DoI:10.1002/14651858. CD001081.

2. Noordzij PG, Poldermans D, Schouten O, *et al*. Postoperative mortality in The Netherlands. *Anethesiology*, 2008; 112: 1105–15.

3. United Kingdom EVAR Trial Investigators. Endovascular versus open repair of abdominal aortic aneurysm. *N Engl J Med* 2010; 362:1863–71.

4. De Bruin JL, Baas AF, Buth J., *et al*. Long-term outcome of open or endovascular repair of abdominal aortic aneurysm. *N Engl J Med* 2010;362: 1881–9.

5. Powell JT, Brady AR, Brown LC, *et al*. (1998). Mortality results for randomised controlled trial of early elective surgery or ultrasonographic surveillance for small abdominal aortic aneurysms. *Lancet* 1998;352: 1649–56.

6. United Kingdom EVAR Trial Investigators. Endovascular repair of aortic aneurysm in patients physically ineligible for open repair. *N Engl J Med* 2010;362:1872–80.

7. Kodama S, Saito K, Tanaka S. Cardiorespiratory fitness as a quantitative predictor of all-cause mortality and cardiovascular events in healthy men and women: a meta-analysis. *JAMA* 2009; 301:2024–5.

8. Myers J, Prakash M, Froelicher V. (2002). Exercise capacity and mortality among men referred for exercise testing. *N Engl J Med* 2002; 346:793–801.

9. Gulati M, Black HR, Shaw LJ, *et al*. The prognostic value of a nomogram for exercise capacity in women. *N Engl J Med* 2005; 353:468–75.

10. Wasserman K, Hansen JE, Sue DY, *et al*. *Principles of Exercise Testing and Interpretation*, 4th Edn. Philadelphia, PA: Lippincott, Williams & Wilkins 2005.

11. Carlisle J, Swart M. Mid-term survival after abdominal aortic aneurysm surgery predicted by cardiopulmonary exercise testing. *Br J Surg* 2007;94:966–9.

12. Prospective Studies Collaboration. Body-mass index and cause-specific mortality in 900 000 adults: collaborative analyses of 57 prospective studies. *Lancet* 2009;373:1083–96.

13. Byrne NM, Hills AP, Hunter GR, *et al*. Metabolic equivalent: one size does not fit all. *J Appl Physiol* 2005;99:1112–19.

14. Lee TH, Marcantonio ER, Mangione CM, *et al*. Derivation and prospective validation of a simple index for prediction of cardiac risk of major noncardiac surgery. *Circulation* 1999;100:1043–9.

15. Fleisher LA, Beckman JA, Brown KA, *et al*. ACC/AHA 2007 guidelines on perioperative cardiovascular evaluation and care for noncardiac surgery: a report of the American College of Cardiology/American Heart Association task force on practice guidelines. *J Am Coll Cardiol* 2007;50:e159–241.

16. Kertai MD, Boersma E, Klein J, van Urk H, Poldermans D. Optimizing the prediction of perioperative mortality in vascular surgery by using a customized probability model. *Arch Int Med* 2005;165:898–904.

17. Beattie WS, Abdelnaem E, Wijeysundera DN, *et al*. A meta-analytic comparison of preoperative stress echocardiography and nuclear scintigraphy imaging. *Anesth Analg* 2006;102:8–16.

18. Kertai MD, Boersma E, Bax JJ, *et al*. A meta-analysis comparing the prognostic accuracy of six diagnostic tests for predicting perioperative cardiac risk in patients undergoing major vascular surgery. *Heart* 2003;89:1327–34.

19. Doust JA, Pietrzak E, Dobson A, *et al*. (2005). How well does B-type natriuretic peptide predict death and cardiac events in patients with heart failure: systematic review. *BMJ* 2005;340:b5526.

20. McKie PM, Cataliotti A, Lahr BD, *et al*. The prognostic value of N-terminal pro-B-type natriuretic peptide for death and cardiovascular events in healthy normal and stage A/B heart failure subjects. *J Am Coll Cardiol* 2010;55:2140–7.

Co-existing disease in vascular surgery patients

John Carlisle

Chapter 1 discusses the epidemiology and pathophysiology of arterial disease. In this chapter we detail this and other diseases that contribute to preoperative risk assessment and can alter perioperative care. General preoperative risk assessment is summarized in Chapter 2 and further detailed in chapters specific to particular operations.

In Chapter 3 we discuss how general population survival is independently decreased by ischaemic heart disease, cardiac failure and renal failure. Estimation of preoperative mortality risk is completed by adding the independent risks associated with ischaemic brain disease, peripheral arterial disease, age, sex and objectively measured aerobic fitness. Hypertension, smoking, hypercholesterolaemia, diabetes mellitus (DM) and chronic obstructive pulmonary disease (COPD) are less important. These variables do not reliably affect general survival estimation once the eight variables listed previously have been summated. However, hypertension, DM and COPD make patients susceptible to particular perioperative morbidities. In addition severe COPD might have an independent effect on survival that has not been captured in models of survival. We discuss these three variables at the end of the chapter.

In large observational studies the rates of non-lethal strokes and non-lethal heart attacks have each been about half the mortality rate. For instance if the mortality rate is 1 in 1000 per month then the rate of non-lethal stroke will be 1 in 2000. Acute coronary syndromes (ACS) – and the other major morbidities – contribute to the postoperative mortality rate. The relationship between the rate of all-cause mortality and major non-lethal morbidity probably holds in the postoperative period: the total rate of ACS may be higher than the mortality rate, but the rate of non-lethal ACS is not.

All these morbidities interact with one another and mortality risk. A patient with one of these morbidities, for instance renal impairment, will be more likely to have another, for instance ischaemic heart disease (IHD) (and vice versa), than a patient whose renal function is normal. Deteriorating function in one organ system threatens compound deterioration in other systems.

It is simplest to consider each morbidity in its relationship with overall mortality, both as a contributor to that mortality and as an association with a given all-cause mortality.

Coronary artery disease

Acute coronary syndromes

History of an acute coronary syndrome (ACS), with or without ST-segment elevation, permanently increases risk of dying 1.5 times [1–4]. For instance the monthly mortality risk for a 65-year-old man who had an ACS 5 years ago is increased from the UK average of 1 in 800 to 1 in 530. It takes about 2 years for the mortality risk in survivors of ACS to settle at 1.5 times above the base rate for the population. Relative risk (RR) falls from an early extreme of 50 times base rate in the first 2 weeks following an ST-elevation myocardial infarction (STEMI), to a RR of about 13 at 3 months, 6 at 6 months, 3 at 1 year to 1.5 at 2 years. This fall in risk is shown in Figure 3.1 for a population of men suffering a STEMI on their 60th birthdays (a 60-year-old man without prior major morbidity would be representative of this population).

The base rate mortality increases with age whilst the relative risk after an ACS falls. The lowest composite risk occurs about 2 years following an ACS. In the example in Figure 3.1 the monthly mortality

Core Topics in Vascular Anaesthesia, ed. Carl Moores and Alastair F. Nimmo. Published by Cambridge University Press. © Cambridge University Press 2012.

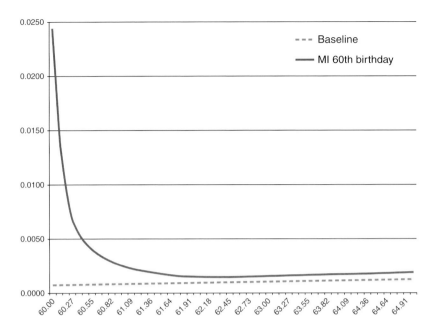

Figure 3.1 Relative risk of mortality. Dotted line: gradually rising monthly mortality rate as a 60 year-old man ages. Solid line: very high mortality rate after a STEMI, followed by a rapid fall in rate to a nadir 2 years later.

immediately following the STEMI is 2.5%, 0.5% at 6 months, 0.25% at 1 year and 0.14% at 2 years. The shape of the curve depicted in Figure 3.1 will be the same for all populations, with the relative mortality risk falling rapidly. The only difference between populations will be the absolute mortality risk, i.e. the vertical scale. For instance the respective mortality rates for a population of 74-year-old men after a STEMI would be 10%, 2%, 1% and 0.5%. Acute myocardial infarction (MI) interacts directly with a patient's background risk, whether that risk is composed solely of age-specific and sex-specific average risks, or is also composed of comorbidities. For example the relative mortality after ACS increases by 0.85% (RR 0.0085) for each 1 ml/min fall in estimated glomerular filtration rate (eGFR), as it does for the background population (see Chapter 2) [5]. These mortality estimates might be about 20% less after primary percutaneous coronary interventions (PCI) than after fibrinolysis for the treatment of ACS, although the nadir will still occur at 2 years [6]. There is probably no long-term difference in mortality between bare metal stents (BMS) and drug-eluting stents (DES) inserted for acute MI. [7, 8] Clopidogrel is used to reduce the risk of thromboses within DES. The risk of DES thrombosis and death increases when clopidogrel is stopped. These risks probably persist whenever clopidogrel is discontinued, whether less or more than 12 months after DES implantation (see Chapter 4).

- Timing of elective procedures should default to the lowest base rate mortality, which is about 2 years following an ACS. Patients should actively decide to have surgery before 2 years, usually in an attempt to alleviate the symptoms of surgical pathology.

Angina pectoris in the absence of an ACS is associated with a lower long-term mortality risk, about 1.2 times the base rate for the population. New chest pain, or a change in chest pain, is associated with a higher risk, partly because ACS is not excluded. However excess mortality gradually falls towards a relative risk of 1.2 once angina is established and stable.

Coronary revascularisation

Chapter 4 discusses perioperative coronary artery bypass grafting (CABG) and PCI. Here we discuss patients presenting for vascular surgery who have already had either. Management of clopidogrel and other thienopyridines is discussed in Chapters 4 and 8.

Both CABG and PCI are palliative procedures. They can relieve angina and ischaemic shortness-of-breath that have not responded to optimal medical treatment and lifestyle changes; PCI does not increase survival in patients with stable ischaemic symptoms (Figure 3.2) [9].

The outcome of CABG has been compared with medical therapy in eight randomised controlled trials

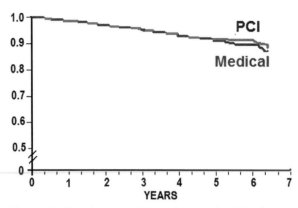

Figure 3.2 Equivalent survival in populations with stable ischaemic heart disease randomly allocated to early percutaneous coronary intervention, PCI (red line), of drugs (blue line). Reproduced with permission from reference [9]. See plate section for colour version.

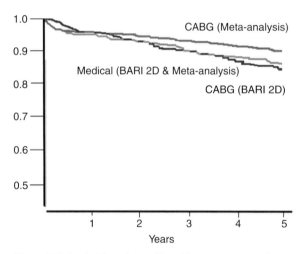

Figure 3.3 Survival in patients with stable coronary artery disease treated with drugs (blue line) or coronary artery bypass grafting (CABG). The red CABG survival curve is reproduced with permission from an early meta–analysis [10] and the orange CABG survival curve is reproduced with permission from reference [11]. See plate section for colour version.

(RCTs) for treatment of angina and shortness-of-breath induced by myocardial ischaemia. Results are presented in two publications. In one meta-analysis of seven RCTs, 2649 participants with IHD were allocated to initial CABG or medical therapy between 1972 and 1984 [10]. In the second publication 763 patients with type II diabetes and IHD were allocated to either CABG or medical therapy between 2001 and 2005 (the BARI 2D study)[11]. CABG caused early deaths (3.2% and 1.4% within 30 days respectively). CABG did not improve population survival in the long term in BARI 2D. CABG increased survival in

the meta-analysis, but not until 3 years after allocation. Survival 5 years following allocation for both publications is shown in Figure 3.3. The survival curves for participants allocated to the medication arm of each trial are coincident, i.e. one curve serves both publications. Some of the subsequent apparent reduction in mortality in the CABG group in the meta-analysis was due to Darwinian selection of fitter patients by surgery (see Chapter 2), contrasted with mortality associated with medical participants having CABGs (25% at 5 years, 33% at 7 years and 41% at 10 years). CABG meaningfully extended long-term survival for only the 6% of participants who had left main stem disease (from 80 months to 100 months at 10 years). HMG CoA reductase inhibitors ('statins') and ACE inhibitors were not used in the seven meta-analysis RCTs.

- In planning vascular surgery the default delay after CABG should be at least 6 months to avoid the period of increased mortality. A similar default delay follows PCI with BMS, whereas delay following DES implantation might be extended. Again balance has to be made with other factors that increase mortality and morbidity with time.

Hypertension, hypercholesterolaemia, smoking and diabetes

There is a strong continuous correlation of mortality and cardiovascular morbidity with age, sex, fitness, blood pressure, smoking, hypercholesterolaemia (low-density lipoprotein), male fat distribution, renal dysfunction and diabetes. However strong univariate associations between these factors and survival are weakened or lost in multivariate analyses. Important multivariate factors are: age, sex, fitness, major cardiovascular events, renal dysfunction (see Chapter 2). This observation does not necessarily conflict with the decrease in mortality and cardiovascular morbidities afforded by interventions that reduce the other univariate factors. Conversely exercise reduces mortality and morbidity, and also reduces blood pressure, cholesterol, central obesity, diabetes and smoking.

- All modifiable risk factors should be reduced by primary care before referral. However, delaying surgery after referral in an attempt to reduce risk factors may not reduce mortality or morbidity.

Interference by secondary care preoperative assessment services can be counter-productive, particularly in regard to blood pressure assessment and management.

Hypertension

Hypertension is arbitrarily defined as persistent systolic blood pressures (SBP) above 140 mm Hg in primary care (mortality and morbidity correlate with SBP). Studies of interventions to reduce mortality and morbidity through SBP reduction have usually been conducted in populations with hypertension, usually with SBP of 160 mm Hg or more, and often with co-existent risk factors (older than 50 years, male, smoker, diabetic, hypercholesterolaemic). Reduction of SBP by 10 mm Hg reduces relative mortality (RR 0.90) and the incidences of coronary heart disease (RR 0.75) and stroke (RR 0.60) [12–14]. These risk reductions also probably occur by treating 'normotensive' people, for instance reducing SBP with treatment from 130 mm Hg to 120 mm Hg, or from 120 mm Hg to 110 mm Hg. The absolute reduction in risk will depend upon the level of risk before treatment, itself dependent upon age, sex, fitness and comorbidities (see Chapter 2).

The current evidence is that attempts to reduce SBP in patients with hypertension by more than 15 mm Hg (or below 135 mm Hg) do not further reduce mortality or morbidity, despite many guidelines recommending greater reductions in SBP in higher-risk patients (age, major cardiovascular events, diabetes). There is some evidence that targeting SBP below 140 mm Hg increases mortality and morbidity in patients with peripheral arterial disease and patients with heart failure. [15–17]. Confirmation of hypertension takes about 3 months after it is suspected [18]. Once treatment response is established further SBP checks in primary care overestimate SBP and have no prognostic value [19–21].

Chapters 5 and 6 and the surgery-specific chapters discuss intraoperative blood pressure monitoring and control. Whilst the role of perioperative interventions remains uncertain preoperative preparation should extend principles derived from studies of hypertension and its treatment in primary care.

(1) Long-term risk of death and morbidity correlates with many variables.

(2) Antihypertensive medications will reduce these risks in all patients being considered for vascular surgery, irrespective of SBP, except patients with peripheral arterial disease (PAD) or heart failure (HF) with SBP <140 mm Hg (importantly on repeated measurement in primary care or at home) (see 'Heart failure' below).

(3) Primary and secondary care should agree to start antihypertensive medication on anyone being referred to vascular surgeons (except PAD and HF): this action does not depend upon either SBP or diastolic blood pressure (DBP). The only reasons to measure SBP (in primary care) are: to calculate absolute risk (to inform patient decision-making); to determine whether patients with PAD or HF are prescribed antihypertensive medication; to determine how much more medication can be introduced. These can only be determined by SBP measurements and blood tests in primary care or at home. It takes about 3 months for SBP to fall by 10–15 mm Hg after antihypertensive medication is first started. In one-third of patients more than one drug is needed to establish this reduction in SBP.

(4) Therefore SBP should not be measured in hospital before surgery, but should be measured in primary care (National Service Frameworks support GPs doing this irrespective of surgery).

(5) Resting SBP should not be checked in primary care if effective treatment has been established in the previous 2 years: only ambulatory 24-hour monitoring has prognostic value in resistant hypertension.

(6) The primary role of secondary care is to encourage patients to take their medications, including antihypertensives: it is not to measure SBP or to prescribe medication. The only exceptions are patients with PAD or HF who have SBP <140 mm Hg (measured in primary care): these patients should be encouraged *not* to change their compliance, i.e. they should not start to take medications that lower SBP, even if they have been prescribed.

(7) For long-term benefit vascular surgery patients whose risk factors have not been assessed in primary care should be referred to their general practitioners. Importantly abdominal aortic aneurysm (AAA) screening services should do this for all the people they screen, particularly those found to have a widened aorta.

(8) Timing of surgery depends upon patient preference and balance of risk and benefit. The absolute risk of dying in the month after surgery depends upon a patient's preoperative risk (see Chapter 2). One of these factors is age. Even though risk factor reduction always reduces relative risk, delaying surgery to instigate antihypertensive medication could increase absolute risk (ageing increases mortality risk × 1.0083, or RR by nearly 1%, each month). It therefore takes 11 months for risk to increase by 10%, compared to 6 months for antihypertensive medication to reduce risk by 10% (see point 3).

(9) This is why risk-reduction strategies are implemented by default in primary care or triggered by referral to hospital.

The principles of risk reduction for hypertension also apply to cholesterol, smoking, diabetes and physical fitness. Secondary care can assist primary care by motivating patients to exercise, stop smoking and take medication as prescribed. Primary care should be leading primary and secondary risk reduction. In addition to starting antihypertensive medication after discussion with patients, referral to a vascular surgeon should trigger:

(10) Reinforcement of exercise advice and help (RR 0.87 for each MET – see Chapter 2) [22];

(11) Reinforcement of smoking cessation advice and help (RR 0.65, but might take up to 2 years) [23];

(12) Reassessment of HbA1c levels (target 7% – less than this is harmful or not beneficial) [24];

(13) A HMG CoA reductase inhibitor for all patients who have had a cardiovascular event (RR 0.90, unclear how long the effect takes);

(14) A HMG CoA reductase inhibitor for all patients who have PAD (RR 0.90);

(15) A HMG CoA reductase inhibitor for all diabetic patients (RR 0.90) [25].

Heart failure

In 2000 about 40% of patients discharged with a diagnosis of heart failure died within 3 years, three-quarters the mortality rate in 1988, when 55% patients died within 3 years (Figure 3.4) [26]. Between 1988 and 2000 heart failure mortality fell annually to 95% of the previous year's rate, whereas in the general population mortality fell to 98% of the previous year's

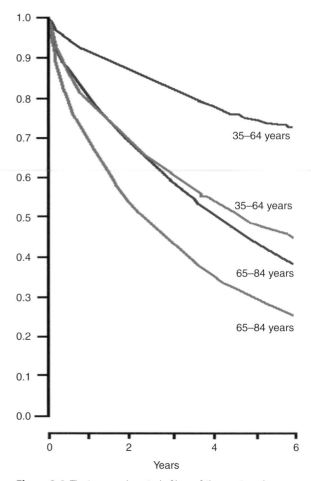

Figure 3.4 The improved survival of heart failure patients between 1988 and 2000 (lower and upper curves respectively), categorised according to age group (35–64 years in blue, 65–84 years in red). Reproduced with permission from reference [26]. See plate section for colour version.

(see Chapter 2). One might expect that in 2010 the 3-year mortality would have fallen to 25%. However the authors of the observational paper from Sweden thought that the year-on-year improvement in heart failure survival may have slowed or stopped, in which case the current 3-year mortality rate might be closer to 33% (survival 67%).

Survival may have improved more in the heart failure population compared to the general population because of the increased use of interventions that reduce heart failure mortality:

- cardiac-specific beta-blockade (Figure 3.5) [27];
- ACE inhibition (Figure 3.6) [28];
- aldosterone blockade (Figure 3.7) [29];
- resynchronisation (Figure 3.8) [30].

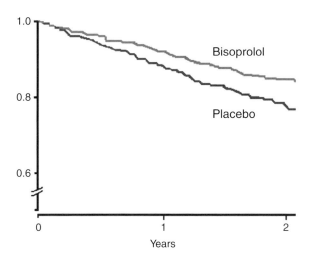

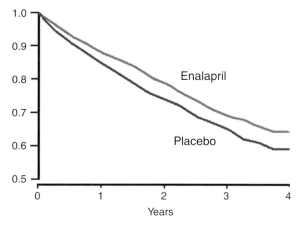

Figure 3.5 Survival improved by bisoprolol in heart failure patients with reduced ejection fractions. Reproduced with permission from reference [27]. See plate section for colour version.

Figure 3.6 Survival improved by enalapril in heart failure patients with reduced ejection fractions. Reproduced with permission from reference [28]. See plate section for colour version.

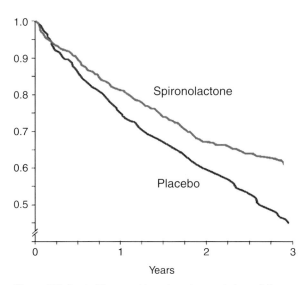

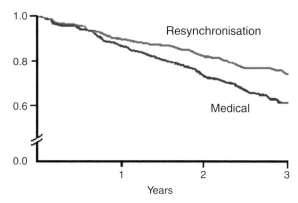

Figure 3.8 Survival improved by cardiac resynchronisation in heart failure patients with reduced ejection fractions (<25%). Reproduced with permission from reference [30]. See plate section for colour version.

Figure 3.7 Survival improved by spironolactone in heart failure patients with reduced ejection fractions. Reproduced with permission from reference [29]. See plate section for colour version.

whether mortality rates for populations with PSF are similar or less than those with reduced ejection fraction (REF)[31,32] The reduction in mortality seen in populations with REF has not been observed in those with PSF, probably because there is no effective treatment [33].

Unfortunately both drugs and resynchronisation only reduce mortality in half of the patients with heart failure – those with reduced ejection fractions (<35% in most RCTs). Half of patients who die with heart failure have preserved systolic function (PSF), with ejection fractions >45%. Currently no intervention has been shown to improve their survival. Patients with PSF are more likely to be hypertensive women without ischaemic heart disease. It is unclear

- The preoperative clinic should support primary care in helping reduce long-term mortality and morbidity in patients with heart failure. In patients with REF this means checking that appropriate drugs have been prescribed and are being taken: ACE inhibitors, cardioselective beta-blockers and spironolactone. These drugs take about 6 months to reduce mortality in REF heart failure patients.

Preserved systolic function heart failure

Preserved systolic function (PSF) patients are clinically indistinguishable from patients with REF. They have a mean age of 72 and most are short of breath on minimal exertion, but have a mean resting ejection fraction of 60% [34]. In the preoperative assessment clinic resting echocardiography will miss half the patients with undiagnosed heart failure, unless the echocardiographer is familiar with the ratio between mitral early velocity and mitral annular velocity[35]. Diagnosis of heart failure – of either subtype – helps estimation of median life expectancy and postoperative mortality and morbidity, all necessary for estimating how likely vascular surgery is to benefit or harm a patient (see Chapter 2). Steps to limit the harm of vascular surgery depend upon these estimations. Therefore anaesthetists must consider how they intend to identify and quantify cardiorespiratory compromise. Cardiopulmonary exercise testing (CPET) elicits pathognomonic patterns in both PSF and REF heart failure, diagnostically and prognostically dominated by raised ventilatory equivalents for carbon dioxide (see Chapter 2) [36]. CPET allows one to distinguish the fat breathless hypertensive woman with PSF from the fat breathless hypertensive woman without heart failure. Anaesthetists without access to CPET diagnosis and prognosis should consider 'low-tech' exercise tests, such as pedalling against increasing resistance without measurement of CPET respiratory variables, perhaps combined with measurement of B-type natriuretic peptide (BNP). In the breathless, higher SBP measurements during exercise confer a better prognosis than lower SBP. Peak power, heart rate and SBP during ramped exercise offer a 'low-tech' option that might provide some prognostic value [37].

Chronic obstructive pulmonary disease

Pulmonary vascular disease combined with cardiac dysfunction partly mediates the decreased survival experienced by patients with chronic obstructive pulmonary disease (COPD), along with airway obstruction. Resting spirometric measurements are not particularly good mortality predictors until abnormalities are severe, partly because they do not tightly correlate with deterioration in ventilation/perfusion matching.

Mortality can be predicted in COPD patients if basic exercise tests, such as the 6-minute walk test (6MWT), are integrated with other historical variables [38]. However peak power or peak oxygen consumption, either measured in a 6MWT, ramped treadmill or cycle CPET, incompletely capture available prognostic information. As detailed in Chapter 2, the ratio of gas flow to exchange, particularly for carbon dioxide ($\dot{V}_E/\dot{V}CO_2$), adds to prognostic precision [39]. It is more likely that inclusion of $\dot{V}_E/\dot{V}CO_2$ for risk estimation will make a clinically important difference in patients with either pulmonary vascular disease and heart failure, as $\dot{V}_E/\dot{V}CO_2$ values are raised. Mortality increases by 6% for each unit increase in $\dot{V}_E/\dot{V}CO_2$. The label 'COPD' does not appear to have additional prognostic significance after $\dot{V}_E/\dot{V}CO_2$ has been combined with $\dot{V}O_2$ in the risk estimation strategy described in Chapter 2.

Renal impairment

Chapter 2 details the continuous relationship between renal impairment and mortality. In summary risk of death increases 0.85% (RR 1.0085) for each 1-ml fall in eGFR. The 'normal' eGFR changes with age and is different for men and women. Chapter 2 details these expected values and how to adjust risk estimations based upon renal impairment.

Management of comorbidity in vascular patients

Chapters 4 to 7 discuss in part anaesthetic management of coincident disease. I have suggested above default delays before vascular surgery after: acute coronary syndromes, coronary artery bypass grafting and percutaneous stenting.

I have suggested that preoperative and anaesthetic services should check prescription and encourage compliance for those drugs that improve survival in patients with comorbidities. However, this is for long-term patient benefit, rather than for short-term perioperative benefit. New medications can be introduced following preoperative assessment, but with an eye on general survival and health. The utility of introducing new medication will depend upon how long before vascular surgery you are assessing patients. Patients with incidental or screened AAAs less than 5 cm diameter should have a general health review, by both primary and secondary care, with introduction of new drugs as indicated. In the past non-cardiac surgery has been viewed as an additional reason to consider new drugs or coronary revascularisation. The pendulum of evidence and opinion appears to have swung to a point where non-cardiac surgery is either irrelevant or considered a relative contraindication to either intervention. Please see the discussion of blood pressure control above.

Perioperative management of diabetes, ischaemic heart disease, heart failure and renal impairment for vascular surgery is fundamentally the same as any other surgery. Postoperative risks of death and morbidity are greater after vascular operations than after many other operations, but unfortunately there are no special interventions known to reduce their incidence. What is probably true is that patients will benefit from rapid identification of perioperative physiological derangement. The emphasis should be on intraoperative and postoperative surveillance and response rather than on extreme intervention.

Postoperative morbidity and mortality are most easily limited by the most vulnerable patients deciding to avoid surgery. Senior anaesthetists should help surgical colleagues quantify background mortality and morbidity risks, including median life expectancy, and then estimating the risks of temporary or permanent harm and benefit (see Chapter 2). An informed group discussion can then take place, exploring the merits of futures with and without surgery. Patients should not proceed to surgery until they *understand* these risks: whether a patient is 'well-informed' cannot be defined on the basis of how much information they have been given. We should consign to historical regret misunderstanding patients submitting themselves to any medical intervention, particularly high-risk procedures like vascular surgery.

References

1. Fox KAA, Carruthers KF, Dunbar DR, *et al.* Underestimated and under-recognized: the late consequences of acute coronary syndrome (GRACE UK-Belgian Study). *Eur Heart J* 2010; DOI:10.1093/eurheartj/ehq326.

2. Brindle P, Beswick A, Fahey T, *et al.* Accuracy and impact of risk assessment in the primary prevention of cardiovascular disease: a systematic review. *Heart* (2006); **92**:1752–9.

3. Empana JP, Ducimetière P, Arveiler D. Are the Framingham and PROCAM coronary heart disease risk functions applicable to different European populations? The PRIME study. *Eur Heart J* 2004; **24**:1903–11.

4. Clayton TC, Lubsen J, Pocock SJ, *et al.* Risk score for predicting death, myocardial infarction, and stroke in patients with stable angina, based on a large randomised trial cohort of patients. *BMJ* 2005; **331**: 869–74.

5. Anavekar NS, McMurray JJV, Velazquez EJ, *et al.* Relation between renal dysfunction and cardiovascular outcomes after myocardial infarction.

N Engl J Med 2004; **351**: 1285–95.

6. Huynh T, Perron S, O'Loughlin J, *et al.* Comparison of primary percutaneous intervention and fibrinolytic therapy in ST-segment-elevation myocardial infarction: Bayesian hierarchical meta-analyses of randomized controlled trials and observational studies. *Circulation* 2009; **119**:3101–9.

7. Kastrati A, Dibra A, Spaulding C, *et al.* Meta-analysis of randomized trials on drug-eluting stents vs bare-metal stents in patients with acute myocardial infarction. *Eur Heart J* 2007;**28**:2706–13.

8. Kaltoft A, Kelbæk H, Thuesen L, *et al.* Long-term outcome after drug-eluting versus bare-metal stent implantation in patients with ST-segment elevation myocardial infarction. *J Am Coll Cardiol* 2010; **56**:641–5.

9. Boden WE, O'Rourke RA, Teo KK, *et al.* Optimal medical therapy with or without PCI for stable coronary disease. *N Engl J Med* 2007; **356**:1503–16.

10. Yusuf S, Zucker D, Peduzzi, P, *et al.* Effect of coronary artery bypass graft surgery on survival: overview of 10-year results from

randomised trials by the Coronary Artery Bypass Graft Surgery Trialists Collaboration. *Lancet* 1994; **344**: 563–70.

11. Frye L, August P, Brooks MM, *et al.* A randomized trial of therapies for type 2 diabetes and coronary artery disease. *N Engl J Med* 2009; **360**:2503–15.

12. Gu Q, Dillon CF, Burt VL, *et al.* (2010). Association of hypertension treatment and control with all-cause and cardiovascular disease mortality among US adults with hypertension. *Am J Hypertens* 2010;**23**:38–45.

13. Arguedas JA, Perez MI, Wright JM. Treatment blood pressure targets for hypertension. *Cochrane Database Syst Rev* 2009; **CD004349.**

14. Law MR, Morris JK, Wald NJ. Use of blood pressure lowering drugs in the prevention of cardiovascular disease: meta-analysis of 147 randomised trials in the context of expectations from prospective epidemiological studies. *BMJ* **338**:b1665.

15. Cushman WC, Evans GW, Byington RP, *et al.* Effects of intensive blood-pressure control

in type 2 diabetes mellitus. *N Engl J Med* 2010;**362**:1575–85.

16. Bejan-Angouvant T, Saadatian-Elahi M, Wright, J.M., *et al.* Treatment of hypertension in patients 80 years and older: the lower the better? A meta-analysis of randomized controlled trials. *Hypertens* 2010; **28**:1366–72.

17. Pladevall M, Brotons, C, Gabriel R, *et al.* Multicenter cluster-randomized trial of a multifactorial intervention to improve antihypertensive medication adherence and blood pressure control among patients at high cardiovascular risk (the COM99 study). *Circulation* 2010; **122**:1183–91.

18. Bavry AA, Anderson D, Gong Y, *et al.* Outcomes among hypertensive patients with concomitant peripheral and coronary disease: findings from the International VErapamil-SR/Trandolapril Study (INVEST). *Hypertension* 2010; **55**:48–53.

19. Selby JV, Lee J, Swain BE, *et al.* Trends in time to confirmation and recognition of new-onset hypertension, 2002–6. *Hypertension* 2010; **56**:605–11.

20. Keenan K, Hayen A, Neal BC, *et al.* Long term monitoring in patients receiving treatment to lower blood pressure: analysis of data from placebo controlled randomised controlled trial. *BMJ* 2009; **338**:b1492.

21. Niiranen TJ, Hanninen MR, Johansson J, *et al.* Home-measured blood pressure is a stronger predictor of cardiovascular risk than office blood pressure: the Finn-Home study. *Hypertension* 2010; **55**:1346–51.

22. Kokkinos P, Doumas M, Myers J, *et al.* A graded association of exercise capacity and all-cause mortality in males with high-normal blood pressure. *Blood Press* 2009; **18**:261–7.

23. Critchley JA, Capewell S. Smoking cessation for the secondary prevention of coronary heart disease. *Cochrane Database Syst Rev* 2003;**CD003041**.

24. Marso SP, Kennedy KF, House, JA, *et al.* The effect of intensive glucose control on all-cause and cardiovascular mortality, myocardial infarction and stroke in persons with type 2 diabetes mellitus: a systematic review and meta-analysis. *Diabetes Vasc Dis Res* 2010; 7:119–30.

25. Cholesterol Treatment Trialists' (CTT) Collaborators. Efficacy of cholesterol-lowering therapy in 18 686 people with diabetes in 14 randomised trials of statins: a meta-analysis. *Lancet* 2008; **371**:117–25.

26. Shafazand M, Schaufelberger M, Lappas G., *et al.* Survival trends in men and women with heart failure of ischaemic and non-ischaemic origin: data for the period 1987–2003 from the Swedish Hospital Discharge Registry. *Eur Heart J* 2009; **30**:671–8.

27. Dargie HJ, Lechat P, and the CIBIS-II investigators. The cardiac insufficiency bisoprolol study II (CIBIS-II): a randomised trial. *Lancet* 1999; **353**:9–13.

28. Yusuf S, and the SOLVD investigators. Effect of enalapril on survival in patients with reduced left ventricular ejection fractions and congestive heart failure. *N Engl J Med* 1991; **325**: 293–302.

29. Pitt B, Zannad F, Remme WJ, *et al.* The effects of spironolactone on morbidity and mortality in patients with severe heart failure. *N Engl J Med* 1999; **341**:709–17.

30. Cleland JGF, Daubert J-C, Erdmann E, *et al.* The effect of cardiac resynchronization on morbidity and mortality in heart

failure. *N Engl J Med* 2005; **352**:1539–49.

31. Somaratne JB, Berry C, McMurray JJV, *et al.* The prognostic significance of heart failure with preserved left ventricular ejection fraction: a literature-based meta-analysis. *Eur J Heart Fail* 2009; **11**:855–62.

32. Fonarrow GC, Stough WG, Abraham WT, *et al.* Characteristics, treatments, and outcomes of patients with preserved systolic function hospitalized for heart failure: a report from the OPTIMIZE-HF registry. *J Am Coll Cardiol* 2008; **50**:768–77.

33. Shamagian LG, Gonzalez-Juanetey JR, Roman AV, *et al.* The death rate among hospitalized heart failure patients with normal and depressed left ventricular ejection fraction in the year following discharge: evolution over a 10-year period. *Eur Heart J* 2005; **26**:2251–8.

34. McMurray JJV, Carson PE, Komajda M, *et al.* (2008). Heart failure with preserved ejection fraction: clinical characteristics of 4133 patients enrolled in the I-PRESERVE trial. *Eur J Heart Fail* 2008; **10**:149–56.

35. Guazzi M, Myers J, Arena R. Cardiopulmonary exercise testing in the clinical and prognostic assessment of diastolic heart failure. *J Am Coll Cardiol* 2005; **46**:1883–90.

36. Guazzi M, Myers J, Peberdy MA, *et al.* Cardiopulmonary exercise testing variables reflect the degree of diastolic dysfunction in patients with heart failure-normal ejection fraction. *J Cardiopulm Rehabil Prev* 2010; **30**:165–72.

37. Corra U, Mezzani A, Giordano A, *et al.* Exercise haemodynamic variables rather than ventilatory efficiency indexes contribute to risk assessment in chronic heart failure patients treated with

carvedilol. *Eur Heart J* 2009; **30**:3000–6.

38. Cote CG, Pinto-Plata VM, Marin JM, *et al.* The modified BODE index: validation with mortality in COPD. *Eur Respir J* 2008; **32**:1269–74.

39. Torchio R, Guglielmo M, Giardino R, *et al.* Exercise ventilatory inefficiency and mortality in patients with chronic obstructive pulmonary disease undergoing surgery for non-small-cell lung cancer. *Eur J Cardiothorac Surg* 2010; **38**:14–9.

Chapter 4

Reducing perioperative cardiac risk

Craig Beattie and Bruce Biccard

Introduction

Patients undergoing non-cardiac surgery who have or are at risk of cardiac disease have a 4% risk of suffering a major perioperative cardiac event (cardiac death, non-fatal myocardial infarction (MI) and non-fatal cardiac arrest) with an associated in-hospital mortality rate after MI of 15% to 25% [1]. Perioperative MI is most likely to occur in patients with significant coronary artery stenoses characteristic of vascular surgical patients [2]. Supply–demand MIs occur in the first few postoperative days. These patients probably have a relative flow-mediated hypoperfusion which precedes MI, most commonly at the site of significant stenoses. Hypoperfusion may be aggravated by hypotension, or intracoronary thrombosis secondary to hypercoagulability and inflammation, possibly further aggravated by an increased myocardial oxygen demand associated with surgery, pain and sympathetic stimulation.

In contrast, perioperative MIs following plaque rupture resemble medical MIs and are evenly distributed throughout the postoperative period. Plaque may rupture secondary to intrinsic factors related to the plaque morphology, with a large necrotic lipid pool, characterised by neovascularisation and many inflammatory cells or extrinsic factors such as circumferential stress or haemodynamic shear stress.

Therapies targeting inflammation, coagulation, oxygen supply–demand and coronary anatomy in vascular surgical patients are therefore potentially cardioprotective. Due to the multiple factors involved in perioperative cardiac events, it is perhaps unlikely that any single intervention will produce a very large relative risk reduction.

Antiplatelet drugs

Disruption of endothelium at the site of unstable plaques, inflammation, platelet activation and aggregation are fundamental to the formation of arterial thromboses. Antiplatelet drugs form the mainstay of treatment to prevent these thrombotic events in patients with coronary artery disease. Despite this they are frequently stopped before surgery because of the perceived risks of bleeding.

Antiplatelet drugs are indicated for primary and secondary prevention of atherosclerotic disease and most commonly include aspirin, dipyridamole and clopidogrel. They may be used alone or in combination. Their use raises a number of issues for the perioperative care of the vascular surgical patient. It is important to identify the clinical indication to allow informed risk–benefit analysis. In practical terms this means balancing the risk of thrombosis versus the risks of bleeding [3]. There are limited data in the perioperative setting on which to base these decisions.

Aspirin

Aspirin or acetylsalicylic acid is an irreversible cyclo-oxygenase-1 inhibitor. It blocks the breakdown of arachidonic acid to thromboxane A2, a potent vasoconstrictor and stimulator of platelet aggregation. Platelet function takes 7–10 days to return to normal. Meta-analysis suggests that aspirin reduces cardiovascular death by 15% and non-fatal cardiovascular events by 30% in high-risk patients. Among patients with peripheral arterial disease, aspirin reduces the risk of adverse cardiovascular events by 23% [4]. While it is likely these effects are secondary to an antiplatelet effect, aspirin also induces the synthesis of nitric oxide in endothelial cells, inhibits prostaglandin production and has an anti-inflammatory effect. These actions may all contribute to the vascular protective effect. All patients with peripheral arterial disease, in the absence of contraindications, should be taking aspirin.

Core Topics in Vascular Anaesthesia, ed. Carl Moores and Alastair F. Nimmo. Published by Cambridge University Press.
© Cambridge University Press 2012.

Risk of thrombosis

In patients with stable coronary artery disease stopping aspirin is associated with up to a fourfold increase in risk of death or MI [5]. In the perioperative period interruption of aspirin precedes more than 10% of acute coronary syndromes in the wider surgical population [6]. A randomised controlled trial in intermediate and high-risk patients having surgery comparing aspirin with placebo demonstrated a 7% absolute risk reduction in major adverse cardiovascular events [7]. It is possible in study that those patients taking aspirin who were randomised to placebo group may have been placed at additional risk because of aspirin withdrawal. A meta-analysis of 10 randomised controlled trials in patients undergoing infrainguinal bypass surgery suggested a reduction in serious vascular events and death in those patients taking aspirin although benefit did not reach statistical significance [8]. In patients undergoing carotid endarterectomy, aspirin reduced stroke rate but not MI or mortality [9]. In a cohort of 181 patients presenting with acute lower limb ischaemia, 6.1% had stopped their aspirin recently [10]. This apparent increase in thrombotic risk associated with stopping aspirin may be due to platelet recovery or a rebound elevation in thromboxane A2 or both. Experimental data to answer this question are lacking.

Risk of haemorrhage

It is the perceived risks of bleeding complications that drive patients and clinicians to stop aspirin before surgery. In a meta-analysis of nearly 50 000 patients having a wide range of surgeries, almost 15 000 of which were taking aspirin, the rate of bleeding complications was increased by a factor 1.5 [6]. The bleeding complication rate for the subset undergoing vascular surgery was less than 2.5% [11]. The increased bleeding rate did not lead to more severe bleeding complications with the exception of intracranial surgery and possibly transurethral prostatectomy. In two randomised controlled trials looking at vascular surgical patients the odds ratio of requiring re-operation for bleeding complications in those on aspirin was 1.4 for carotid endarterectomy and 1.9 for femoral popliteal bypass [9,12].

Recommendation

Based on current literature, we would recommend that aspirin should be continued throughout the perioperative period in vascular surgery patients, until such time as the results of the PeriOperative ISchemic Evaluation-2 (POISE-2) trial are known.

Dipyridamole

Dipyridamole is a pyrimidopyrimidine derivative that increases intracellular 3'-5'-cyclic adenosine monophosphate by phosphodiesterase inhibition and blockage of adenosine reuptake by platelets, endothelial cells and erythrocytes. It increases concentrations of cyclic guanosine monophosphate and potentiates the local effects of nitric oxide. The absorption of dipyridamole is variable. The drug has a terminal half-life of approximately 10 hours though modified release preparations are available. Recovery of platelet function is seen with clearance of the drug. Excretion is biliary and is subject to enterohepatic circulation.

Dipyridamole is indicated with aspirin for the secondary prevention of cerebrovascular disease and is frequently encountered in those patients presenting for carotid endarterectomy. It is not used as a sole agent for the primary or secondary prevention of atherosclerotic disease.

Dipyridamole in the perioperative period

There is little in the literature to quantify the risk of thrombosis versus risk of bleeding in patients taking dipyridamole alone or in combination.

Recommendation

Based on current literature, dipyridamole should be continued throughout the perioperative period in vascular surgery patients. Where it is used in combination and stopped before surgery it should be restarted as soon as possible following surgery.

Clopidogrel

Clopidogrel is a thienopyridine pro-drug rapidly oxidised by the cytochrome P450 system to an active metabolite. Inhibition of platelet effect is seen within 2 hours of a loading dose by inhibiting adenosine diphosphate induced activation of platelets. Platelet activity is blocked for the lifespan of the individual platelets with normal function 7–10 days after last dose. The only large trial comparing aspirin and clopidogrel in patients with a history of MI, stroke or peripheral arterial disease found that clopidogrel reduced serious vascular events by 8.7% versus 16.5% with aspirin [13]. The absolute risk reduction was 1.9% versus 3.2% over 1.8 years. Subgroup analysis of patients with peripheral arterial disease indicated a 23.8% relative risk reduction in favour of clopidogrel. Clopidogrel is more frequently prescribed as a single agent to those patients that are intolerant of aspirin and is prescribed in combination with aspirin after acute coronary syndromes and percutaneous coronary revascularisation. Combination therapy is discussed later.

Risk of thrombosis

While there is evidence of a modest reduction in frequency of thromboembolic events in patients at risk who are changed from aspirin to clopidogrel, there are no data quantifying the thrombotic risks of stopping it in the perioperative period. Given that in many cases clopidogrel is prescribed in patients at high risk, stopping the drug in the perioperative period is likely to place the patient at increased risk of thrombotic complications.

Risk of haemorrhage

There are few studies in the non-cardiac surgical population assessing the risk of haemorrhage in patients taking clopidogrel alone. While it does have a potent effect on platelet function in the laboratory there is little evidence that perioperative bleeding rates are any higher than in those patients taking aspirin alone.

Recommendation

In the absence of good evidence describing the risks of thrombosis against the risk of bleeding in patients taking clopidogrel alone, each case must be considered individually. It is important to know the indication for treatment before a decision weighing the risk–benefit of stopping the drug before surgery.

Dual antiplatelet therapy

Aspirin and dipyridamole

These drugs are indicated in combination for the secondary prevention of transient ischaemic attacks or ischaemic cerebrovascular accidents and may be continued indefinitely [14]. They are frequently encountered in those patients presenting for carotid endarterectomy but may also be taken together in the vascular patient presenting for other surgery. Where the risk of bleeding is thought to be high, dipyridamole may be stopped briefly to allow surgery

to proceed and restarted as soon as possible after surgery.

Aspirin and clopidogrel

Dual antiplatelet therapy with aspirin and clopidogrel is indicated for the treatment of acute coronary syndromes (ACS) and after coronary artery stenting. While the optimal duration of dual therapy is not well established, recommendations suggest dual therapy for 12 months following ACS while for patients with coronary artery stents the duration of therapy depends on the type of stent placed. Patients with coronary artery disease at high risk of developing ACS may also be on dual therapy indefinitely.

Aspirin and clopidogrel in the perioperative period
Risks of thrombosis

In the non-surgical population stopping a patient's clopidogrel prematurely following an acute coronary syndrome places them at high risk of recurrent ACS and cardiac death [5]. While not quantified in a surgical population, risk is likely to be greater given the inflammatory and prothrombotic response to surgery.

Risk of haemorrhage

The addition of low-dose clopidogrel to aspirin reduces platelet aggregation and increases bleeding time in drug responders [15]. There are case series in the non-cardiac surgical population describing increased blood loss and transfusion rates but no increase in mortality. In those patients on aspirin and clopidogrel undergoing coronary artery bypass grafting bleeding rates requiring re-operation are greater than in those patients on aspirin alone [16]. It would seem likely that bleeding rates in the vascular surgical population are higher in those patients who are on aspirin and clopidogrel therapy. There is however currently no evidence that this increases mortality.

Recommendation

Where a patient is on both aspirin and clopidogrel it is likely that this patient is at high risk of thrombotic events and stopping either drug would place the patient at high risk of an adverse cardiac event. Where the risks of bleeding are thought to be high, surgery should be postponed until dual therapy can be safely discontinued. Where patients on aspirin or clopidogrel develop severe or life-threatening bleeding platelet transfusion is required.

Glycoprotein IIb/IIIa receptor antagonists

These drugs block glycoprotein IIb/IIIa receptors on the platelet surface, the final common pathway of platelet activation. They are indicated in acute coronary syndromes and coronary stenting. While oral preparations are in development the drugs in current clinical use are given intravenously as a loading dose followed by infusion.

Abciximab has a rapid onset of action and although it has a short plasma half-life platelet aggregation may take 48 hours to return to 50% of baseline values in some patients.

Tirofiban has a rapid onset of action and normal coagulation is restored within 4–8 hours of the end of an infusion in patients with normal renal function.

Eptifibatide has a rapid onset of action and normal coagulation is restored within 4–8 hours of the end of an infusion in patients with normal renal function.

There are case reports of these drugs being used in the perioperative period as a 'bridging strategy' in patients at high thrombotic risk [17]. These cases require close collaboration with cardiology colleagues.

Other perioperative issues in patients on antiplatelet drugs
Neuraxial blocks

Spinals and epidurals are widely performed in patients on aspirin alone. The American Society of Regional Anaesthesia recommends against performance of these blocks in patients taking clopidogrel. While there are case series describing neuroaxial blockade in patients taking clopidogrel the magnitude of risk is uncertain. If neuraxial block is undertaken it is important to monitor for complications suggesting haematoma formation. Prompt diagnosis and treatment within 8 hours of symptoms is essential to give the best chance of neurological recovery [18,19]. In the case of dual antiplatelet therapy it is very likely that there is an increased risk of epidural haematoma.

Variable response to antiplatelet agents

It is increasingly recognised that not all patients respond equally to aspirin and clopidogrel. There is an expanding understanding of the genetic polymorphisms that may affect the metabolism of antiplatelet agents. Recent advances in reliable platelet function testing outside of the laboratory may change prescribing practice and our perioperative management of antiplatelet therapy in the future.

Statins

Statins inhibit 3-hydroxy-3-methylglutaryl coenzyme A (HMG CoA) reductase and thus decrease cholesterol synthesis. A second effect is decreased L-mevalonic acid synthesis which inhibits synthesis of isoprenoid intermediates which are necessary for post-translation modification of various proteins essential for cellular signalling and intracellular trafficking which include anti-inflammatory, vasodilatory and antithrombogenic effects.

Statins show the greatest relative risk reduction for mortality associated with MI and major coronary events (non-fatal MI or coronary heart disease death) in medical patients. Current medical guidelines recommend that patients with known coronary heart disease or coronary artery disease equivalents (peripheral vascular disease, aortic aneurysm and cerebrovascular disease) should receive statin therapy for secondary prevention [20].

Statins in the perioperative period
The efficacy of statin therapy in surgical patients

Currently, two meta-analyses have shown a significant reduction in mortality and improved cardiac outcomes following non-cardiac surgery [21,22]; however, both meta-analyses concluded that the evidence base was inadequate to recommend routine administration, as the majority of the studies were retrospective and the heterogeneity was large.

There are currently three prospective, randomised peer-reviewed studies of acute perioperative statin therapy in non-cardiac surgical patients [23–25]. The two vascular surgical studies show exceedingly large relative risk reductions for major adverse cardiac events (52% to 75%) [24,25]. The third study reported on a mixed group of non-cardiac nonvascular elective surgical patients (DECREASE-IV study) [23] over 40 years of age with a predicted cardiovascular death rate

Study or sub-category	Statin n/N	Control n/N	OR (fixed) 95% CI	Weight %	OR (fixed) 95% CI
Durazzo	4/50	10/50		14.85	0.35 [0.10, 1.20]
DECREASE-IV	17/354	26/532		40.70	0.64 [0.34, 1.19]
DECREASE-III	14/250	29/247		44.45	0.45 [0.23, 0.87]
Total (95% CI)	834	829		100.00	0.51 [0.33, 0.78]

Total events: 35 (Statin), 65 (Control)
Test for heterogeneity: Chi^2 = 1.04, df = 2 (P = 0.60), I^2 = 0%
Test for overall effect: Z = 3.10 (P = 0.002)

0.1 0.2 0.5 1 2 5 10
Favours statin   Favours placebo

Figure 4.1 Combined 30-day all-cause mortality and non-fatal myocardial infarction in prospective randomised trials of statin therapy in non-cardiac surgical patients.

exceeding 1%. There was a reported 35% relative risk reduction (3.2% versus 4.9%) for the combined endpoint of 30-day cardiac death and non-fatal MI [23]. A meta-analysis of these three studies shows a significant decrease in the composite outcome of 30-day death and non-fatal MI (odds ratio (OR) 0.51, 95% confidence interval (CI) 0.33–0.78, $p = 0.002$) with a relative risk reduction of 46% (7.8% and 4.2% event rates in the control and treatment groups respectively) and a number-needed-to-treat (NNT) of 28 (Figure 4.1). This is much higher than the 18% relative risk reduction seen in medical patients. One should have some reservation about this meta-analysis, as the small sample size in the studies may have resulted in the treatment effect being overestimated.

It is possible however, that the relative risk reduction associated with statin therapy in vascular surgical patients is higher than that of medical (non-surgical) patients or other non-cardiac non-vascular surgical patients, especially as inflammation is potentially important in vascular surgical patients with both plaque rupture and thrombosis. There are three potentially complementary mechanisms of cardioprotection associated with statin therapy in the perioperative period for vascular surgical patients: low-density lipoprotein (LDL) cholesterol reduction, C-reactive protein (CRP) reduction and immunomodulation of the surgical stress response (Figure 4.2). Both LDL cholesterol and CRP are reduced in the perioperative period after initiation of statin therapy with the proviso of a run in time of about 30 days [25] and a high-dose statin regimen for CRP reduction [24].

While LDL cholesterol reduction and CRP reduction are likely to be responsible for the 19% (95% CI 13–25%) risk reduction in medical (non-surgical) patients with peripheral vascular disease further

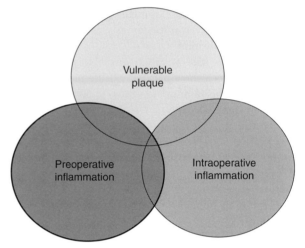

Figure 4.2 The potential mechanisms of perioperative statin cardioprotection.

cardioprotection may be afforded by modification of the preoperative CRP and immunomodulation of the surgical inflammatory response [26].

A marked pre-existing inflammatory response may be reflected in an increased CRP, which would put the patient at risk of coronary plaque rupture, or coronary thrombosis. How much difference does a high CRP make to outcome in surgical patients? It was shown that for 30-day major adverse cardiac events (MACE) following vascular surgery a low CRP is associated with a 43% risk reduction when compared to a high CRP, defined as a CRP > 3 mg/dl, although this was not statistically significant due to the small sample size [27]. When considering long-term MACE, vascular surgical patients with a high CRP had an event rate of 20.7% and patients with a normal CRP had an event rate of 9.5%, giving a risk reduction of 54% associated with a low CRP. Should one be able to decrease the CRP from the high to normal group preoperatively, it would then be theoretically possible that a relative risk reduction of 50% might be possible with perioperative statin therapy in high-risk vascular patients. It is important to note that in all the studies discussed, the control event rate for MACE at 30 days exceeded 10% [24,25] and approached 20% [27] at 1 to 2 years and hence one would only expect this additional cardioprotection in patients of a similar risk profile.

It is possible that the inflammatory response to surgery may precipitate both plaque rupture and coronary thrombosis in the presence of complex coronary atherosclerotic plaque. The inflammatory response in the perioperative period is correlated with the extent of surgical trauma and perioperative statin therapy may decrease the inflammatory response to major surgery, which may result in less plaque disruption and coronary thrombosis, although there are no data which have evaluated this hypothesis in vascular surgical patients.

The safety of statins

Statin-associated rhabdomyolysis in the perioperative period is uncommon. Its incidence has been estimated at between 0.1% and less than 0.5%. Withdrawal of statin therapy in response to elevated creatinine kinase (CK) levels after surgery may often be unnecessary and is potentially harmful, as omission of therapy for more than 4 days postoperatively has also been identified as an independent predictor of cardiac myonecrosis following infrarenal aortic vascular surgery [28]. Although statin therapy may be associated with an elevated CK in vascular surgical patients, there are a number of other factors associated with an elevated CK, including the surgical procedure (embolectomy, fasciotomy and aortic surgery), the duration of surgery, the medical condition of the patient (renal dysfunction) and complicating cardiac events which are potentially more important for patient outcome, than the rare occurrence of statin-associated rhabdomyolysis and CK elevation [29]. The presence of statin therapy has been associated with improved survival in vascular surgical patients [29].

Recommendations

All patients with medical indications for statin therapy should receive statins in the perioperative period. Statins should not be withdrawn perioperatively.

Beta-blockers and other rate-limiting drugs

The central premise of the cardioprotective efficacy of beta-blocker therapy is based upon heart rate reduction, resulting in an optimisation of myocardial oxygen supply–demand, which decreases myocardial ischaemia, improving cardiac outcome. However, beta-blockers may also prevent plaque rupture and reduce inflammation. Other cardioprotective mechanisms of beta-blockers (which are also mediated independently of the heart rate) include alteration of apoptosis, anti-arrhythmic properties, modulation of coagulation, mechanical unloading of the heart and alteration of bioenergetics [30].

Perioperative myocardial ischaemia, heart rate and reported morbidity

The following principles have been identified which are important when considering perioperative cardiac outcome associated with heart rate. Postoperative myocardial ischaemia is more common than pre- and intraoperative myocardial ischaemia and of longer duration than pre- or intraoperative myocardial ischaemia [31]. Myocardial ischaemia associated with postoperative MI is usually prolonged (between 30 minutes to >120 minutes) [31]. Many studies report an association between an increasing and an elevated perioperative heart rate and myocardial ischaemia. The observations of these studies are shown in Table 4.1.

Table 4.1 suggests that the absolute change and the lability of the heart rate appear to be important determinants of myocardial ischaemia. An increase in intraoperative heart rate in vascular surgical patients has been shown to be independently associated with troponin release and long-term mortality (OR 1.57 and OR 1.37 respectively) [32].

Perioperative myocardial ischaemia has been associated with adverse short- and long-term outcomes. Postoperative MI was shown to be strongly correlated with postoperative myocardial ischaemia in vascular surgical patients. When postoperative myocardial ischaemia lasted >10 minutes and was associated with ST depression or elevation of >1 mm, the peak troponin level was correlated with both the duration and the cumulative myocardial ischaemia time ($r = 0.83$ and $r = 0.78$ respectively) [33].

Table 4.1 Intraoperative heart rate and myocardial ischaemia

First author, year	Surgery	Percentage of patients with ischaemia	Absolute heart rate at time of ischaemia (beats per minute)	Significance when comparing with group with no ischaemia	Absolute change in heart rate from baseline to ischaemia	Significance of change in heart rate
Ouyang, 1989	Vascular	63%	107 ± 12	NS	NR	NR
Landesberg, 2001	Vascular	21%	106 ± 18	NR	84 ± 12 to 106 ± 18	$p < 0.0001$
Fleisher, 1995	Vascular or ≥2 cardiac risk factors	26%	98 ± 21	NR	NR	NR
Groves, 1999	Thoracic	24%	93 ± 19	$p < 0.05$	76.7 ± 9.8 to 93 ± 19	$p < 0.05$
Raby, 1999	Vascular	50%	Postoperative HR within 20% of preoperative ischaemic threshold	RR 12.0, 95% CI 1.81–79.4, $p<0.0001$	NR	NR
Feringa, 2006	Vascular	31%	NR	NR	10 beats per minute increase	OR 1.75, 95% CI 1.25–2.45, $p < 0.001$

NR, not reported; NS, not significant; OR, odds ratio; RR, relative risk; CI, confidence interval; HR, heart rate.
Source: Biccard BM. Heart rate and outcome in patients with cardiovascular disease undergoing major noncardiac surgery. *Anaesth Intens Care* 2008;**36**:489–501.

The evidence for acute perioperative beta-blockade

The current evidence suggests that acute perioperative beta-blockade is associated with beneficial, neutral and adverse effects. Beneficial effects include decreased non-fatal MI (OR 0.65, 95% CI 0.54–0.79) and decreased myocardial ischaemia (OR 0.36, 95% CI 0.26–0.50) [34]. However, no benefit has been shown with all-cause mortality, cardiovascular mortality and heart failure, and beta-blockers have been associated with an increased risk of stroke (OR 2.01, 95% CI 1.27–3.68) [34]. Drug-associated side-effects are significantly increased: hypotension requiring treatment (OR 1.62, 95% CI 1.44–1.82) and bradycardia requiring treatment (OR 2.74, 95% CI 2.29–3.29) [34]. Importantly, these drug-associated side-effects are associated with major morbidity. In the Peri-Operative Ischemic Evaluation (POISE) trial, both bradycardia and hypotension were independent predictors of mortality with a population attributable risk (PAR) of 7.9% (95% CI 3.9–15.3%) and 37.3% (95% CI 29.5–45.8%) respectively [35]. Hypotension was also an independent predictor of stroke (PAR 14.7%, 95% CI 5.2–35.4%) [35].

Heart rate considerations when using perioperative beta-blockers

The current data suggests that in the perioperative period a J-shaped relationship probably exists between heart rate and outcome. POISE showed that beta-blocker-associated bradycardia was an independent predictor of all-cause mortality (hazard ratio (HR) 1.99, 95% CI 1.35–2.92). Higher heart rates result in an exponential increase in adverse outcomes in vascular surgical patients. A meta-analysis of prospective perioperative beta-blocker studies divided the studies into two groups as defined by a maximum heart rate either below or above 100 beats per minute. Studies where the maximum heart rate did not exceed 100 were associated with cardioprotection (OR 0.23, 95% CI 0.08–0.65), while the studies exceeding a 100 beats per minute were not (OR 1.17, 95% CI 0.79–1.80) [36]. This meta-analysis confirms that the maximum heart rate is an important determinant of outcome.

Clearly, the challenge for anaesthetists is to determine the most appropriate method of acute perioperative beta-blocker administration, in order to optimise perioperative short- and possibly long-term outcome, while eliminating any increase in morbidity.

Are perioperative beta-blockers preferable in certain select populations?

It is tempting to consider that the cardioprotective efficacy differs between different patient population groups. However, the current data is conflicting. In the subgroup analysis of POISE, only two subgroups had a significant reduction in the primary outcome of cardiovascular death, non-fatal MI and non-fatal cardiac arrest. These were vascular patients (high-risk surgical patients) and patients with two Lee's risk factors. However, none of the interaction p values were significant in this study, which suggests that there is no subgroup effect based on the evidence available [35].

The patients with three or four Lee's risk factors had a trend to a worse outcome [35]. It is possible however, that only a very select group of patients with inducible ischaemia in this very high-risk group may benefit. This is supported by a large observational study of over 780 000 patients that showed that the most benefit associated with perioperative beta-blockade was seen in the highest risk group, defined as four or more Lee's Revised Cardiac Risk Index factors (OR 0.58 for mortality, 95% CI 0.50–0.67) [37], which is contrary to the POISE data.

Conversely, randomisation of patients at low risk (no Lee's risk factors) may be associated with morbidity and mortality. In the same observational study, patients with no Lee's risk factors who were beta-blocked had an associated increased mortality (OR 1.36, 95% CI 1.29–1.58) [37]. Certainly identification of the patients most likely to benefit from acute perioperative beta-blockade needs further investigation.

Finally beta-receptor polymorphisms may modify the response to beta-blocker therapy. A recent study of vascular surgical patients randomised to placebo or bisoprolol found that the only independent predictor of a composite outcome of cardiovascular death, non-fatal MI, unstable angina, heart failure and stroke was an adrenergic receptor polymorphism. Patients with at least one glycine allele at Arg389 of the beta-adrenergic receptor had a significantly higher risk of the primary outcome (HR 1.87, 95% CI 1.04–3.35) [38]. This is an issue which has not previously been considered in any of the perioperative beta-blocker studies.

Chronic beta-blockade

A history of chronic beta-blockade has been associated with a significantly increased incidence of perioperative MI in non-cardiac surgical patients (OR 2.14, 95% CI 1.29–3.56) probably following perioperative withdrawal [39]. Case series that have documented withdrawal of chronic beta-blockade following mixed vascular surgical procedures have reported extremely poor outcomes; with an in-hospital mortality of 24% to 50%, an early cardiovascular mortality of 29%, a perioperative MI rate of 50% and a 1-year mortality following surgery of 38% [40,41]. It is therefore critical that chronic beta-blockade is continued in the perioperative period.

Recommendations

Chronic beta-blockers should be continued in the perioperative period. Acute beta-blockade should be individualised considering the risk of stroke versus the risk of acute cardiac events secondary to tachycardia and myocardial ischaemia.

Other cardioprotective drugs

When considering the cardioprotective effects of drugs there are two questions to consider:

(1) Should the drug be started as part of a perioperative risk reduction strategy?
(2) Should the drug be given in the perioperative period where it is part of chronic drug therapy?

Alpha-2-adrenergic agonists

Alpha-2-adrenergic agonists including clonidine, dexmeditomidine and mivazerol may have anti-ischaemic properties. These drugs reduce postganglionic noradrenaline release and theoretically may moderate the catecholamine response to surgery. Clonidine has been shown to reduce myocardial ischaemia in vascular patients and in one small study to reduce perioperative mortality in patients with or at risk of coronary artery disease undergoing non-cardiac surgery [42]. Mivazerol, an intravenous alpha-2-agonist, has been studied in high-risk patients with coronary artery disease who were undergoing major vascular or orthopaedic procedures. Overall there was no survival benefit but in the vascular surgical population rates of MI and cardiac death were reduced [43]. Meta-analysis of 23 trials incorporating nearly 3500 patients taking alpha-2-adrenergic agonist studies in the perioperative period suggests a decrease in mortality in patients having vascular surgery [44]. The efficacy and safety of these agents in relation to beta-blocker and statin therapy in reducing cardiovascular risk is unclear as is their effect, if any, on longer-term mortality. They are rarely started as part of a risk reduction strategy. It is unusual to encounter patients taking these drugs for other indications but there is nothing in the literature to guide best practice. Again the results of the POISE-2 trial are eagerly awaited.

Calcium channel blockers

These include dihydropyridines (nifedipine, amlodipine) and the non-dihydropyridines (verapamil, diltiazem) which may reduce heart rate. Trials are limited by small size, different patient groups and drugs. Meta-analysis of this mixed group of studies suggests that they may reduce perioperative ischaemia and supraventricular tachycardia. The majority of the benefit was attributable to diltiazem and in the single study with nifedipine no benefit was seen [45]. In aortic aneurysm surgery dihydropyridine use is independently associated with increased mortality. This could simply suggest these patients were high risk to begin with or were not started on other cardioprotective medication such as beta-blockers [46]. There are no guidelines to suggest that calcium channel blockers should be started as a risk reduction strategy. It seems reasonable to continue diltiazem and verapamil in the perioperative period after careful preoperative assessment and with close perioperative monitoring.

Nitrates

Nitrates are used routinely for the treatment of angina and myocardial ischaemia although there is no evidence that they reduce the rate of MI or cardiac death. These drugs have the potential to cause hypotension and tachycardia and must be used with caution perioperatively. Like calcium channel blockers, based on current literature these drugs should not be started as a risk reduction strategy; however, it seems reasonable to continue them in the perioperative period after careful preoperative assessment and with close perioperative monitoring.

Angiotensin-converting-enzyme inhibitors/angiotensin receptor blockers

There are limited data to guide best perioperative practice. Both angiotensin-converting-enzyme inhibitors and angiotensin blockers are associated with hypotension and a requirement for vasopressor therapy throughout the perioperative period. Hypotension is exacerbated by diuretics, beta-blockers and hypovolaemia [47]. Angiotensin-converting-enzyme inhibitors have been associated with perioperative renal dysfunction [48], and a recent study suggested that these agents were associated with increased mortality in aortic vascular surgical patients [49]. It is common practice to omit these drugs before aortic surgery. However, in stable patients who are taking these drugs for left ventricular dysfunction or heart failure as opposed to hypertension it may be prudent to either continue or interrupt the drugs for as short a time as possible in aortic surgery. Close perioperative monitoring for hypotension and renal dysfunction is important.

Ivabradine

Ivabradine acts directly at the sinoatrial node to slow conduction and reduce heart rate. It does not act via the sympathetic nervous system and has no direct effect on blood pressure or myocardial contractility. In one randomised controlled trial in vascular surgical patients it reduced both ischaemia and MI [50]. Further work is required with this drug that may favourably affect myocardial oxygen balance in the perioperative period without some of the unwanted effects of beta-blocker therapy.

Preoperative coronary artery revascularisation

Introduction

The initial series of predominantly retrospective studies examining the role of coronary artery bypass grafting (CABG) in reducing cardiac events in high-risk patients undergoing vascular surgery showed a potential for reduction of both morbidity and mortality from myocardial events. However, the two prospective randomised trials of preoperative revascularisation (by coronary stenting or CABG) versus medical therapy, the Coronary Artery Revascularization Prophylaxis (CARP) [51] and the Dutch Echocardiographic Cardiac Risk Evaluation Applying Stress Echo – V (DECREASE-V) pilot study [52], failed to show any benefit. These studies were associated with significantly increased 30-day mortality, and the 30-day and late composite outcome of death and non-fatal MI. Thirty-day non-fatal MI showed a trend to a worse outcome [53].

Why the difference in reported outcomes between the retrospective and prospective studies?

Firstly, some of the accepted indications for preoperative CABG were exclusion criteria in the prospective trials. It is important that patients with accepted indications for preoperative coronary revascularisation are still considered for preoperative coronary revascularisation. The findings from the CARP study regarding left main stem pathology should be highlighted. In the 4.6% of patients identified with >50% left main stem stenosis they found that coronary revascularisation prior to non-cardiac surgery significantly improved long-term survival (82% versus 52%, $p < 0.01$) [51].

Secondly, patients who had percutaneous coronary interventions had their subsequent non-cardiac surgery relatively early at a median of 41 days [51] and 29 days [52] following the percutaneous intervention which may be associated with a worse outcome. Indeed in the CARP study, CABG and percutaneous coronary intervention have been subsequently compared and perioperative MI was found to be significantly decreased in the CABG group ($p = 0.024$) [54]. A meta-analysis comparing CABG and percutaneous coronary intervention in the prospective studies showed that CABG had a trend to a better composite outcome at 30 days, which was subsequently statistically significant for the late composite outcome of death and myocardial infarction [53].

Coronary artery bypass grafting

A meta-analysis of the prospective studies found that CABG was associated with a trend to a worse outcome than medical therapy for all 30-day events, but a trend to a better late composite outcome although the meta-analysis was underpowered to adequately address this issue [53]. Coronary artery bypass grafting has been associated with improved long-term survival in patients undergoing non-cardiac vascular surgery. Hertzer et al. showed in a prospective cohort of 1000 patients with peripheral vascular disease that CABG was associated with superior 5-year survival compared to medical management (72% versus 21%, $p = 0.0001$ respectively) [55]. Since then CABG has shown improved outcomes in the majority of early observational studies, with an improved long-term survival in patients with severe coronary artery disease following aortic surgery and peripheral vascular surgery.

A clinical survival score to predict which vascular patients will benefit from preoperative coronary revascularisation suggests that only intermediate-risk patients are likely to benefit in the long term from preoperative coronary revascularisation (moderate to severe ischaemia on thallium scanning with two to three of the following risk factors: diabetes, age ≥ 65 years, ischaemic heart disease, renal disease, congestive heart failure, ST depression on preoperative ECG) [56].

Coronary artery stents and anaesthesia for vascular surgery

Percutaneous intervention has developed exponentially since the first percutaneous coronary angioplasty was performed in 1977. Approximately 80 000 percutaneous coronary interventions (PCI) were performed in the United Kingdom in 2009, more than three times as frequently as CABG. Percutaneous coronary intervention is indicated for patients with unstable coronary syndromes and in some cases stable coronary disease. With stent and antiplatelet drug development more than 90% of all PCIs now involve placement of a coronary artery stent. It is estimated that approximately 5% of the 2 million patients undergoing PCI annually in Western countries present for non-cardiac surgery within 1 year [57]. As a result there is an increasing cohort of patients with coronary artery disease treated with a coronary artery stent presenting for surgery. Given the prevalence of coronary disease in the vascular surgery population they are likely to represent an increasing cohort of high-risk patients.

Types of coronary artery stents

Coronary angioplasty is limited by complications such as immediate vessel closure, dissection and constrictive remodelling resulting in restenosis in up to 80% of cases. Bare metal stents (BMS) provide a rigid scaffold to prevent this. Placement of the stent itself, however, causes vessel injury and a cascade of inflammatory reactions that produce scarring and vessel restenosis in up to 30% of patients in the 3–6 months following BMS insertion. Restenosis occurs gradually and treatment options include balloon angioplasty, intracoronary irradiation (brachytherapy) and re-stenting. Restenosis of BMS limited the cost effectiveness of PCI and exposed patients to the risk of additional procedures [58].

Drug-eluting stents (DES) were developed to prevent restenosis by using a drug bound to a polymer on the stent surface to inhibit the inflammation and cell proliferation that result in restenosis. A number of these stents were developed and they have been very successful in reducing the incidence of restenosis and the need for repeated procedures to less than 5% [58]. As a result in 2005 more than 60% of all stents inserted in the UK and more than 95% in the United States were DES. Concerns have emerged regarding the longer-term safety profile of DES and the potential for late stent thrombosis [59]. Drug-eluting stents delay re-endothelialisation of the stent surface and present a prolonged thrombogenic risk in the coronary circulation. This can result in sudden, catastrophic thrombosis and vessel occlusion termed stent thrombosis. In the case of BMS re-endothelialisation is complete within 6 weeks; however, in the case of DES there is no easy way of determining when re-endothelialisation has occurred. Different drugs are released from DES at different rates such that the optimal duration of dual antiplatelet therapy to prevent thrombosis is unknown for the individual patient. Risk factors for stent thrombosis include stopping antiplatelet drugs, long complex coronary lesions requiring multiple stents, renal failure, diabetes mellitus and low ejection fraction [60].

A number of newer stents are in clinical trials including stents with novel coatings to reduce the need for long courses of antiplatelet drugs and to reduce the risk of late and very late stent thrombosis.

Antiplatelet drugs and coronary artery stents

The evolution of coronary artery stenting has only been possible with parallel developments in antiplatelet drug therapy. Exposed thrombogenic metal stents in the coronary circulation meant that early stents were plagued by both thrombotic episodes and haemorrhagic complications because of complex anticoagulant regimes that included combinations of heparin, warfarin and antiplatelet drugs. The development of clopidogrel and glycoprotein IIb/IIIa receptor blockers used in combination with aspirin reduced the risk of these complications. Early interruption of aspirin and clopidogrel therapy is the biggest single risk factor for stent thrombosis [60].

Implications for anaesthesia

In deciding when to undertake surgery in patients with coronary artery stents, and whether or not to continue antiplatelet medications, both the elapsed *time* since stent insertion and the *type* of stent are important factors. In a retrospective study of nearly 200 patients with both BMS and DES there was an association between early surgery, interruption of antiplatelet therapy and adverse outcomes [61]. More than 13% of patients who had early surgery (within 6 weeks for BMS and 12 months for DES) died or had a non-fatal MI compared with only 0.6% of patients in the group where surgery was delayed. Very early surgery after coronary stent insertion appears to be associated with even greater risks of thrombotic complications. A number of case series have documented extremely high mortality rates (26–32%) in patients undergoing surgery within 2–3 weeks of stent insertion [62,63]. This is supported by a prospective study where the risks of surgery were greatest within 35 days of stenting, with more than twice the complication rate (44.7%) compared with operations after 90 days [57].

The type of stent used is also an important factor to consider as the risk of risk of late stent thrombosis appears to be greater for DES than for BMS. Case reports describe patients who have suffered perioperative MI secondary to DES occlusion many months (4–14) after original stent insertion where antiplatelet agents have been stopped [64,65]. Not all reports describe such poor outcomes in patients with DES. In a retrospective series where 38 patients had surgery within 9 months (median) of DES placement (in most cases aspirin was continued, whilst clopidogrel use was about 40%) there were no major adverse events or deaths reported [66]. Likewise, in the only prospective study of patients with DES, 96 patients underwent surgery on average 14 months after stent insertion. There were only four deaths including one DES thrombosis and one BMS thrombosis. It is possible that the low mortality rate reported in this study reflected the delayed timing of surgery and continuation of antiplatelet therapy (75% continued aspirin and 50% continued clopidogrel).

Haemorrhage versus thrombosis

As has already been discussed most studies of *dual* antiplatelet therapy have been conducted in patients undergoing cardiac surgery where bleeding, re-operation rates and days spent in hospital are higher in those on dual therapy [16]. Case series in vascular surgery have not shown increased mortality in those on clopidogrel despite moderate increases in surgical blood loss and transfusion rate [3]. Patients with stents clearly present a high thrombotic risk where surgery is performed early and when antiplatelet drugs are stopped. A prospective study of over 2000 patients with DES reported that a third of those who stopped antiplatelet therapy early (in some cases for surgical procedures) developed stent thromboses with an associated mortality rate of 45% [60]. Furthermore, a prospective study of patients on antiplatelet therapy who underwent non-cardiac surgery within 12 months of BMS or DES insertion found that 96% of all complications were *thrombotic* in nature whilst only 4% were haemorrhagic [57]. None of the bleeding episodes were life-threatening. From this, albeit limited, evidence the perceived risk and consequences of haemorrhage may be overstated. Suggested strategies to reduce perioperative stent thrombosis are shown in Table 4.2.

Recommendations

Based on current literature, where a patient is on dual anti-platelet therapy following coronary artery stenting then elective surgery should be postponed until the patient has completed the period of prescribed dual anti-platelet therapy. Guidelines suggest postponing elective surgery for 2 weeks following angioplasty alone, for 4–6 weeks following BMS insertion and for 1 year following DES insertion. Aspirin therapy should never be stopped [67,68].

Where a patient is on dual antiplatelet therapy following coronary artery stenting and presents for surgery that cannot be delayed then consideration should be given to continuing dual antiplatelet therapy throughout perioperative period. Where this is

Table 4.2 Suggested strategies for preventing perioperative stent thrombosis

Do not stent patients before elective surgery

Where patients require revascularisation and likely to need surgery within 12 months do not use DES

Where stent in situ consider balance of risk of thrombosis vs. haemorrhage

Delay surgery until patient has completed period of prescribed dual antiplatelet therapy for stent type

Plan antiplatelet drug therapy after multidisciplinary consultation

Perioperative risk reduction strategies

Monitor for perioperative ischaemia

Close collaboration with cardiology colleagues

not possible clopidogrel should be stopped for as short a time as possible, aspirin continued and the patient managed as high cardiac risk. Early diagnosis and treatment of stent thrombosis is essential. While there is no evidence that heparin or glycoprotein IIb/IIIa inhibitors prevent perioperative stent thrombosis, case reports have been published suggesting a role for a glycoprotein IIb/IIIa drugs that are short-acting being used as a 'bridging' strategy [17].

The future of preoperative coronary revascularisation

It is too early to consider that there is no place for preoperative coronary revascularisation in vascular surgical patients. Routine preoperative coronary angiography in preoperative vascular aortic surgical patients with a Revised Cardiac Risk Index (RCRI) of ≥ 2 risk factors and subsequent preoperative coronary revascularisation was associated with an improved outcome in 30-day MACE and intermediate-term outcome when compared to a selective strategy based on preoperative special investigation results [69]. All the patients were started on beta-blocker therapy with a heart rate titrated to <60 beats per minute and statin therapy. Significantly more patients in the routine coronary angiography group were found to have significant coronary atherosclerosis ($p = 0.02$). This study also confirmed that intermediate-term survival is improved with preoperative coronary revascularisation in vascular surgical patients [69]. This study suggests that the greatest limitation to our success in the application of appropriate preoperative coronary revascularisation may not be the procedure itself, but rather the inability of our risk stratification processes to select appropriate patients who may benefit from coronary revascularisation.

References

1. Devereaux PJ, Goldman L, Cook DJ, et al. Perioperative cardiac events in patients undergoing noncardiac surgery: a review of the magnitude of the problem, the pathophysiology of the events and methods to estimate and communicate risk. Can Med Ass J 2005;173:627–34.

2. Biccard BM, Rodseth RN. The pathophysiology of perioperative myocardial infarction. Anaesthesia 2010;65:733–41.

3. Chassot PG, Delabays A, Spahn DR. Perioperative antiplatelet therapy: the case for continuing therapy in patients at risk of myocardial infarction. Br J Anaesth 2007;99:316–28.

4. Collaborative meta-analysis of randomised trials of antiplatelet therapy for prevention of death, myocardial infarction, and stroke in high risk patients. BMJ 2002;324:71–86.

5. Collet JP, Montalescot G, Blanchet B, et al. Impact of prior use or recent withdrawal of oral antiplatelet agents on acute coronary syndromes. Circulation 2004;110:2361–7.

6. Burger W, Chemnitius JM, Kneissl GD, Rucker G. Low-dose aspirin for secondary cardiovascular prevention: cardiovascular risks after its perioperative withdrawal versus bleeding risks with its continuation – review and meta-analysis. J Intern Med 2005;257:399–414.

7. Oscarsson A, Gupta A, Fredrikson M, et al. To continue or discontinue aspirin in the perioperative period: a randomized, controlled clinical trial. Br J Anaesth 2010; 104:305–12.

8. Robless P, Mikhailidis DP, Stansby G. Systematic review of antiplatelet therapy for the prevention of myocardial infarction, stroke or vascular death in patients with peripheral vascular disease. Br J Surg 2001;88:787–800.

9. Lindblad B, Persson NH, Takolander R, Bergqvist D. Does low-dose acetylsalicylic acid prevent stroke after carotid surgery? A double-blind, placebo-controlled randomized trial. Stroke 1993;24:1125–8.

10. Albaladejo P, Geeraerts T, Francis F, et al. Aspirin withdrawal and acute lower limb ischemia. Anesth Analg 2004;99:440–3.

11. Neilipovitz DT, Bryson GL, Nichol G. The effect of perioperative aspirin therapy in peripheral vascular surgery: a decision analysis. Anesth Analg 2001;93:573–80.

12. McCollum C, Alexander C, Kenchington G, Franks PJ, Greenhalgh R. Antiplatelet drugs in femoropopliteal vein bypasses: a multicenter trial. J Vasc Surg 1991;13:150–61; discussion 161–2.

13. CAPRIE Steering Committee. A randomised, blinded, trial of clopidogrel versus aspirin in patients at risk of ischaemic events (CAPRIE). Lancet 1996;348:1329–39.

14. Halkes PH, van Gijn J, Kappelle LJ, Koudstaal PJ, Algra A. Aspirin plus dipyridamole versus aspirin alone after cerebral ischaemia of arterial origin (ESPRIT): randomised controlled trial. Lancet 2006;367:1665–73.

15. Payne DA, Hayes PD, Jones CI, et al. Combined therapy with clopidogrel and aspirin significantly increases the bleeding time through a synergistic antiplatelet action. J Vasc Surg 2002;35:1204–9.

16. Chen L, Bracey AW, Radovancevic R, et al. Clopidogrel and bleeding in patients undergoing elective coronary artery bypass grafting. J Thorac Cardiovasc Surg 2004;128:425–31.

17. Savonitto S, D'Urbano M, Caracciolo M, et al. Urgent surgery in patients with a recently implanted coronary drug-eluting stent: a phase II study of 'bridging' antiplatelet therapy with tirofiban during temporary withdrawal of clopidogrel. Br J Anaesth 2010;104:285–91.

18. Horlocker TT, Wedel DJ, Benzon H, et al. Regional anesthesia in the anticoagulated patient: defining the risks (the second ASRA Consensus Conference on Neuraxial Anesthesia and Anticoagulation). Reg Anesth Pain Med 2003; 28:172–97.

19. Spahn DR, Howell SJ, Delabays A, Chassot PG. Coronary stents and perioperative antiplatelet regimen: dilemma of bleeding and stent thrombosis. Br J Anaesth 2006;96:675–7.

20. National Institute for Health and Clinical Excellence. Statins for the Prevention of Cardiovascular Events, Technology Appraisal 94. London: NICE, 2006. Available from www.nice.org.uk/page.aspx?o=TA094guidance.

21. Hindler K, Shaw AD, Samuels J, et al. Improved postoperative outcomes associated with preoperative statin therapy. Anesthesiology 2006;105:1260–72; quiz 1289–90.

22. Kapoor AS, Kanji H, Buckingham J, Devereaux PJ, McAlister FA.

Strength of evidence for perioperative use of statins to reduce cardiovascular risk: systematic review of controlled studies. *BMJ* 2006;**333**:1149.

23. Dunkelgrun M, Boersma E, Schouten O, *et al.* Bisoprolol and fluvastatin for the reduction of perioperative cardiac mortality and myocardial infarction in intermediate-risk patients undergoing noncardiovascular surgery: a randomized controlled trial (DECREASE-IV). *Ann Surg* 2009;**249**:921–6.

24. Schouten O, Boersma E, Hoeks SE, *et al.* Fluvastatin and perioperative events in patients undergoing vascular surgery. *N Engl J Med* 2009;**361**:980–9.

25. Durazzo AE, Machado FS, Ikeoka DT, *et al.* Reduction in cardiovascular events after vascular surgery with atorvastatin: a randomized trial. *J Vasc Surg* 2004;**39**:967–75; discussion 975–6.

26. Heart Protection Study. Randomized trial of the effects of cholesterol-lowering with simvastatin on peripheral vascular and other major vascular outcomes in 20 536 people with peripheral arterial disease and other high-risk conditions. *J Vasc Surg* 2007;**45**:645–53; discussion 653–4.

27. Padayachee L, Rodseth RN, Biccard BM. A meta-analysis of the utility of C-reactive protein in predicting early, intermediate-term and long term mortality and major adverse cardiac events in vascular surgical patients. *Anaesthesia* 2009;**64**:416–24.

28. Le Manach Y, Godet G, Coriat P, *et al.* The impact of postoperative discontinuation or continuation of chronic statin therapy on cardiac outcome after major vascular surgery. *Anesth Analg* 2007;**104**:1326–33.

29. Biccard BM. Investigation of predictors of increased creatine kinase levels following vascular surgery and the association with perioperative statin therapy. *Cardiovasc J Afr* 2009;**20**:187–91.

30. Zaugg M, Tagliente T, Lucchinetti E, *et al.* Beneficial effects from beta-adrenergic blockade in elderly patients undergoing noncardiac surgery. *Anesthesiology* 1999;**91**:1674–86.

31. Landesberg G. Monitoring for myocardial ischemia. *Best Pract Res Clin Anaesthesiol* 2005;**19**:77–95.

32. Feringa HH, Bax JJ, Boersma E, *et al.* High-dose beta-blockers and tight heart rate control reduce myocardial ischemia and troponin T release in vascular surgery patients. *Circulation* 2006; **114**(1 Suppl):I344–9.

33. Landesberg G, Mosseri M, Zahger D, *et al.* Myocardial infarction after vascular surgery: the role of prolonged stress-induced, ST depression-type ischemia. *J Am Coll Cardiol* 2001;**37**:1839–45.

34. Bangalore S, Wetterslev J, Pranesh S, *et al.* Perioperative beta blockers in patients having non-cardiac surgery: a meta-analysis. *Lancet* 2008;**372**:1962–76.

35. PeriOperative ISchaemic Evaluation. Effects of extended-release metoprolol succinate in patients undergoing non-cardiac surgery (POISE trial): a randomised controlled trial. *Lancet* 2008;**371**:1839–47.

36. Beattie WS, Wijeysundera DN, Karkouti K, McCluskey S, Tait G. Does tight heart rate control improve beta-blocker efficacy? An updated analysis of the noncardiac surgical randomized trials. *Anesth Analg* 2008;**106**:1039–48.

37. Lindenauer PK, Pekow P, Wang K, *et al.* Perioperative beta-blocker therapy and mortality after major noncardiac surgery. *N Engl J Med* 2005;**353**:349–61.

38. Zaugg M, Bestmann L, Wacker J, *et al.* Adrenergic receptor genotype but not perioperative bisoprolol therapy may determine cardiovascular outcome in at-risk patients undergoing surgery with spinal block: the Swiss Beta Blocker in Spinal Anesthesia (BBSA) study – a double-blinded, placebo-controlled, multicenter trial with 1-year follow-up. *Anesthesiology* 2007;**107**:33–44.

39. Giles JW, Sear JW, Foex P. Effect of chronic beta-blockade on perioperative outcome in patients undergoing non-cardiac surgery: an analysis of observational and case control studies. *Anaesthesia* 2004;**59**:574–83.

40. Shammash JB, Trost JC, Gold JM, *et al.* Perioperative beta-blocker withdrawal and mortality in vascular surgical patients. *Am Heart J* 2001;**141**:148–53.

41. Hoeks SE, Scholte Op Reimer WJ, van Urk H, *et al.* Increase of 1-year mortality after perioperative beta-blocker withdrawal in endovascular and vascular surgery patients. *Eur J Vasc Endovasc Surg* 2007;**33**:13–19.

42. Wallace AW, Galindez D, Salahieh A, *et al.* Effect of clonidine on cardiovascular morbidity and mortality after noncardiac surgery. *Anesthesiology* 2004;**101**:284–93.

43. Oliver MF, Goldman L, Julian DG, Holme I. Effect of mivazerol on perioperative cardiac complications during non-cardiac surgery in patients with coronary heart disease: the European Mivazerol Trial (EMIT). *Anesthesiology* 1999; **91**:951–61.

44. Wijeysundera DN, Naik JS, Beattie WS. Alpha-2 adrenergic agonists to prevent perioperative cardiovascular complications: a meta-analysis. *Am J Med* 2003;**114**:742–52.

45. Wijeysundera DN, Beattie WS. Calcium channel blockers for reducing cardiac morbidity after

noncardiac surgery: a meta-analysis. *Anesth Analg* 2003;**97**:634–41.

46. Kertai MD, Westerhout CM, Varga KS, Acsady G, Gal J. Dihydropiridine calcium-channel blockers and perioperative mortality in aortic aneurysm surgery. *Br J Anaesth* 2008;**101**:458–65.

47. Kheterpal S, Khodaparast O, Shanks A, O'Reilly M, Tremper KK. Chronic angiotensin-converting enzyme inhibitor or angiotensin receptor blocker therapy combined with diuretic therapy is associated with increased episodes of hypotension in noncardiac surgery. *J Cardiothorac Vasc Anesth* 2008;**22**:180–6.

48. Cittanova ML, Zubicki A, Savu C, *et al.* The chronic inhibition of angiotensin-converting enzyme impairs postoperative renal function. *Anesth Analg* 2001;**93**:1111–15.

49. Railton CJ, Wolpin J, Lam-McCulloch J, Belo SE. Renin–angiotensin blockade is associated with increased mortality after vascular surgery. *Can J Anaesth* 2010;**57**:736–44.

50. Shchukin I V, Vachev AN, Surkova EA, *et al.* [The role of beta-adrenoblockers and If-inhibitor ivabradine in lowering of rate of development of cardiac complications after carotid endarterectomy.] *Kardiologiia* 2008;**48**:56–9.

51. McFalls EO, Ward HB, Moritz TE, *et al.* Coronary-artery revascularization before elective major vascular surgery. *N Engl J Med* 2004;**351**: 2795–804.

52. Poldermans D, Schouten O, Vidakovic R, *et al.* A clinical randomized trial to evaluate the safety of a noninvasive approach in high-risk patients undergoing major vascular surgery: the DECREASE-V Pilot Study.

J Am Coll Cardiol 2007;**49**: 1763–9.

53. Biccard BM, Rodseth RN. A meta-analysis of the prospective randomised trials of coronary revascularisation before noncardiac vascular surgery with attention to the type of coronary revascularisation performed. *Anaesthesia* 2009;**64**:1105–13.

54. Ward HB, Kelly RF, Thottapurathu L, *et al.* Coronary artery bypass grafting is superior to percutaneous coronary intervention in prevention of perioperative myocardial infarctions during subsequent vascular surgery. *Ann Thorac Surg* 2006;**82**:795–800; discussion 800–1.

55. Hertzer NR, Young JR, Beven EG, et al. Late results of coronary bypass in patients with infrarenal aortic aneurysms: The Cleveland Clinic Study. *Ann Surg* 1987;**205**:360–7.

56. Landesberg G, Berlatzky Y, Bocher M, *et al.* A clinical survival score predicts the likelihood to benefit from preoperative thallium scanning and coronary revascularization before major vascular surgery. *Eur Heart J* 2007;**28**:533–9.

57. Vicenzi MN, Meislitzer T, Heitzinger B, *et al.* Coronary artery stenting and non-cardiac surgery: a prospective outcome study. *Br J Anaesth* 2006;**96**:686–93.

58. Serruys PW, Kutryk MJ, Ong AT. Coronary-artery stents. *N Engl J Med* 2006;**354**:483–95.

59. Lagerqvist B, James SK, Stenestrand U, *et al.* Long-term outcomes with drug-eluting stents versus bare-metal stents in Sweden. *N Engl J Med* 2007;**356**:1009–19.

60. Iakovou I, Schmidt T, Bonizzoni E, *et al.* Incidence, predictors, and outcome of thrombosis after successful implantation of

drug-eluting stents. *JAMA* 2005;**293**:2126–30.

61. Schouten O, van Domburg RT, Bax JJ, *et al.* Noncardiac surgery after coronary stenting: early surgery and interruption of antiplatelet therapy are associated with an increase in major adverse cardiac events. *J Am Coll Cardiol* 2007;**49**:122–4.

62. Kaluza GL, Joseph J, Lee JR, Raizner ME, Raizner AE. Catastrophic outcomes of noncardiac surgery soon after coronary stenting. *J Am Coll Cardiol* 2000;**35**:1288–94.

63. Sharma AK, Ajani AE, Hamwi SM, *et al.* Major noncardiac surgery following coronary stenting: when is it safe to operate? *Catheter Cardiovasc Interv* 2004;**63**:141–5.

64. Auer J, Berent R, Weber T, Eber B. Risk of noncardiac surgery in the months following placement of a drug-eluting coronary stent. *J Am Coll Cardiol* 2004;**43**:713; author reply 714–15.

65. McFadden EP, Stabile E, Regar E, *et al.* Late thrombosis in drug-eluting coronary stents after discontinuation of antiplatelet therapy. *Lancet* 2004;**364**:1519–21.

66. Compton PA, Zankar AA, Adesanya AO, Banerjee S, Brilakis ES. Risk of noncardiac surgery after coronary drug-eluting stent implantation. *Am J Cardiol* 2006;**98**:1212–13.

67. Fleisher LA, Beckman JA, Brown KA, *et al.* ACC/AHA 2007 Guidelines on perioperative cardiovascular evaluation and care for noncardiac surgery: executive summary: a report of the American College of Cardiology/ American Heart Association Task Force on Practice Guidelines (Writing Committee to Revise the 2002 Guidelines on Perioperative Cardiovascular Evaluation for Noncardiac Surgery): Developed in Collaboration With the American Society of

Echocardiography, American Society of Nuclear Cardiology, Heart Rhythm Society, Society of Cardiovascular Anesthesiologists, Society for Cardiovascular Angiography and Interventions, Society for Vascular Medicine and Biology, and Society for Vascular Surgery. *Circulation* 2007;**116**:1971–96.

68. Poldermans D, Bax JJ, Boersma E, *et al.* Guidelines for pre-operative cardiac risk assessment and perioperative cardiac management in non-cardiac surgery: the Task Force for Preoperative Cardiac Risk Assessment and Perioperative Cardiac Management in Non-cardiac Surgery of the European Society of Cardiology (ESC) and endorsed by the European Society of Anaesthesiology (ESA). *Eur Heart J* 2009; **30**:2769–812.

69. Monaco M, Stassano P, Di Tommaso L, *et al.* Systematic strategy of prophylactic coronary angiography improves long-term outcome after major vascular surgery in medium- to high-risk patients: a prospective, randomized study. *J Am Coll Cardiol* 2009;**54**:989–96.

Anaesthesia in the vascular surgery patient

Carl Moores

Anaesthesia for patients undergoing vascular surgery is challenging for a number of reasons. The high incidence of intercurrent cardiac and pulmonary disease, the relatively elderly vascular population and the often major surgical interventions which are undertaken all mean that vascular patients are at relatively high risk of major complications in comparison to other surgical patients.

Throughout this book, a number of authors have described anaesthetic techniques for a range of vascular surgical procedures. This chapter, however, is concerned with a few general principles concerning the anaesthetic management of vascular patients and the extent to which anaesthetic techniques can influence postoperative outcome. The role and possible benefits of regional versus general anaesthesia are discussed, both in terms of the avoidance of perioperative major adverse events and in terms of the possible effects on surgical outcome in lower limb procedures. The relative benefits of total intravenous anaesthesia and volatile anaesthesia for major vascular surgery are also discussed. Finally, the role of the vascular anaesthetist in the postoperative period is discussed.

Regional versus general anaesthesia

There has been much debate over the years as to the relative merits of regional anaesthesia versus general anaesthesia in vascular anaesthetic practice. Vascular patients are at high risk of serious postoperative cardiac and pulmonary complications, and it has been tempting to think that outcome might be improved by the use of regional techniques. The superior pain relief provided by postoperative epidural analgesia could conceivably improve outcome, as could the avoidance of a general anaesthetic in high-risk vascular patients. Regional techniques could also, in theory,

improve the results of lower limb revascularisation procedures as a result of the sympathetic blockade that they produce. And the debate among vascular anaesthetists as to whether carotid endarterectomy is best performed with a regional or general technique has been going on for some years now. It is not considered in this chapter, but is discussed in detail in Chapter 16.

Epidural analgesia and aortic surgery

Epidural anaesthesia, both as part of the anaesthetic technique during aortic surgery and to provide analgesia into the postoperative period, is well established. There is ample evidence that epidural analgesia provides superior pain relief compared to other forms of postoperative analgesia, particularly when patients are required to move, cough or comply with physiotherapy. Whether or not epidural analgesia confers other advantages, such as reducing the incidence of respiratory complications, cardiac complications, deep venous thrombosis, renal failure or death in patients undergoing aortic surgery has been studied by a number of authors over the years, often with conflicting results.

Respiratory complications

By obtaining better pain relief, it might be anticipated that patients receiving epidural analgesia would have a better pattern of ventilation, decreasing the risk of postoperative respiratory complications.

In a meta-analysis looking at a heterogenous group of patients, Ballantyne found that epidural anaesthesia decreased the incidence of postoperative atelectasis and pulmonary infections, compared to systemic opioids used for analgesia [1]. In addition, two recent large, multicentre, prospective trials have confirmed that epidural analgesia reduces the incidence of postoperative respiratory complications.

Core Topics in Vascular Anaesthesia, ed. Carl Moores and Alastair F. Nimmo. Published by Cambridge University Press.
© Cambridge University Press 2012.

The MASTER trial of patients undergoing major abdominal surgery demonstrated a reduced incidence of respiratory failure (prolonged intubation, or the requirement for reintubation) in patients receiving epidural analgesia, compared to those receiving systemic opioids [2], and the Veterans Affairs Medical Centre study noted a decreased incidence of postoperative respiratory failure, but only in patients undergoing aortic surgery [3]. A *Cochrane Review* of 2006 which analysed studies comparing epidural analgesia to other forms of postoperative analgesia in patients undergoing aortic surgery concluded that epidural analgesia reduced the incidence of prolonged postoperative mechanical ventilation [4].

Cardiac complications

Good analgesia, and possibly the effects of sympathetic blockade in epidural analgesia, might be expected to reduce the incidence of postoperative ischaemia and myocardial infarction. This effect may possibly be more apparent in aortic patients, given the relatively high prevalence of coronary artery disease in these patients.

In 2001, Beattie performed a meta-analysis of studies which compared epidural anaesthesia with other forms of analgesia for up to 24 hours postoperatively [5]. He found that epidural analgesia was associated with a reduced incidence of postoperative myocardial infarction. Subgroup analysis suggested that this effect was confined to patients who had been given a thoracic epidural. The Veterans Affairs study showed that epidural analgesia did confer a benefit in terms of reducing the incidence of postoperative myocardial infarction only if patients undergoing aortic surgery were considered; there appeared to be no benefit in patients undergoing other forms of abdominal surgery. The MASTER study found no benefit of epidural analgesia in preventing postoperative myocardial events; however the 2006 *Cochrane Review* concluded that epidural analgesia was effective in reducing the incidence of myocardial events in patients undergoing abdominal aortic surgery.

Other complications

In addition to the benefits listed above the 2006 *Cochrane Review* also concluded that in aortic patients, epidural analgesia reduced the incidence of postoperative renal insufficiency and gastrointestinal complications. In both these cases, the effect seemed to be limited to thoracic epidural analgesia.

Mortality

Of the modern studies looking at the effect of epidural analgesia on outcome in high-risk patients, none have concluded that epidural analgesia improves postoperative mortality. This is despite its apparent beneficial effect in reducing potentially fatal postoperative complications. In part, this is because postoperative mortality is low, and only a very large study would be able to demonstrate a statistically significant effect of an analgesic technique on postoperative mortality. Good analgesia forms only part of a package of postoperative care and it would be difficult to show the benefit that one single part of this package has on mortality. Furthermore, epidural analgesia may not benefit all patients equally: epidurals may help to prevent myocardial infarctions in fitter patients (who are more likely to survive a myocardial infarction), but could have a smaller benefit on sicker patients (in whom a myocardial infarction is more likely to be fatal).

For providing postoperative analgesia, epidural blocks are usually superior to other forms of analgesia and, in vascular patients in particular, may also have the effect of reducing the incidence of serious postoperative cardiac, pulmonary and renal complications. Whether this translates into an effect on postoperative mortality is less clear.

Peripheral revascularisation and regional anaesthesia

A number of studies in the past concluded that regional anaesthesia for peripheral limb revascularisation offered an advantage over general anaesthesia in that it led to a decreased incidence of postoperative graft occlusion. Presumably this effect is mediated via changes in lower limb blood flow that accompany regional anaesthesia, although some authors suggested that regional anaesthesia may have an effect on blood coagulation. For example Tuman [6] and Christopherson [7] both found that reintervention rates for graft failure were lower in patients receiving epidural anaesthesia compared to those receiving general anaesthesia. However, larger studies carried out later failed to confirm these findings [8]. A recent *Cochrane Review* on the subject of regional versus general anaesthesia concluded only that the rate of amputation post lower limb revascularisation was not influenced by the choice of anaesthetic, although only four studies were rated highly enough to be included in the review [9]. The review also concluded that there was no effect of anaesthetic technique on the incidence of cardiac complications, although the incidence of pneumonia did appear to be lower in the regional anaesthesia group. Further discussion on this topic can be found in Chapter 14.

Volatile versus intravenous anaesthesia

Both volatile-based and intravenous-based techniques are suitable for the maintenance of anaesthesia during vascular surgery. Total intravenous anaesthesia (TIVA) has the advantage of offering a degree of flexibility in that it can be used for anxiolysis, sedation and general anaesthesia. Thus, it may be used to help relax a patient during the insertion of epidural, arterial and other lines, before the plasma concentration is increased to induce general anaesthesia. Following surgery it can be used to provide sedation for transfer to intensive care if necessary.

It must be remembered, though, that the metabolism of propofol takes place primarily in the liver. For example, during thoracoabdominal aortic aneurysm repair, when the period of visceral ischaemia means there is little or no hepatic perfusion, the rate of infusion of propofol should be decreased to take this into account. Monitoring with a depth of anaesthesia monitor (such as Bispectral Index or analysis of entropy) is helpful in this situation in order to ensure an adequate level of anaesthesia without leading to excessively high plasma concentrations of propofol which could result in cardiovascular instability.

Volatile anaesthetic agents may have the advantage of providing the heart with a degree of protection against ischaemic/reperfusion injury. Given their high incidence of coronary heart disease, this may be of benefit in vascular patients. There are numerous animal studies to suggest that the effect is real, but it has been more difficult to establish whether the use of volatile anaesthetic drugs, in preference to intravenous ones, has any significant benefit in humans in terms of protecting the myocardium [10, 11]. Nearly all of the research in this field has been carried out in patients undergoing cardiac surgery on cardiopulmonary bypass. The results of studies looking at, for example, postoperative troponin levels, myocardial function and overall mortality have been conflicting. In addition, questions remain concerning the timing and duration of volatile administration and the possible effects of patients' age and beta-blocker usage on the putative benefit of these drugs. It remains questionable, therefore, whether the use of volatile agents, either throughout the operation or for short periods of 'preconditioning', has any beneficial effects in vascular surgery patients.

Postoperative care and the vascular anaesthetist

Finally, for a successful postoperative outcome, vascular patients need optimum postoperative care. The vascular anaesthetist can play an important role in the postoperative management of their patients, for example by:

- Ensuring that adequate postoperative monitoring is carried out. For example, many monitors in critical care units can monitor ST segments on the ECG trace, although this capability is often switched off.
- Ensuring that clinical goals are clearly documented and adhered to, for example blood pressure limits.
- Ensuring adequate analgesia. This is of obvious importance. Vascular patients are a group who have been shown to benefit from good epidural analgesia.
- Ensuring patients receive appropriate postoperative drug therapy. There is good evidence that the sudden withdrawal of beta-blockers or statins can lead to harm. If a patient is not able to take drugs by mouth, beta-blockers can be given intravenously. Although no intravenous formulation of a statin is currently available, tablets can be crushed and administered nasogastrically.
- After major thoracoabdominal surgery, playing a pivotal role in the management of cerebrospinal fluid drainage in order to reduce the incidence of paraplegia.

References

1. Ballantyne JC, Carr DB, deFerranti S, *et al.* The comparative effects of postoperative analgesic therapies on pulmonary outcome: cumulative meta-analyses of randomized, controlled trials. *Anesth Analg* 1998;**86**: 598–612.

2. Rigg JR, Jamrozik K, Myles PS, *et al.* Epidural anaesthesia and analgesia and outcome of major surgery: a randomised trial. *Lancet* 2002;**359**:1276–82.

3. Park WY, Thompson JS, Lee KK. Effect of epidural anesthesia and analgesia on perioperative outcome: a randomized, controlled Veterans Affairs cooperative study. *Ann Surg* 2001;**234**:560–9; discussion 569–71.

4. Nishimori M, Ballantyne JC, Low JH. Epidural pain relief versus systemic opioid-based pain relief for abdominal aortic surgery. *Cochrane Database Syst Rev* 2006; **CD005059**.

5. Beattie WS, Badner NH, Choi P. Epidural analgesia reduces postoperative myocardial infarction: a meta-analysis. *Anesth Analg* 2001;**93**:853–8.

6. Tuman KJ, McCarthy RJ, March R J, *et al.* Effects of epidural anesthesia and analgesia on coagulation and outcome after major vascular surgery. *Anesth Analg* 1991;**73**:696–704.

7. Christopherson R, Beattie C, Frank SM, *et al.* Perioperative morbidity in patients randomized to epidural or general anesthesia for lower extremity vascular surgery. Perioperative Ischemia Randomized Anesthesia Trial Study Group. *Anesthesiology* 1993;**79**:422–34.

8. Pierce ET, Pomposelli FB, Jr, Stanley GD, *et al.* Anesthesia type does not influence early graft patency or limb salvage rates of lower extremity arterial bypass. *J Vasc Surg* 1997;**25**:226–32; discussion 32–3.

9. Barbosa FT, Cavalcante JC, Juca MJ, Castro AA. Neuraxial anaesthesia for lower-limb revascularization. *Cochrane Database Syst Rev* 2010; **CD007083**.

10. Van Rompaey N, Barvais L. Clinical application of the cardioprotective effects of volatile anaesthetics: CON – total intravenous anaesthesia or not total intravenous anaesthesia to anaesthetise a cardiac patient? *Eur J Anaesthesiol* 2011;**28**:623–7.

11. Bein B. Clinical application of the cardioprotective effects of volatile anaesthetics: PRO – get an extra benefit from a proven anaesthetic free of charge. *Eur J Anaesthesiol* 2011;**28**:620–2.

Monitoring in the vascular surgery patient

Chapter 6

Suzy O'Neill and Chris P. Snowden

Introduction

Patients undergoing vascular procedures are at high risk of perioperative complications, particularly cardiac events, due to the inherent nature of the vascular disease process. The Association of Anaesthetists of Great Britain and Ireland have published minimum standards for patient monitoring whilst undergoing general anaesthesia. Perioperative monitoring in the vascular population should focus mainly on the cardiovascular system but may also be integrated within protocols to optimise oxygen delivery and reduce perioperative morbidity. In vascular surgical procedures where large fluid shifts, excess blood loss and arrhythmias are likely, more advanced monitoring techniques, concentrating on the detection of cardiac ischaemia and acute haemodynamic changes are essential to allow early identification and prompt intervention in problems that may subsequently lead to increased morbidity and mortality. The present chapter outlines the monitoring entities available to the anaesthetist concerned with the care of vascular patients and the rationale for their use.

Electrocardiogram

The electrocardiogram (ECG) is included as an important component of the minimum monitoring standards and should be routinely used in all patients undergoing vascular surgery. In the general surgical population it is particularly useful in determining the presence of arrhythmias, whilst it has increased relevance to the vascular population as the most practical and validated monitor of cardiac ischaemia. In a review of studies involving more than 2400 patients between 1990 and 2003, the relative risk of suffering a postoperative cardiac event, in patients with ischaemic ECG changes, ranged between 2.2% and 73%.

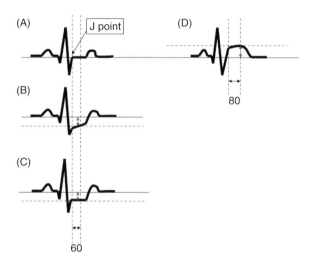

Figure 6.1 Changes in ST segments remain the most sensitive method of detecting ischaemia. (A) The changes are measured from the J point, which represents the end of depolarisation and the beginning of repolarisation. (B) Horizontal or down-sloping ST segment depression of ≥ 1 mm (0.1 mV) occurs during myocardial ischaemia. (C) Ischaemic changes are measured 60 milliseconds from the J point. (D) ST elevation of ≥ 1.5 mm (0.15 mV) measured 80 milliseconds from the J point indicates myocardial ischaemia and potential infarction, secondary to proximal coronary artery occlusion.

Early detection and treatment of perioperative myocardial ischaemia may improve the subsequent outcome of these events.

Changes in ECG that may be associated with myocardial ischaemia include T wave changes, dysrhythmias and atrioventricular blocks. However, these changes are inconsistent and often demonstrated preoperatively. Changes in ST segments remain the most sensitive method of detecting ischaemia (Figure 6.1). The changes in ST segment criteria often used to detect myocardial ischemia are ≥ 1 mm (0.1 mV) of horizontal or down-sloping ST segment

Core Topics in Vascular Anaesthesia, ed. Carl Moores and Alastair F. Nimmo. Published by Cambridge University Press.
© Cambridge University Press 2012.

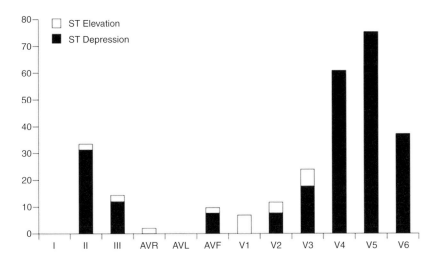

Figure 6.2 The distribution of intraoperative ischaemic ST segment changes in each of the 12 ECG leads is shown. The estimated sensitivity was calculated from the number of changes in a single lead as a percentage of the total number of episodes. The sensitivity was highest in lead V5 (75%).

depression (measured 60 milliseconds from the J point) and up sloping ST segment elevation of ≥ 1.5 mm (0.15 mV) measured 80 milliseconds from the J point. Down sloping ST depression is more serious than horizontal depression, whereas ST elevation is associated with proximal coronary artery obstruction. Changes in the ST segment may also be seen with changes in acid base balance, temperature, intrathoracic pressure and the administration of drugs (e.g. naloxone, digoxin). Changes in ECG may also be difficult to interpret in patients with pre-existing bundle branch blocks and patients who have implantable pacemakers.

The detection of early myocardial ischaemia requires careful positioning of the ECG electrodes and optimum lead selection. Continuous periopera-tive 12-lead ST segment analysis and cardiac troponin levels have been compared with the incidence of ECG changes detected by individual precordial leads, in patients undergoing major vascular surgery [1]. When used in isolation, Lead V5 detects 75% of the intraoperative ischaemic episodes seen on 12-lead monitoring (Figure 6.2). However, it has also been shown that lead V5 is more likely to have baseline ST depression or T wave inversion on the preoperative resting ECG and lead V4 may be even more sensitive in the early detection of ischaemic changes. When leads are used in combination, monitoring ECG leads II and V5 detect 80% of ischaemic changes whilst combining leads V4 and V5 increases the sensitivity to 90%.

A simple three-lead configuration allows only the standard leads I, II and III to be visualised and

therefore is of limited use in detecting early ischaemia (Figure 6.3A). The CM5 and CB5 configurations pos-ition the right arm electrode on the manubrium (CM5) or the right scapula (CB5), the left arm electrode in the fifth intercostal interspace (anterior axillary line) and the third lead on the left clavicle (Figure 6.3B). These configurations give an early and sensitive detection of myocardial ischaemia when compared to preoperative lead V5. Ideally, a five-lead configuration is used to monitor all standard leads (I, II, III AVF, AVR and AVL) and one precordial lead (usually V4 or V5). This configuration allows a more complex and sensitive detection of ischaemia and is preferred in all vascular patients (Figure 6.3C).

More recently, most monitoring systems have the capability to output computerised ST segment analy-sis, which allows for continuous display of ischaemic trends and response to treatment. The algorithms on which these systems output trends may be different. Where some systems derive changes relative to the ST deviation from the reference resting ECG, others acti-vate alarms based on the absolute ST deviation from the isoelectric level. It is important to select the cor-rect appropriate filter and bandwidth gain. Filters are added to the ECG to reduce drift and interference. However, a low-frequency filter can distort the ST segment and a high-frequency filter can distort pacing spikes. Also it is important to remember that change in the gain may amplify or reduce ST segment changes [2].

The duration of ECG monitoring is also crucial in vascular patients. A study of 151 consecutive patients undergoing major vascular surgery showed that there

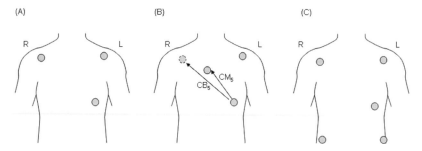

Figure 6.3 (A) Simple three-lead configuration: two leads act as positive and negative electrodes, third lead is neutral electrode. (B) CM5 and CB5 three-lead configurations (monitor set to lead I). The left arm electrode is at the V5 position, fifth intercostal space, in the anterior axillary line. For CM5, the right arm electrode is on the manubrium; for CB5 the right arm electrode is placed posteriorly over the right scapula. CM5 and CB5 have a high sensitivity for detection of intraoperative ischaemia compared to lead V5. (C) Five-lead set up: allows recording of five standard ECG leads, including one precordial lead, usually V5. The addition of two electrodes allows monitoring of regions of the myocardium supplied by right coronary artery, left anterior descending and circumflex coronary arteries.

were 342 ischaemic episodes and 48% of these occurred in the postoperative period. The postoperative ischaemic episodes were mainly silent, rate-related ST depression. Postoperative ST segment changes with a prolonged duration (greater than 30 minutes per episode or greater than 2 hours cumulative length) were the only independent predictors of postoperative cardiac events.

Arterial blood pressure

Non-invasive blood pressure monitoring is also included in the minimal monitoring standards. Systolic and mean arterial pressures are measured directly using an automated oscillotonometric device, whilst diastolic pressure is derived. Since this method of measurement is inaccurate under extremes of pressure, where cardiac arrhythmias exist and wherever rapidly changing haemodynamics occur, the use of this modality is limited in many vascular surgical procedures. In addition, since the relationship between blood pressure and cardiac output is not linear, a 'normal' blood pressure does not always equate with adequate organ blood flow.

Direct arterial pressure measurement via cannulae positioned in a distal artery has the potential for complications. However, the risk of arterial occlusion and atheromatous or air embolisation is minimal and overall there is a low complication rate from invasive monitoring. As a result, many vascular anaesthetists prefer direct arterial pressure measurement in the majority of vascular procedures, allowing beat-to-beat assessment of blood pressure. Indeed, direct arterial pressure monitoring should be considered wherever

there is likely to be haemodynamic instability, either related to the patient's comorbidities or the surgical procedure and when vasoactive agents are being utilised. Analysis of the arterial waveform may give indirect information on cardiac contractility, stroke volume and systemic vascular resistance, whilst access to arterial blood also allows for sampling for arterial blood gases, haemoglobin and thromboelastography. Usually, distal positioning of the arterial cannula is preferred in either radial artery. However, selection of the monitoring site will depend on knowledge of the surgical procedure. For example, during some aortic surgery, the proximal occlusion clamp may involve the left subclavian artery. In this instance the cannula should be placed in the right arm and a second arterial cannula may be used in a femoral vessel to measure the retrograde perfusion pressure below the clamp. There are potential limitations with direct arterial pressure measurement. Patients with vascular disease may have reduced peripheral arterial compliance with reduced vessel compliance occurring at an increasing distance from the aortic valve. Direct blood pressure measurements are higher at the periphery, with a widened pulse pressure and lower diastolic pressure. This reverses when arterial wall compliance is increased, for example due to vasodilatation secondary to removal of an aortic cross-clamp. In these conditions, blood pressure readings may lead to false assumptions about need for vasopressor drugs.

Central venous pressure

Central venous pressure (CVP) is commonly used as a measure of preload. The force of cardiac contraction depends on the myocardial length at end-diastole, and the length of fibres depends on the end-diastolic ventricular volume. If the right ventricular function is normal, then central venous pressure may give an indirect estimation of right ventricular end-diastolic volume (RVEDV) and right ventricular preload. This is then used to guide fluid replacement and where ventricular compliance is normal, to allow estimation of left heart pressures. However, there are several limitations to CVP interpretation in this context. Isolated CVP measurements are difficult to interpret and should be assessed rather as a trend analysis in the context of the patient's haemodynamic variables and overall condition. Factors unrelated to preload changes can alter the CVP including raised intrathoracic and intra-abdominal pressure. Importantly, the changes in the CVP following a fluid challenge do not parallel changes in ventricular end-diastolic volumes. As such, CVP cannot identify patients who are likely to be responsive to fluid challenges. For these reasons, central venous pressure monitoring per se is now often cited as a useful adjunct to the insertion of the cannula for central venous access, allowing the safe use of vasoactive drugs and rapid transfusion requirements, and facilitating pulmonary artery catheter and transvenous pacemaker insertion if required [3].

Pulmonary artery diastolic pressure and pulmonary artery occlusion pressure

The benefits of pulmonary artery catheterisation must outweigh the risks and should be made on an individual patient basis. Routine use of a pulmonary artery catheter (PAC) in patients at low risk of developing haemodynamic disturbances is not recommended. Numerous studies have failed to show outcome benefits of pulmonary artery catheterisation in postoperative patients over standard care. More specifically, although early studies were supportive of the preoperative insertion of PAC in vascular patients, subsequent studies have demonstrated that it does not appear to prevent postoperative cardiac, respiratory or renal failure in these patients. Furthermore, other studies have shown a higher incidence of intraoperative complications and postoperative pulmonary thromboembolic complications, and the risk of pulmonary artery rupture and pulmonary infarction. As a corollary to this data, international guidelines have been produced for the insertion of PAC, based on three parameters: patient comorbidity, surgical

procedure and previous physician experience in the management of PAC. Patients with significant cardiac disease, impaired left ventricular function, severe aortic stenosis and severe pulmonary hypertension may benefit from PAC insertion, where the data obtained may change their management and cannot be achieved by safer means. Surgical procedures associated with unpredictable changes in preload, afterload or cardiac contractility may also necessitate pulmonary artery pressure monitoring. Contraindications to PAC insertion include the presence of prosthetic tricuspid or pulmonary valves, endocarditis of tricuspid or pulmonary valves and the presence of right heart thrombus.

There are several potential benefits, whenever a PAC is inserted for measurement of pulmonary artery pressures;

- Alterations in the pulmonary arterial pressure waveform may occur in the presence of incipient myocardial ischaemia. Prominent A and V waves occur (an A wave greater than 15 mm Hg or V wave greater than 20 mm Hg) indicating early ischaemia-related myocardial dysfunction (Figure 6.4). Mitral regurgitation can also be seen in ischaemia, with a tall left atrial V wave on the pulmonary arterial pressure tracing. These changes may also be accompanied by increases in left ventricular end-diastolic pressure (LVEDP) and a consequent increase in the pulmonary arterial diastolic pressure (PADP) and pulmonary artery occlusion pressure (PAOP). However, these secondary pressure changes have a low sensitivity and specificity for ischaemia, only detecting 25% episodes of ischaemia detected on a 12-lead ECG or transoesophageal echocardiography.

- Early systolic dysfunction may be detected when reduced ejection fraction results in an increased left ventricular end-systolic volume, leading to an increase in left ventricular end-diastolic volume. The enlarged chamber has a higher pressure, LVEDP, which will result in an increased PAOP. Diastolic dysfunction can occur in myocardial ischaemia due to impaired relaxation of the ventricle and can be detected as an increased LVEDP and PAOP.

- The PAOP has been targeted as a static measure of left ventricular preload. When the PAC is in the wedged position, there is an uninterrupted column of blood between the distal lumen of the

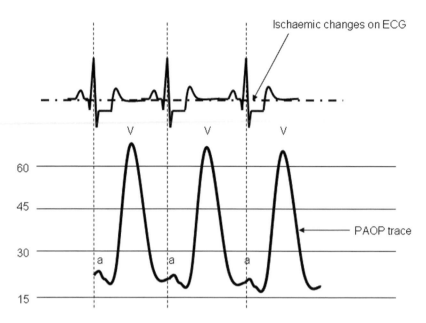

Ischaemic changes on ECG

PAOP trace

Figure 6.4 Changes in pulmonary artery pressure trace during ischaemia. Myocardial ischaemia impairs left ventricular relaxation and produces diastolic dysfunction, with an increase in mean pulmonary artery pressure and PAOP. Tall A and V waves may appear in the PAOP trace. The tall A wave is produced by atrial contraction at the end of diastole into a stiff, incompletely relaxed ventricle. Acute mitral valve regurgitation can occur during ischaemia due to ischaemia-induced structural changes in papillary muscles, chordae tendineae and myocardium. This results in 'functional mitral regurgitation' and the appearance of new regurgitant V waves in the PAOP trace.

catheter and the left atrium. At the end of diastole, the mitral valve opens and the pressure in the left ventricle is transmitted along the column of fluid. Under conditions of normal left ventricular function and constant afterload, the PAOP can be used as a marker of left ventricular preload at the end of expiration. However, there is little evidence that static PAOP measurements identify patients who are likely to respond to fluid loading. Moreover, the linear relationship between PAOP and LVEDP measurements may be affected by poor left ventricular compliance, high intrathoracic pressures, incorrect catheter positioning, high alveolar pressure and increased pulmonary vascular resistance.

- The pulmonary artery pressure waveform can also be monitored for the development of pulmonary hypertension, which can be seen following application of thoracic aortic cross-clamping. Modifications of the PAC also allow for temporary cardiac pacing, and continuous monitoring of mixed venous oxygen saturations to monitor the adequacy of global oxygen delivery.
- Presence of a PAC allows for an invasive method of measuring cardiac output. However, newer less invasive methods have shown adequate measurement of this parameter and may be preferred in this regard, given the aforementioned complications imposed by the PAC (see below).

Cardiac output measurement

Changes in cardiac output during vascular procedures are important in determining the initial haemodynamic status of the patient, the effect of surgical manipulations (e.g. aortic clamping) and the response to vasoactive drugs including inotropes, vasodilators and vasoconstrictors. The thermodilution method of cardiac output assessment used in conjunction with the PAC is often assumed to be a 'gold standard' of cardiac output measurement. This method requires an injection of 5–10 ml of cold dextrose or saline at end expiration through the proximal port of the PAC. The temperature change is measured by a thermistor at the distal end of the catheter. A plot of temperature against time is produced and cardiac output is established using a well-validated algorithm (Stewart–Hamilton). A modification of this technique can also be used for continuous cardiac output measurement. A heating coil within the PAC sits in the right atrium and ventricle. Every 30–60 seconds this heats a bolus of blood and temperature changes are measured by a thermistor, giving a rapid assessment of the changes in cardiac output. Measurements may be inaccurate in the presence of tricuspid regurgitation, intracardiac shunts or variation in the speed or volume of injectate, and if the thermistor is lodged against a vessel wall.

Another method of cardiac output determination uses pulse contour analysis and requires the presence of both central venous and arterial pressure cannulae. In essence, the method converts an arterial pressure waveform (pressure–time curve) into a volume–time curve, thereby allowing the estimation of stroke volume and cardiac output. Calibration of the waveform is achieved by intermittent transpulmonary thermodilution, whereby cold saline is injected through a central venous catheter and dispersed into the intravascular and extravascular pulmonary spaces. Downstream temperature changes are detected via a specific thermodilution tipped arterial catheter. The thermodilution is then used to calibrate the arterial pressure waveform, to give a beat to beat measurement of cardiac output. LiDCO^{TM} is a variant of pulse contour analysis where calibration relies on an injection of lithium rather than cold saline. Haemoglobin, plasma sodium levels and neuromuscular blocking agents may interfere with the lithium electrode. In addition, a requirement for regular recalibration wherever there are rapid changes in haemodynamics may limit its use during vascular surgical procedures. However, the LiDCO system does not require central venous access and is less invasive than the PiCCO® system.

A further cardiac output system (FloTrac/Vigileo) analyses the arterial waveform, without the need for frequent recalibration. It incorporates a transducer which can be connected to any functioning arterial access. Each arterial waveform is analysed for the upstroke and down-slope of curve, and arterial compliance and resistance. Each waveform is then analysed separately and compared with former and subsequent waveforms. From this the average curve is calculated every 20 seconds, and cardiac output can be calculated from the stroke volume and heart rate.

Less invasive measurements of cardiac output include oesophageal Doppler (CardioQ^{TM}). A flexible ultrasound probe placed in the oesophagus displays a continuous velocity–time curve of blood flow in the descending aorta. The CardioQ^{TM} calculates the aortic cross-sectional area from a nomogram based upon the patient's age, height and weight. The oesophageal Doppler can then measure a number of haemodynamic variables which can be used to guide treatment, including peak velocity, stroke volume, cardiac output and corrected flow time (FTc). In addition the appearance of the velocity–time curve may be diagnostic of different fillings states which can occur under anaesthesia, including hypovolaemia, increased afterload or ventricular failure. The trends

of readings in response to treatment are more useful than single readings. In particular if there is less than a 10% increase in stroke volume with a fluid bolus, this suggests that the patient is adequately filled. An FTc less than 330 milliseconds despite fluid may represent hypovolaemia or increased vasoconstriction. A low peak velocity and low FTc represent increased systemic vascular resistance. There are few contra-indications to insertion, which include deranged coagulopathy for nasally inserted probes, oesophageal varices and recent oesophageal surgery. Some circumstances during vascular anaesthesia may limit the intraoperative and perioperative use of the probe: for example in the presence of a thoracic aneurysm the aortic cross-sectional area estimated from the normogram will be inaccurate, and the application of an aortic cross-clamp will interfere with the Doppler waveform trace. An assumption is also made that there is a constant ratio between blood flow in the descending thoracic aorta and to the coronary arteries, which may change in the presence of arterial occlusive disease. Practical considerations include the need to frequently readjust and focus the probe and that oral probes are tolerated poorly by awake patients. However the oesophageal Doppler has a good safety benefit profile and is easy to use. There is increasing evidence to support its use in goal-directed protocols for fluid optimisation, which may reduce perioperative morbidity.

Transoesophageal echocardiography

The American Heart Association and American Task Force Practice guidelines recommend that intraoperative transoesophageal echocardiography (TOE) should be considered where the nature of the surgery or the patient's known or suspected cardiovascular pathology may result in severe haemodynamic, pulmonary or neurological compromise. Benefits of intraoperative TOE include real-time monitoring of left ventricular preload, estimates of ventricular systolic and diastolic function and measurement of cardiac output. Some studies have reported the use of intraoperative TOE in patients undergoing open and endovascular aortic surgery, both as a monitoring and diagnostic tool. It has been used to guide fluid management and optimise blood flow to vascular beds; and to demonstrate abnormal pathology in aortic disruption and dissection. During endovascular aortic aneurysm repair, intraoperative TOE can be used not

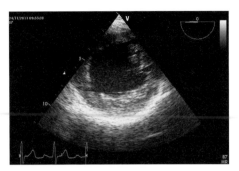

Figure 6.5 The transgastric mid papillary short axis view is used most often as it demonstrates a portion of the myocardium perfused by all three main coronary arteries.

only to demonstrate anatomy, but also to identify the loading zone and deployment of the stent.

Another reason that TOE is used in the operative setting is to provide direct visual assessment of changes in ventricular wall motion, which may be related to ischaemia. This may be important in the setting of vascular anaesthesia. The transgastric short-axis views and the mid oesophageal left ventricular views are the best views for detecting abnormal wall motion. The transgastric mid papillary short axis view is used most often as it demonstrates a portion of the myocardium perfused by all three main coronary arteries: right, circumflex and left anterior descending (Figure 6.5). During a normal contraction, the myocardium, seen on two-dimensional echocardiography, thickens and its endocardial surface moves towards the centre of the chamber. A partially ischaemic myocardial segment has less thickening and motion than normal and is said to be *hypokinetic*. A severely ischaemic or scarred region which does not thicken or move at all is called *akinetic*. A segment which actually gets thinner and moves away from the centre of the chamber during systole is termed *dyskinetic*, a condition that is usually due to an acute, complete interruption of blood flow to previously normally contracting myocardium. Based on the qualitative assessment of its motion, a semi-quantitative numerical wall motion score is usually assigned to each region of the left ventricle: 1, normal; 2, mildly hypokinetic; 3, severely hypokinetic; 4, akinetic; and 5, dyskinetic. Changes in this wall motion score of two or more grades have been shown to have reasonable intra-observer and inter-observer reproducibility.

The detection of abnormal thickening is more specific than the endocardial wall motion for myocardial ischaemia. The changes in endocardial wall motion occur quickly in the setting of ischaemia and may occur before ischaemic changes are seen on the ECG. The incidence of wall motion abnormality (WMA) detected by TOE is 27% to 100% when there is ECG evidence of ischaemia; and 56% to 85% when there is no evidence of ischaemia on ECG. The use of TOE is associated with a low incidence of complications, such as oesophageal perforation and dental injury, and its benefits should outweigh the risks. There are few absolute contraindications to TOE, including patients with oesophageal strictures or varices, and patients post oesophageal surgery.

However, even given the direct views of the myocardium produced by the TOE, not all studies have shown a good correlation between WMA, ST segment changes and elevated enzymes indicative of postoperative myocardial infarction. Moreover, TOE combined with clinical data and information from CM5 ECG has shown to have little incremental value in identifying patients at high risk for perioperative ischaemia. There are also practical limitations. It is not possible to use the transoesophageal probe during induction or emergence, which may be associated with the highest cardiac stress. The entire ventricle cannot be seen in a single view, so an area of ischaemia may be missed. It is not practical to monitor images continuously and there is significant inter-observer variability in the detection of WMA, even in experienced hands. Other factors may cause changes in endocardial wall motion, including myocardial stunning, conduction abnormalities and sudden changes in cardiac preload and afterload. Furthermore, WMA may occur during induction and be attributed as baseline, so decreasing the sensitivity [4].

Functional haemodynamic monitoring (fluid responsiveness): stroke volume variation, pulse pressure variation

Given the magnitude and variability in fluid shifts during vascular procedures, the ability of a vascular surgical patient to produce an adequate response to fluid replacement is an important component of anaesthetic management. It is well established that static markers of preload such as CVP and PAOP measurements are not an indication of fluid responsiveness. Indeed, not all patients are fluid-responsive and optimising their filling status can prove to be challenging. Overzealous use of fluids may be

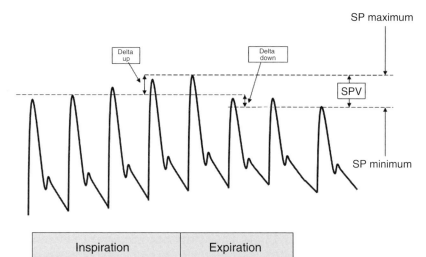

Figure 6.6 Schematic of changes in blood pressure during mechanical ventilation. Systolic pressure variation is divided into components. Delta up represents the systolic pressure increase during inspiration. Delta down represents the systolic pressure decrease during expiration. SP maximum; maximum systolic pressure; SP minimum; minimum systolic pressure. SPV represents the difference between SP maximum and SP minimum. The magnitude of SPV during mechanical ventilation is predictive of fluid responsiveness and can be used to guide targeted intraoperative fluid and inotropic management.

associated with worsening oxygenation and cardiac function, especially where cardiac function is pre-load-independent (i.e. in cardiac failure) [5,6].

It follows that a measurement related to fluid responsiveness is important to anaesthetic management. Under positive pressure ventilation, there are cyclical changes in the right and left ventricular stroke volume. During inspiration, venous return falls, right ventricular preload falls and right ventricular stroke volume falls. Left ventricular preload is increased due to the emptying of pulmonary veins. A fall in transmural pressure reduces left ventricular afterload and left ventricular stroke volume increases. During expiration left ventricular stroke volume then falls, secondary to the reduced left ventricular preload. The magnitude of these changes in stroke volume during mechanical ventilation is predictive of fluid responsiveness. If both of the ventricles are preload-responsive, then the cyclical changes in stroke volume are increased. These changes can be measured and used to guide targeted intraoperative fluid and inotropic management.

The changes in stroke volume can be measured in various ways, including stroke volume variation (SVV), systolic pressure variation (SPV) and pulse pressure variation (PPV). Systolic pressure variation is the difference between the maximal and minimal values of systolic pressure during one mechanical breath (Figure 6.6). The delta down change in the systolic pressure waveform is the downward deflection of the waveform from the baseline. It reflects the expiratory decrease in left ventricular preload and stroke volume related to inspiratory decrease in right

ventricular stroke volume. Under conditions of hypovolaemia secondary to blood loss, the delta down component of the waveform has been shown to correlate with blood loss.

Pulse pressure variation is the difference between systolic and diastolic pressure during the respiratory cycle. During positive pressure ventilation, PPV increases at the end of inspiration and decreases at the end of expiration. The PPV before volume expansion can predict the effect of volume expansion on cardiac output. Patients with a baseline PPV value of more than 13% are likely to respond to volume expansion by increasing $CO > 15\%$ (positive predictive value 94%). Patients with a baseline PPV value of less than 13% are unlikely to respond to fluid challenges.

Stroke volume variation can be measured by pulse contour analysis using the PiCCO and LiDCO. The PiCCO Pulsion Medical system provides two estimates of preload: global end-diastolic volume index (GEDVI) and intrathoracic blood volume index (ITBVI). The GEDVI represents the volume of blood in all the heart chambers at the end of diastole and is a marker of preload. An increase in GEDVI during fluid loading correlates with the increase in ventricular stroke volume. It has been shown that GEDVI is a more reliable indicator of preload than CVP and PAOP, and is not affected by changes in intrathoracic pressure during positive pressure ventilation. However GEDVI cannot distinguish between left ventricular and right ventricular preload. Similarly, ITBVI represents the total volume of blood in the thorax. It is estimated by the single thermodilution method from GEDVI measurements (ITBV = GEDV × 1.25), so measurements of GEDVI are more commonly used in practice. Fluids may be targeted to a GEDVI and ITBVI values of 650–1000 ml/m^2 and 800–1000 ml/m^2 respectively.

Overall PPV is a better predictor of fluid responsiveness than SVV and SPV. There are however limitations to these methods of assessing fluid responsiveness. They do not predict fluid responsiveness in patients who are breathing spontaneously or who have arrhythmias. Also changes in tidal volume and intrathoracic pressure may affect the cyclical changes in ventricular stroke volume.

Perioperative cardiac biomarker surveillance

Cardiac biomarkers can be monitored during the perioperative period and may yield both diagnostic and prognostic information for perioperative cardiac morbidity and mortality [7]. Studies have shown that up to 21% of patients undergoing major vascular surgery have a perioperative cardiac troponin (cTn) rise. The release of cTn is highly specific for myocardial damage and even microscopic areas of necrosis. An elevated troponin has short- and long-term prognostic significance independent of other variables including renal failure. A study of patients undergoing major vascular surgery found that a raised cTnI was associated with a 6-fold increased risk of death and a 27-fold increased risk of myocardial infarction in the 6 months following surgery. There was a dose–response relationship between postoperative cTn concentration and the duration of ischaemia on continuous ECG monitoring and mortality. Both cardiac troponin I (cTnI) and cardiac troponin T (cTnT) were associated with equivalent risk. Further work showed that even minor elevations of troponin are associated with increased cardiac risk at 5 years.

International guidelines recommend postoperative troponin measurements in patients with ECG changes or chest pain typical of acute coronary syndrome. The measurement of postoperative troponin is not well established in patients who are clinically stable and have undergone vascular and intermediate risk surgery. Troponin measurements are not recommended in asymptomatic patients who have undergone low risk surgery. The European Society of Cardiology/American College of Cardiology define an elevated troponin as the maximal concentration of troponin

T or I exceeding the 99th percentile of the values for a reference control group, on at least one occasion in the first 24 hours after an ischaemic event.

The actual timing of troponin measurements may also be significant. Troponin T and I concentrations demonstrate a biphasic release following myocardial injury. Levels rise at 4–6 hours and peak 12–24 hours following myocardial injury. There is a second peak from the second to fourth day after injury, due to release of unbound troponin from cells. In a series of 1136 patients undergoing aortic surgery, 9% of patients had a cTnI concentration of less than 1.5 ng/ml, and 5% of patients had a cTnI concentration greater than 1.5 ng/ml, in keeping with myocardial ischaemia and myocardial infarction respectively. Some 2% of patients had an early peak in cTnI within the first 24 hours. However 3% of patients had a delayed peak in cTnI after 24 hours, which was preceded by a period when cTnI measurements were abnormal but below the infarction threshold. Timely and repeated troponin measurements are necessary to identify patients with ongoing myocardial injury and guide aggressive intervention to prevent postoperative infarction.

There are limitations to troponin measurements. The exact cut-off value for myocardial injury or infarction in the perioperative setting remains contentious and may vary depending on the assay kit. Troponin cannot be used in isolation to diagnose a myocardial infarction and has to be used in conjunction with other criteria, including typical ischaemic pain, the development of pathological Q waves and ECG changes of ischaemia. Cardiac troponins do not explain the mechanism for myocardial damage, so other investigations including ECG and echocardiography are necessary. Cardiac troponins do not differentiate between patients with a ruptured atheromatous plaque and an occluded vessel, and patients with an imbalance in myocardial oxygen demand and supply. Finally other factors can cause an elevated cTn, including ventricular failure, myocarditis, pericarditis, pulmonary embolism, pulmonary hypertension, stroke, renal dysfunction and sepsis.

Other cardiac biomarkers include creatinine kinase (CK) and B-type natriuretic peptide (BNP). Creatinine kinase MB (CK-MB) is released 4–6 hours after the onset of myocardial infarction, peaks at 24 hours and returns to normal at 36–73 hours. Using conventional cut-off values alone, CK-MB has low sensitivity and specificity for the diagnosis of myocardial infarction. Creatinine kinase is also released from ischaemic muscle during aortic and peripheral vascular surgery. The biomarkers BNP and its N-terminal propeptide (NT-proBNP) are released from cardiac myocytes in response to myocardial stretch and ischaemia. In patients undergoing major vascular surgery, preoperative BNP values >35 pg/ml are associated with a 3.5-fold increased risk of death and 6.9-fold increased risk of cardiac events. An elevated preoperative BNP and postoperative cTnI is associated with a 20 times increased risk compared with patients with a normal preoperative BNP, regardless of the troponin value. An elevated postoperative BNP is associated with cardiac death (odds ratio, OR 7.6), non-fatal myocardial infarction (OR 6.24) and major cardiac events (OR 17.3) at 30 days. However the optimal threshold value for BNP has not been established and may depend on the assay used. Further, BNP is not specific for myocardial ischaemia, and may be elevated whenever there is ventricular pressure or volume overload, for example ventricular failure, diastolic dysfunction, pulmonary embolus, pulmonary hypertension, arrhythmias and sepsis.

Integrated monitoring

Myocardial ischaemia in patients undergoing vascular surgery is frequently an imbalance between myocardial oxygen supply and demand. This results in a continuum of haemodynamic abnormalities including ischaemic ECG changes, arrhythmias, hypotension and cardiac failure. Preoperative risk stratification and an awareness of the timing of possible complications during the perioperative period are important when choosing both which monitors to use and the duration of monitoring. The ideal monitor should be safe, versatile, accurate and rapidly responsive and show beneficial effects on outcome for each patient. In reality no individual monitor fulfils these criteria. However an integrated approach, using individual monitors which when combined provide information on ventricular function and fluid responsiveness and allow for early detection of ischaemia may allow timely intervention to prevent complications. Haemodynamic monitoring may be integrated within protocols to optimise fluids and inotropic therapy to meet the increased oxygen demand throughout the perioperative period, and reduce perioperative morbidity and mortality in these high-risk patients.

Summary

Monitoring the vascular patient is heavily targeted towards the cardiovascular system. Basic monitoring standards should be supplemented with more advanced techniques as the comorbidity and complexity of the case necessitates. The detection of myocardial ischaemia is important but must be performed alongside other components of cardiovascular monitoring including ventricular function, fluid responsiveness and adequacy of haemodynamic optimisation. The introduction of biochemical markers of cardiovascular damage provides a novel approach to monitoring. However, it is unlikely that a single monitor will provide all the information required in the more complex vascular procedures especially with the increased degree of patient comorbidity that is likely to occur in the future. Therefore, the choice of appropriate monitoring in individual patients will always be the domain of an experienced vascular anaesthetist.

References

1. London MJ, Hollenberg M, Wong MG, et al. Intraoperative myocardial ischemia: localization by continuous 12-lead electrocardiography. *Anesthesiology* 1988;**69**:232–41.

2. Mark JB. Multimodal detection of perioperative myocardial ischemia. *Tex Heart Inst J.* 2005;**32**:461–6.

3. Magder S. Central venous pressure monitoring. *Curr Opin Crit Care* 2006;**12**: 219–27.

4. Mahmood F, Christie A, Matyal R. Transesophageal echocardiography and noncardiac surgery. *Semin Cardiothorac Vasc Anesth* 2008;**12**:265–89.

5. Slagt C, Breukers RM, Groeneveld AB. Choosing patient-tailored hemodynamic monitoring. *Crit Care* 2010;**14**:208.

6. Monnet X, Teboul JL. Invasive measures of left ventricular preload. *Curr Opin Crit Care* 2006;**12**:235–40.

7. Barry J, Barth JH, Howell SJ. Cardiac troponins: their use and relevance in anaesthesia and critical care medicine. *Contin Educ Anaesth Crit Care Pain* 2008;**8**:62–6.

Chapter 7

Intravenous fluid therapy

Michael F. M. James and Ivan A. Joubert

Intravenous fluid therapy remains surprisingly contro-versial in modern anaesthetic and critical care practice. Although there has been little direct research on fluid therapy specifically in vascular anaesthesia, much of the work that has been conducted has been in major surgical procedures in which vascular surgery has been included and many of the lessons to be gained from these studies are entirely applicable to the vascular surgical patient. The most significant shift in fluid therapy for major surgical procedures has been the questioning of the so-called 'third space' with the realisation that the studies on which this concept was based probably used flawed methodology [1]. This has led to a reappraisal of volume therapy, particularly with crystalloids, during major surgical procedures. Several studies in major abdominal surgery have concluded that generous fluid loading during major surgical procedures may increase the risk of postoperative tissue oedema and consequently the risk of postoperative complications [2]. Other studies have suggested that moderate fluid loading with crystalloids for intermediate surgery such as abdominal laparoscopic or peripheral procedures may improve recovery but larger volumes carried the risk of post-operative hypoxaemia [3]. It is clear from these studies that provision of appropriate volume requirements is beneficial but that recipe-driven fluid regimens for major surgical procedures are inappropriate and that a more rational approach to fluid therapy must be sought. The modern objective is to provide the patient with precisely the amount and type of fluid therapy required without either fluid overload or inadequate volume replacement and consequent impaired tissue perfusion.

Crystalloids versus colloids

The crystalloid/colloid debate has ranged far and wide in the literature over many years. Current consensus opinion is that no outcome advantage has been shown for colloid therapy. This is quite specifically related to mortality as an end-point. A definitive finding on this stance is published in a *Cochrane Review* meta-analysis [4].

What are the implications of such a finding for the vascular anaesthesiologist? When one considers the variables determining outcome for vascular surgery, such as duration and extent of procedure, overall blood loss, total ischaemic time and baseline organ function, it is highly probable that the small signal that may exist with respect to fluid choice is drowned out. The conduct and extent of the procedure are the prime determinants of mortality rather than the choice of fluid type and mortality may thus be an inappropriate end-point. One has to look at other end-points such as morbidity to evaluate fluid choice and here the literature is more revealing. Overall, end organ-specific morbidity may indeed be related to choice of fluid therapy.

It is currently undisputed that patients who receive colloids as fluid therapy receive less fluid than those receiving crystalloid alone. While the ratio of crystalloid to colloid was originally thought to be in the order of 3 or 4 to 1, recent data suggest that, in resuscitation, this may be closer to 1.5 to 1 [5]. Irrespective of the actual ratio, colloid fluid therapy is associated with substantially less total volume of fluid administered.

Recent data argue strongly that the total volume of fluid administered has an impact on outcome. The fact that administration of large volumes of fluid leads to increased morbidity is currently unquestioned. Impaired pulmonary, cardiac and gastrointestinal function, are linked to fluid excess, as are increased tissue oedema, wound dehiscence and wound infection. The term hospital-acquired generalized interstitial

Core Topics in Vascular Anaesthesia, ed. Carl Moores and Alastair F. Nimmo. Published by Cambridge University Press.
© Cambridge University Press 2012.

Table 7.1 Approximate constituents of some common electrolyte solutions (mmol/l) (vary from country to country)

Solution	Na	K	Ca	Mg	Cl	Lactate	Bicarbonate	Acetate	Gluconate	Osmolarity	Osmolality
0.9% saline	154	154	–	–	–	–		–	–	308	287
Ringer's lactate	131	5	1.8	–	111	27		–	–	274	256
Plasmalyte B	131	5	1.8	1.5	111		29			276	nd
Plasmalyte A	140	5		1.5	98			27	23	294	nd

nd, no data.

oedema (HAGIE) has been coined to describe the tissue oedema associated with excessive crystalloid administration. The development of pulmonary oedema has been linked to positive fluid balance. Of particular importance is the association between the development of abdominal compartment syndrome and fluid balance.

The risk factors for the development of abdominal compartment syndrome have been described. Chief among the risk factors is a large fluid volume administered (>3.5 l in 24 hours). Raised intra-abdominal pressure has been shown to have a direct effect on gastrointestinal mucosal saturation and there is little question that raised intra-abdominal pressure has an impact on outcome [6]. In this study raised intra-abdominal pressure was significantly associated with organ failure (respiratory and renal) and independently predicted mortality. Excessive fluid administration predicts the development of raised intra-abdominal pressure and is associated with worse survival.

There is, thus, a strong argument for limiting crystalloid loading in favour of volume support with colloids.

Balanced electrolyte solutions

The use of so-called 'balanced' crystalloid solutions as part of perioperative fluid strategy is under scrutiny. Whilst it seems empirically correct to infuse intravenous solutions that closely resemble the electrolyte composition of extracellular fluid (ECF), producing such solutions in practice is difficult. A solution that resembles ECF requires replacement of the bicarbonate with a more stable alternative and the provision of other, physiologically safe anions. The simplest answer is 0.9% sodium chloride solution which has an approximately physiological osmolarity. Although the calculated osmolarity of such a solution is

308 mOsm/l (Na^+ 154 mmol/l and Cl^- 154 mmol/l), the osmotic coefficient of this solution is 0.926; consequently, the osmolality is 287 mosm/kg, similar to that of plasma. If a solution with an ideal osmolality is the prime requirement, then 0.9% saline is an acceptable preparation. None of the currently available balanced salt solutions is ideal. Ringer's lactate or acetate and other similar solutions are frequently low in sodium ($\pm$130 mmol/l) and are thus hypotonic which may be disadvantageous in certain circumstances, particularly when the brain is at risk. The composition of some commercially available solutions is given in Table 7.1. There is a remarkable absence of evidence confirming the safety of the various anions (acetate, malate, gluconate) that are frequently added to balanced salt solutions. There is no experimental or scientific support for the widespread assumption that acetate is safer than lactate. There is a possibility that the more rapid metabolism of acetate may result in a greater degree of postinfusion metabolic alkalosis. Using lactate infusions may impair the value of lactate measurements as an assessment of tissue perfusion. Where lactate measurements are important, or in diabetics taking metformin, there is a possible argument for avoiding lactate.

Hyperchloraemic acidosis

The excessive use of saline will result in hyperchloraemic acidosis which has been identified as a potential side effect of saline-based solutions [7]. There is debate about the morbidity associated with this condition, with no clear evidence of harm from short-duration mild hyperchloraemia [8].

Effects on renal function

Animal studies suggest that chloride may have adverse effects on the kidney including renal vasoconstriction, increase in renal vascular resistance, decrease in glomerular filtration rate (GFR) and decrease in renin activity. Delayed production of urine following fluid loading in volunteers has also been described with saline as compared to Ringer's lactate [9]. However, these volunteer studies have not been translated into postoperative renal dysfunction and it may well be that these observations are more related to the osmolality of the infused fluids than to evidence of renal dysfunction.

O'Malley *et al.* compared Ringer's lactate with isotonic saline in patients undergoing renal transplantation. In this study it was found that recipients undergoing kidney transplants had greater acidosis and higher potassium concentrations if they were given 0.9% saline as opposed to Ringer's lactate [10]. This is the consequence of acidosis mobilising potassium from the intracellular space in patients where renal function is unable to compensate for these changes. It is worth noting that there was no adverse effect of isotonic saline on renal function. There is no evidence of this effect in other studies comparing isotonic saline to balanced salt crystalloids in patients with normal renal function.

Overall, there are no clinical studies demonstrating clinically relevant decreases in renal function in patients undergoing surgery where either a balanced salt or saline is used as the major crystalloid component. However, it must be borne in mind that a number of these studies were conducted with both crystalloid and colloid and that the diminution in volume requirements from the colloid mean that the overall chloride load is quite small.

Effects on coagulation

A study of patients undergoing repair of abdominal or thoracoabdominal aortic aneurysms compared the use of Ringer's lactate to isotonic saline. There was a small, non-significant difference in blood loss between the groups and a statistically significant increase in the total volume of blood products administered in the saline group without any effect on outcome [11].

Studies of test-tube dilution of blood with saline or saline-based colloids have shown that balanced solutions containing calcium cause significantly less disturbance of coagulation as measured by thrombelastography using either crystalloid or colloid suspended in a balanced salt solution [12]. However, such in vitro studies artificially decrease ionised

calcium and this can have a profound effect on coagulation in the test-tube that may not reflect clinical reality [13]. There is no evidence that the calcium content of any balanced salt preparation is of any clinical value. However high calcium concentrations (>1 mmol/l of ionised Ca^{2+}) have the disadvantage that they may cause transfused blood or plasma to clot in the administration set if the calcium-containing solution is mixed with citrated blood products.

These studies suggest that large volumes of saline will increase chloride concentration and reduce base excess in a dose-dependent manner, with the peak effect occurring a few hours post infusion. The effect is temporary, and levels generally return to normal within 1 or 2 days. When fluid therapy is based on colloids in an isotonic saline carrier, together with a balanced crystalloid like Ringer's lactate, the effects on acid–base equilibrium appear limited. Where a strategy of moderate crystalloid replacement with Ringer's lactate is used, the use of saline-based colloid for plasma volume replacement would seem to be acceptable.

Colloids

There is a variety of synthetic colloids currently available including the gelatins, the dextrans and the hydroxyethyl starches (HES) in addition to albumin solutions derived from human plasma.

Gelatins

There are two types of gelatins available, the urea-linked form typified by Haemaccel® and the succinylated form as typified by Gelofusin®.

Urea-linked gelatin consists of polypeptides linked through a urea bond giving an average molecular weight (MW) of 35 kDa. The suspending solution is saline-based with additional potassium and a high calcium concentration (approximately 6 mmol/l) making it inadvisable to mix citrated blood in the same giving set as this gelatin.

The succinylated gelatins have a negative charge and an effectively larger molecule for the same molecular weight. This enhances intravascular retention, despite a MW of only 30 kDa. However, there is currently no evidence that these gelatins have a longer duration of action than their older cousins. The electrolyte content of Gelofusin is similar to 0.9% saline, with a slightly lower osmolarity than plasma, and a lower chloride content than that of saline.

The gelatins give short lived plasma volume expansion lasting for 1–3 hours. Consequently, they are useful plasma expanders in circumstances where a short-term increase in volume is desirable, such as during neuraxial blockade, or as an interim measure while waiting for red cell infusions to become available. The gelatins are fully cleared from the body through the kidney. They exert little effect on coagulation, although they may impair clot strength, mainly on a dilution basis. The main adverse effect attributable to the gelatins is that of anaphylaxis. The risk is substantially greater for the urea-linked gelatins than the fluid gelatins.

Dextrans

The dextrans are polydisperse glucose polymers with a wide range of molecular sizes. There is some in vivo metabolism, but the main route of elimination is through the kidney.

There are various dextran preparations, defined by the average molecular weight, ranging from Dextran 1 (MW 1 kDa) to the now obsolete Dextran 110. The dextrans generally enhance tissue plasma flow by reducing blood viscosity, by diminishing red cell aggregation and enhancing endothelial integrity. From a purely pharmacokinetic point of view, Dextran 70 is a near-ideal volume expander as it has a long dwell time, is biodegradable and gives good volume expansion.

Dextran 40 (generally available in a 10%, hyperoncotic preparation) produces greater volume expansion than Dextran 70, but has a shorter duration of action due to the smaller mean molecular size. The smaller dextran molecules are readily filtered in the kidney where they have significant osmotic effects. The most noted side-effect of dextrans is interference with coagulation. Dextran 40 may be beneficial in decreasing the incidence of cerebral embolism and improving cerebral blood flow following carotid endarterectomy and in the management of crescendo ischaemic attacks [14]. It has been suggested that they may be of benefit in various forms of vascular surgery where the perfusion of grafts is precarious [15]. However, these applications should be regarded as pharmacological rather than fluid therapy as the volume recommended is small (500 ml/24 hours).

The dextrans have numerous adverse effects. The osmotic diuresis associated with Dextran 40 may lead to hyperosmotic renal failure. Rarely, adverse reactions including the dextran syndrome and anaphylaxis may occur. However, the risk of anaphylaxis with the dextrans can be almost completely eliminated by pre-treatment with Dextran 1.

Hydroxyethyl starches

The hydroxyethyl starches (HES) are a group of compounds characterised by hydroxyethyl substitution of plant-derived starch molecules. Hydroxyethylation increases the water solubility of the starch and inhibits breakdown of the starch molecule by amylase. Starches used in the manufacture of these products are derived either from waxy corn or potato, producing compounds with somewhat different properties. Hydroxyethyl groups attach to the glucose subunits mainly at the C2 and C6 positions on the molecule. Substitution in the C2 position is the most important in terms of inhibiting the action of amylase. The extent of substitution is described as the molar substitution (MS), which is the average molar mass of hydroxyethyl groups compared to the molar mass of glucose residues.

A variety of different HES products exist, with considerable differences in their pharmacological properties. These HES solutions are classified according to the average in vitro MW into high MW (450–700 kDa), medium MW (100–200 kDa) and low MW (70 kDa). However, further classification is necessary as the starches undergo some metabolism in the plasma which results in changes in the molecular weight. The rate of metabolism is determined by the MS (ranging from 0.4 to 0.7) and the ratio of the carbon atom position at which the substitution occurs (C2/C6). High values for MW, MS and C2/C6 ratio all result in a reduction in metabolism with long-lasting volume effects and extended tissue persistence. Large molecules increase the incidence of bleeding complications and may be associated with an increased risk of pruritis. Since the degree of in vivo metabolism is critical, it is now more common to classify the starches by their molar substitution ratios. The current classification is illustrated in Table 7.2.

The starches, therefore, are characterised by both MW and MS, and typical nomenclature gives both of these values; hence Hespan® is characterised as 450/0.7 while Voluven® is characterised as 130/0.4 and Venofundin® as 130/0.42.

The lower MS of the newer HES products results in more rapid breakdown of the starch in the plasma,

Table 7.2 Classification of hydroxyethyl starch (HES) products

Generic name	Molecular weight (kDa)	Molar substitution (MS)	Suspending solution	Commercial examples
Hetastarch	450	0.7	Saline	Hespan®, Plasmasteril®
Hetastarch	650	0.7	Balanced salt	Hextend®
Hexastarch	260	0.6	Saline	EloHaes®
Pentastarch	200	0.45–0.5	Saline	HAES-Steril®, Pentaspan®, Hemohes®
Tetrastarch	130	0.4–0.45	Saline	Voluven®, Venofundin®
Tetrastarch	130	0.4–0.45	Balanced salt	Tetraspan®, Volulyte®

resulting in lower in vivo MW in the order of 70 kDa. This has resulted in substantial decreases in the major adverse effects of the HES products including coagulopathy [16], tissue accumulation and potential for renal dysfunction [17] However, as the in vivo MW remains above the crucial value of 65 kDa there is minimal loss of efficacy, and tetrastarch has been shown to be as effective and to have similar duration of action as the older HES products [18].

Administration of HES gives plasma expansion that is usually more than 100% of the volume infused, with a relatively long duration of action of 4–8 hours and a possible protective effect of the endothelium. Adverse effects include interference with coagulation through binding and inactivation of the factor VIII/vWF complex, tissue persistence that may result in skin itching and possible renal dysfunction that is probably the result of hyperosmolar states, rather than a direct toxic effect of the starch molecules. All of these effects appear to be related to the higher levels of MS and to be of less importance with the tetrastarches [19].

One of the most attractive class actions of HES is the potential to diminish inflammatory responses. Although evidence of clinical benefit of this effect is limited, there is some evidence of protection of renal and pulmonary function through reduced inflammatory processes following aortic aneurysm surgery when HES is compared to gelatin [20].

Recently, potato-derived starches have been introduced that are substantially different from the waxy corn starch product. Waxy corn starch is almost pure amylopectin, whereas the potato starch contains a significant proportion of amylose. The potato starch also has a significant phosphate content that is not present in the waxy corn starch product. The physical characteristics of the two starch products are different and the pharmacokinetic profiles are similar but not truly bioequivalent. Early clinical use of potato starch 200/0.5 and 130/0.42 was associated with a postoperative increase in bilirubin in both groups [21]. A recent analysis of the corn starch and potato starch HES preparations has demonstrated substantial differences between the products in terms of in vitro MW, MS, amylose content and phosphate content. Whether these differences are clinically important remains to be established, but, at present, these HES preparations should not be regarded as being interchangeable.

The HES starches as a group have the lowest incidence of allergic reactions of all of the colloid preparations, including albumin.

Most starch products are suspended in saline, with the potential for hyperchloraemic acidosis referred to above. Recently, starch solutions containing balanced salts have been introduced. These include a HES 650/0.7 available in the USA (Hextend®), and two products that have recently entered the market containing HES 130/0.4 or HES 130/0.42. Whether or not the replacement of saline with balanced salt-suspending solutions will be of clinical benefit remains to be established.

Human albumin solution

Albumin has been widely regarded as the most appropriate resuscitation and volume support fluid for the critically ill and for patients undergoing major surgical procedures. However, a *Cochrane Review* meta-analysis concluded that for patients with hypovolaemia there is no evidence that albumin reduces mortality when compared with cheaper alternatives such as saline [4].

The most important consideration regarding albumin is the high cost. Although pricing structures vary from country to country, generally albumin preparations cost about 10 times the price of the equivalent synthetic colloids. In addition, albumin may be less of an ideal plasma volume expander than it would at first sight appear to be. As it is derived from human proteins, it carries with it all the risks of allogeneic proteins, including the risks of disease transmission and allergic reactions. It is widely assumed that albumin does not affect coagulation, but this is not entirely true and several studies have found a mild anticoagulant effect from albumin, partly due to its ability to bind calcium, in addition to the dilution of coagulation proteins. Compared to isotonic HES 200/0.5 for plasma volume expansion, 5% albumin showed similar coagulation and renal function effects, blood loss was not significantly different between the groups but the use of HES reduced costs by 35% [22]. In the SAFE study, no survival difference could be demonstrated for albumin when compared to saline for volume of therapy in the intensive care unit, although statistically significant differences in hemodynamic variables could be demonstrated [5].

Why is albumin less effective than had been assumed? Albumin escapes from the vascular compartment much more readily in sepsis than in non-septic patients and an infused bolus of albumin has a substantially reduced duration of effect in septic patients [23]. In critically ill and cardiac surgery patients interstitial fluid volume expansion resulting from the use of albumin was almost identical to that produced by saline [24]. There is little evidence, therefore that the use of albumin, despite its substantially greater cost, confers any outcome benefit on patients undergoing vascular surgical procedures.

Adverse effects of colloids

Effects on coagulation

It is now well established that moderate crystalloid dilution both in vivo and in vitro can enhance the coagulation of whole blood. The mechanism for this phenomenon is probably dilution of circulating anticoagulants, such as antithrombin III. The presence of calcium in diluent fluids is of relevance for in vitro dilution, but has little practical significance in the clinical situation as calcium homoeostasis is extremely well maintained in most circumstances. However, the presence of calcium in balanced electrolyte solutions may cause citrate-containing blood products to form micro-clots in the administration set.

The effects of colloids on coagulation are more complex. The dextrans have the best demonstrated influence on coagulation although, in moderate doses (<15 ml/kg per 24 hours), there is little evidence of increased surgical bleeding. However, the only real indication for dextrans in vascular surgery is as low-dose pharmacological treatment to minimise the risk of cerebral embolism after carotid endarterectomy or possibly to maintain perfusion in critical grafts.

The gelatins are widely regarded as having minimal effects on coagulation, and for this and historical reasons there is no 24-hour dosage limit imposed on these intravenous solutions. As with most colloids, gelatins may impair clot strength particularly at dilutions in excess of 40%, but whether or not this contributes to increased bleeding is not clear.

Hetastarch preparations undoubtedly contributed to increased postoperative bleeding at dosages exceeding 20 ml/kg per 24 hours. This observation is the basis for the volume limit applied to the hetastarches. Subsequent development of lower in vivo MW HES has decreased the impairment of coagulation. Modern tetrastarches are probably not different from albumin and the gelatins in this regard. Both gelatins and tetrastarches impair measured clot strength, but have no influence on perioperative blood loss compared to a crystalloid fluid strategy [25]. In vascular surgical patients, HES was shown to be neutral in terms of coagulation whereas crystalloid infusions increased coagulation enhancing the risk of intravascular clotting [26].

There is little evidence at the present time to base a choice of intravenous fluid therapy on risks of coagulation. All of the modern colloids cause minor disturbances of coagulation that do not appear to enhance perioperative bleeding, whereas large volumes of crystalloid may increase the risk of coagulation, particularly deep vein thrombosis postoperatively.

Effects on renal function

The use of crystalloids to chase a predetermined renal output in an attempt to 'protect' the kidneys will result in substantial fluid overload that may be counter-productive. Saline is frequently recommended for rehydration in patients who have received radiocontrast agents in order to minimise the risk of contrast-induced nephropathy. However, the metabolic acidosis resulting from saline may be harmful and it has been suggested that sodium bicarbonate with or without n-acetyl-cysteine may be preferable. A recent review concluded that bicarbonate infusions were effective at reducing the incidence of contrast-induced nephropathy and appeared to be more consistently protective than n-acetyl-cysteine [27], and it has been reported that the addition of theophylline may further enhance this benefit [28]. For patients undergoing vascular surgery where large volumes of contrast may be used it would seem appropriate to provide crystalloid fluid therapy in the form of a bicarbonate-containing solution.

The colloids maintain central circulating blood volume better than crystalloids and, for this reason, were expected to reduce the risk of renal failure. However, this expectation was not universally met and there has been some concern that individual colloids may increase the risk of renal failure. This problem was first described with hyperoncotic Dextran 40 solutions but has since been described in conjunction with the use of all colloids, particularly when plasma oncotic pressure is allowed to rise and inadequate crystalloid supplementation is given.

Concern regarding the possible effect of HES compounds on renal function was first raised in renal transplant recipients whose donors had been resuscitated with HES and in whom renal biopsies demonstrated an 'osmotic-nephrosis type lesion'. An intensive care study comparing gelatin to HES suggested a higher incidence of renal dysfunction as defined by an increase in creatinine in those patients who had received HES [29]. However, there was no difference in the requirement for renal replacement therapy between the groups, and nor was there any difference in outcome in terms of days in intensive care or mortality. These reports related to the use of a hexastarch (HES 260/0.6, EloHaes®) that is no longer in use.

Numerous studies using tetrastarch have not demonstrated an increased risk of renal dysfunction. A comparison between gelatin, HES 260/0.6 and HES 130/0.4 in patients undergoing aortic aneurysm repair showed better maintained renal function, together with lower inflammatory markers in both groups given HES with the advantage for the tetrastarch persisting for at least 5 days postoperatively [20]. A comparative study of HES and gelatin in surgical patients with prior renal dysfunction found non-inferiority of HES compared to gelatin and concluded that the choice of the colloid had no impact on renal safety parameters [30].

A study using 10% HES 200/0.5 (a hyperoncotic pentastarch) reported dose-related renal injury from the starch [31]. However, repeated administration of hyperoncotic colloid is known to predispose to renal failure, particularly in the absence of adequate crystalloid support. The doses of HES administered frequently exceeded the recommended dose limitations and crystalloid administration appears to have been inadequate. The most reasonable conclusion from this paper is that hyperoncotic colloids pose a renal risk in sepsis and should not be used in critically ill patients, certainly not in repeated doses. A subsequent multicentre, non-randomised, observational study concluded that hyperoncotic colloids, and in particular hyperoncotic albumin, are associated with an increased risk of renal failure, but iso-oncotic colloids were not [32].

It is possible that HES may represent a risk of renal dysfunction under certain circumstances (notably sepsis) particularly with slowly degradable HES. It seems unlikely that the administration of isotonic HES compounds with a low in vivo MW poses a risk of renal dysfunction. There are no publications describing any deterioration of renal function in association with the use of HES 130/0.4 even when administered in doses in well excess of the recommended dose limit in the perioperative and trauma settings. However, it must be emphasised that it is critical to maintain adequate crystalloid administration whenever colloids are used in large volumes or repeatedly over many days. There would seem to be no justification for repeated use of hyperoncotic colloids of any type.

Volume optimisation

Recent challenges to the free use of crystalloids have focussed attention on appropriate volume strategies in major surgery. Static measurements of arterial and venous pressures and changes in heart rate have been shown to be valueless in terms of estimating volume requirements. Dynamic measures of cardiac response to colloid fluid challenges have shown considerable promise in limiting total fluid volumes and ensuring early, appropriate fluid administration with a reduction in perioperative complications. Derived cardiac performance measures from oesophageal Doppler probes have been best validated for this purpose [33], with consistent reductions in hospital length of stay and the incidence of complications. However, other variables derived from a variety of pulse waveform analysis devices have also shown promise and the use of stroke volume variation, pulse pressure variation and corrected flow time have all been shown to provide useful fluid volume guidance [34]. The extra cost of these monitoring devices appears to be offset by the reduction in complication-related expense and, for major surgical procedures, they seem to be well justified.

Conclusions

Vascular surgical patients present a high-risk group in whom accurate and appropriate fluid therapy may have a substantial impact on the incidence of complications and length of hospital stay. Total crystalloid administration should not exceed 40 ml/kg in a 24-hour period unless there are ongoing losses that should be replaced. Such crystalloid should probably be administered as a balanced salt, although the composition of each solution and the purpose for which it is being given should be considered when a prescription is issued. The use of colloid solutions for plasma volume expansion, particularly when targeted against measures of cardiac performance, appears to offer benefit to high-risk patients. Modern synthetic colloids appear to be very safe and effective for this purpose.

References

1. Brandstrup B, Svensen C, Engquist A. Hemorrhage and operation cause a contraction of the extracellular space needing replacement: evidence and implications? A systematic review. *Surgery*, 2006;**139**: 419–32.

2. Nisanevich V, Felsenstein I, Almogy G, *et al.* Effect of intraoperative fluid management on outcome after intraabdominal surgery. *Anesthesiology* 2005;**103**:25–32.

3. Holte K, Foss NB, Andersen J, *et al.* Liberal or restrictive fluid administration in fast-track colonic surgery: a randomized, double-blind study. *Br J Anaesthes* 2007;**99**:500–8.

4. Alderson P, Bunn F, Li WP, *et al.* Human albumin solution for resuscitation and volume expansion in critically ill patients (Review). *Cochrane Database Syst Rev* 2009; **CD001208**.

5. Finfer S, Bellomo R, Boyce N, *et al.* A comparison of albumin and saline for fluid resuscitation in the intensive care unit. *N Engl J Med* 2004;**350**:2247–56.

6. Vidal MG, Ruiz WJ, Gonzalez F, *et al.* Incidence and clinical effects of intra-abdominal hypertension in critically ill patients. *Crit Care Med* 2008;**36**:1823–31.

7. Williams EL, Hildebrand KL, McCormick SA, Bedel MJ. The effect of intravenous lactated Ringer's solution versus 0.9% sodium chloride solution on serum osmolality in human volunteers. *Anesth Analg* 1999;**88**:999–1003.

8. Handy JM, Soni N. Physiological effects of hyperchloraemia and acidosis. *Br J Anaesth* 2008;**101**:141–50.

9. Reid F, Lobo DN, Williams RN, Rowlands BJ, Allison SP. (Ab) normal saline and physiological Hartmann's solution: a randomized double-blind crossover study. *Clin Sci (Lond)* 2003;**104**:17–24.

10. O'Malley CM, Frumento RJ, Hardy MA, *et al.* A randomized, double-blind comparison of lactated Ringer's solution and 0.9% NaCl during renal transplantation. *Anesth Analg* 2005;**100**:1518–24.

11. Waters JH, Gottlieb A, Schoenwald P, *et al.* Normal saline versus lactated Ringer's solution for intraoperative fluid management in patients undergoing abdominal aortic aneurysm repair: an outcome study. *Anesth Analg* 2001;**93**: 817–22.

12. Roche AM, James MF, Grocott MP, Mythen MG. Coagulation effects of in vitro serial haemodilution with a balanced electrolyte hetastarch solution compared with a saline-based hetastarch solution and lactated Ringer's solution. *Anaesthesia* 2002;**57**:950–7.

13. James MFM, Roche AM. Dose–response relationship between plasma ionized calcium concentration and thrombelastography. *J Cardiothor Vasc An* 2004;**18**:581–6.

14. Lennard NS, Vijayasekar C, Tiivas C, *et al.* Control of emboli in patients with recurrent or crescendo transient ischaemic attacks using preoperative transcranial Doppler-directed Dextran therapy. *Br J Surg* 2003;**90**:166–70.

15. Abir F, Barkhordarian S, Sumpio BE. Efficacy of dextran solutions in vascular surgery. *Vasc Endovasc Surg* 2004;**38**:483–91.

16. Kozek-Langenecker SA, Jungheinrich C, Sauermann W, Van der Linden P. The effects of hydroxyethyl starch 130/0.4 (6%)

on blood loss and use of blood products in major surgery: a pooled analysis of randomized clinical trials. *Anesth Analg* 2008;**107**:382–90.

17. Jungheinrich C, Neff TA. Pharmacokinetics of hydroxyethyl starch. *Clini Pharmacokin* 2005;**44**:681–99.

18. James MF, Latoo MY, Mythen MG, *et al.* Plasma volume changes associated with two hydroxyethyl starch colloids following acute hypovolaemia in volunteers. *Anaesthesia* 2004;**59**:738–42.

19. Westphal M, James MF, Kozek-Langenecker S, *et al.* Hydroxyethyl starches: different products – different effects. *Anesthesiology* 2009;**111**:187–202.

20. Mahmood A, Gosling P, Vohra RK. Randomized clinical trial comparing the effects on renal function of hydroxyethyl starch or gelatine during aortic aneurysm surgery. *Br J Surg* 2007;**94**:427–33.

21. Sander O, Reinhart K, Meier-Hellmann A. Equivalence of hydroxyethyl starch HES 130/0. 4 and HES 200/0. 5 for perioperative volume replacement in major gynaecological surgery. *Acta Anaesthesiol Scand* 2003;**47**:1151–8.

22. Vogt N, Bothner U, Brinkmann A, de Petriconi R, Georgieff M. Peri-operative tolerance to large-dose 6% HES 200/0.5 in major

urological procedures compared with 5% human albumin. *Anaesthesia* 1999;**54**:121–7.

23. Margarson MP, Soni NC Changes in serum albumin concentration and volume expanding effects following a bolus of albumin 20% in septic patients. *Br J Anaesth* 2004;**92**:821–6.

24. Ernest D, Belzberg AS, Dodek PM. Distribution of normal saline and 5% albumin infusions in cardiac surgical patients. *Crit Care Med* 2001;**29**:2299–302.

25. Schramko A, Suojaranta-Ylinen R, Kuitunen A, *et al.* Hydroxyethylstarch and gelatin solutions impair blood coagulation after cardiac surgery: a prospective randomized trial. *Br J Anaesth* 2010;**104**:691–7.

26. Ruttmann TG, James MF, Finlayson J. Effects on coagulation of intravenous crystalloid or colloid in patients undergoing peripheral vascular surgery. *Br J Anaesthes* 2002;**89**:226–30.

27. Massicotte A. Contrast medium-induced nephropathy: strategies for prevention. *Pharmacotherapy* 2008;**28**:1140–50.

28. Malhis M, Al-Bitar S, Al-Deen ZK. The role of theophylline in prevention of radiocontrast media-induced nephropathy. *Saudi J Kidney Dis Transpl* 2010;**21**:276–83.

29. Schortgen F, Lacherade JC, Bruneel F, *et al.* Effects of hydroxyethylstarch and gelatin on renal function in severe sepsis: a multicentre randomised study. *Lancet* 2001;**357**:911–16.

30. Godet G, Lehot JJ, Janvier G, *et al.* Safety of HES 130/0.4 (Voluven®) in patients with preoperative renal dysfunction undergoing abdominal aortic surgery: a prospective, randomized, controlled, parallel-group multicentre trial. *Eur J Anaesthesiol* 2008;**25**:986–94.

31. Brunkhorst FM, Engel C, Bloos F, *et al.* Intensive insulin therapy and pentastarch resuscitation in severe sepsis. *N Engl J Med* 2008;**358**:125–39.

32. Schortgen F, Girou E, Deye N, Brochard L. The risk associated with hyperoncotic colloids in patients with shock. *Intens Care Med* 2008;**34**:2157–68.

33. Phan TD, Ismail H, Heriot AG, Ho KM. Improving perioperative outcomes: fluid optimization with the esophageal Doppler monitor, a metaanalysis and review. *J Am Coll Surg* 2008;**207**:935–41.

34. Cannesson M, Musard H, Desebbe O, *et al.* The ability of stroke volume variations obtained with Vigileo/FloTrac system to monitor fluid responsiveness in mechanically ventilated patients. *Anesth Analg* 2009;**108**:513–17.

Haemostasis and thrombosis

Chapter 8

Gary A. Morrison and Alastair F. Nimmo

Vascular surgery involves surgery on blood vessels and it is not surprising that excessive bleeding during and/or after surgery is a common complication. Bleeding may be 'surgical bleeding' resulting from holes in blood vessels too large to be sealed by the formation of blood clots or may be diffuse microvascular bleeding resulting from an impairment of the ability to form stable clot. Both of these causes of haemorrhage may be present simultaneously.

It is important, however, to appreciate that complications involving thrombosis/thromboembolism are common in vascular surgical patients, e.g. myocardial infarction, ischaemic stroke, bypass graft occlusion and deep vein thrombosis. Some strategies which reduce bleeding such as stopping aspirin before surgery or not giving heparin during surgery may increase not only the incidence of thrombotic complications but the overall rates of morbidity and mortality. Therefore it is important to consider the risks of thrombotic complications as well as the risks of haemorrhage.

Vascular surgery patients frequently have an impaired ability to form stable blood clot. Usually this is an acquired rather than congenital abnormality of haemostasis. The commonest causes are the administration of antiplatelet and anticoagulant drugs and the effects of blood loss and shock on the levels and function of platelets, fibrinogen and other coagulation factors. Sometimes, particularly in shocked patients, excessive breakdown of clot (fibrinolysis) may occur. It is important for the vascular anaesthetist to have an understanding of the mechanisms of normal haemostasis, and to know how to diagnose the nature and severity of abnormalities in the formation of stable clot and how to treat these abnormalities.

Normal haemostasis
Clot formation

Blood clots are composed of platelets, fibrin and red blood cells (Figure 8.1). The commonest causes of excessive microvascular bleeding in vascular surgical patients are reduced platelet count and/or function, reduced fibrinogen concentration and reduced conversion of fibrinogen to fibrin as the result of heparin administration.

Our understanding of haemostasis has undergone great changes in recent years. Furie's in vivo studies in mice have demonstrated that rather than primary haemostasis (formation of a platelet plug) being followed by secondary haemostasis (thrombin generation and formation of a fibrin network), both platelet accumulation and fibrin formation occur simultaneously [1,2]. Hoffmann and Monroe's cell-based

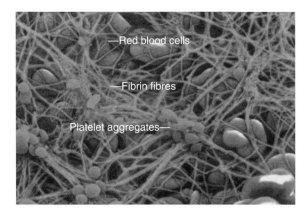

Figure 8.1 Scanning electron micrograph of a blood clot formed in vitro showing fibrin fibres, platelet aggregates and trapped red blood cells. From Veklich Y, Weisel JW. *Nature* 2001;**413**:6855 – cover illustration; with permission. See plate section for colour version.

model of haemostasis describes thrombin generation occurring not as the result of a cascade of proteolytic reactions in the plasma but rather from a series of overlapping initiation, amplification and propagation steps occurring on the surfaces of tissue factor (TF) bearing cells and platelets [3,4].

Cell-based model of coagulation

The cell-based model can be broken down into three overlapping stages (Figure 8.2).

(1) Initiation
(2) Amplification
(3) Propagation.

Initiation

Initiation of coagulation occurs on the surface of TF-bearing cells, typically extravascular monocytes or fibroblasts. Tissue factor is a transmembrane protein which binds factor VII (FVII) converting it to its activated form FVIIa and the resulting FVIIa/TF complex in turn catalyses the activation of factors IX and X. Factor Xa combines with its co-factor FVa to form prothrombinase complexes which convert prothrombin (FII) to small amounts of thrombin (FIIa). Any FXa which moves away from the cell surface is inhibited by tissue factor pathway inhibitor (TFPI) and antithrombin (AT) ensuring that the thrombin-producing process only occurs at the cell surface.

This process occurs continuously on a small scale in the extravascular space in the absence of injury – the coagulation factors are relatively small polypeptides capable of moving between the intra- and extra-vascular spaces. Under normal conditions this initiation process does not lead to clot formation because the larger platelets and von Willebrand factor (vWF) combined with factor VIII are confined within blood vessels.

Amplification

Injury to a blood vessel wall results in the exposure of subendothelial collagen and of tissue factor bearing cells to components of blood from which they are normally separated by an intact endothelium i.e. to platelets and vWF/FVIII. Platelets become attached to the exposed subendothelial connective tissue matrix by interacting with the exposed collagen and with vWF. This leads to the activation of platelets which are also activated by thrombin

produced as described above on the surface of TF-bearing cells. The thrombin produced during the initiation phase has a number of other important roles including the exposure of coagulation factor binding sites on the platelet surface and the activation of FV and FXI on the platelet surface. In addition it acts on the vWF/FVIII complex leading to the activation of FVIII on the platelet surface, and the release of vWF – this free vWF leads to further platelet aggregation and adhesion at the site of vessel injury. Amplification therefore leads to a collection of activated platelets and activated coagulation factors, and provides the basis for the large-scale production of thrombin in a platelet-rich environment at the site of tissue injury.

Propagation

This phase occurs on the platelet surface and leads to the rapid production of thrombin (the 'thrombin burst') and ultimately to the production of fibrin. The amplification phase leads to the activation of a platelet with activated factors V, VIII and XI on its surface. Factor IXa produced in the initiation phase combines with FVIIIa resulting in the formation of the tenase (FVIIIa/FIXa) complex which is required for the activation of FX. In addition FXIa produced during amplification activates more FIX to FIXa. FXa combines with FVa on the platelet surface to produce the prothrombinase complex which converts pro-thrombin (FII) to thrombin.

Conversion of fibrinogen to fibrin

Fibrinogen (factor I) is a 340-kDa protein synthesised by the liver. It is cleaved by thrombin to produce fibrin, which undergoes polymerisation to form a fibrin mesh. The final structure and strength of this mesh depends on a number of factors including pH and the concentrations of fibrinogen, thrombin, and calcium. Thrombin activates FXIII to FXIIIa which stabilises the clot.

Platelet adhesion, activation and aggregation

As described above, when a blood vessel is injured, circulating platelets become attached to the exposed subendothelial connective tissue matrix by interacting with the exposed collagen and with vWF. This *adhesion* and the presence of thrombin lead to an increase in cytosolic calcium levels within the platelet which causes platelet *activation*, leading to the release of ADP and thromboxane A2 (TXA_2) from platelet

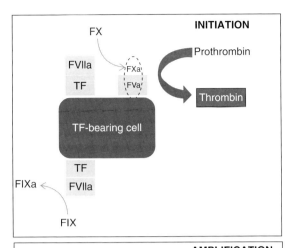

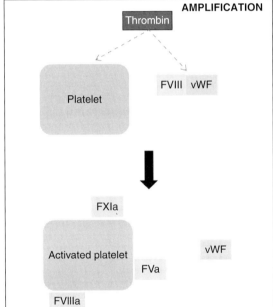

Figure 8.2 Cell-based model of coagulation: initiation, amplification and propagation.

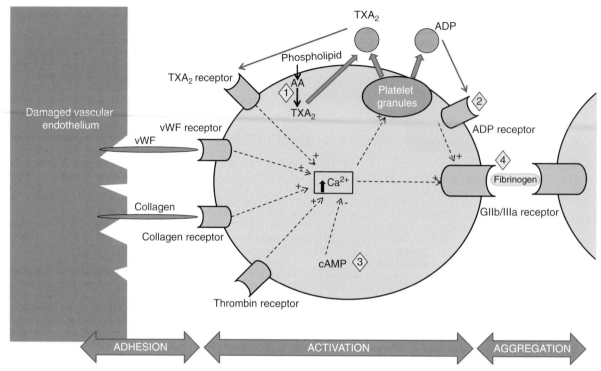

Figure 8.3 Platelet adhesion, activation and aggregation, with site of action of antiplatelet drugs: (1) aspirin, (2) clopidogrel, (3) dipyridamole, (4) glycoprotein IIb/IIIa inhibitors.

granules, the production of additional TXA_2 from platelet membrane phospholipid via the activation of phospholipase A_2, and to the activation of the glycoprotein IIb/IIIa (GIIb/IIIa) receptor which has an important role in platelet-fibrinogen cross-linking. The ADP released from platelet granules acts on platelet surface receptors to cause further activation of GIIb/IIIa receptors, increasing the affinity of the receptor for fibrinogen. Platelet adhesion, activation and aggregation are shown in Figure 8.3.

Platelets and fibrinogen cross-link via the numerous GIIb/IIIa receptors on the platelet surface – each platelet has over 40 000 of these receptors and normally during clot formation there is a large receptor reserve.

Limiting clot formation to site of injury

It would be undesirable for the process of amplification and propagation to continue beyond the site of vessel injury. Some of the thrombin produced moves into the bloodstream and comes into contact with healthy endothelial cells where it forms a complex with thrombomodulin. This complex activates protein C which, in the presence of the co-factor protein

S, inactivates any FVa and FVIIIa in the vicinity. This process occurs on the surface of non-damaged endothelial cells adjacent to the site of injury. In addition, antithrombin (also known as antithrombin III) inactivates and TFPI inhibits activated coagulation factors.

Clot breakdown

Clot breakdown or fibrinolysis is a normal physiological process in which fibrin clots are degraded by the action of plasmin. The system exists in balance with the coagulation system with the purpose of ensuring that clot exists only for as long as is necessary.

Plasmin is the major fibrinolytic protease in the fibrinolytic system and is produced from plasminogen by the enzymatic action of tissue plasminogen activator (tPa). Plasminogen is a large glycoprotein which is synthesised in the liver and circulates in the blood. Plasminogen contains lysine residues which act as a binding site for fibrin. Under normal circumstances plasminogen has a low affinity for tPa but in the presence of fibrin this affinity, and the enzymatic efficiency of tPa, increases significantly leading to the production of plasmin. This plasmin then acts on fibrin leading to the production of fibrin degradation products (FDPs) including D-dimers. Fibrin thus regulates its own breakdown, ensuring the process of fibrinolysis is both localised and augmented at appropriate times.

Drugs affecting haemostasis

Drugs affecting haemostasis can be divided into three main groups:

(1) Antiplatelets
(2) Anticoagulants and their antagonists
(3) Drugs affecting the fibrinolytic system.

Antiplatelets

Antiplatelet drugs reduce platelet aggregation and reduce the risk of thrombotic complications while increasing bleeding. The site of action of the following antiplatelet agents is shown in Figure 8.3.

Aspirin

Aspirin is the most commonly prescribed antiplatelet drug at present. It is used for the primary and secondary prevention of cardiovascular events, in the treatment of acute myocardial infarction and acute coronary syndromes, to prevent thrombotic events after the insertion of coronary stents and in atrial fibrillation. It is commonly continued throughout the perioperative period in patients having vascular surgery to reduce the incidence of thrombotic events.

Mechanism

Aspirin irreversibly inhibits cyclo-oxygenase (COX 1 isoenzyme) in platelets by acetylation. This prevents the formation of prostaglandin precursors from arachadonic acid, ultimately reducing the production of the platelet activator/aggregator TXA_2.

Clinical notes

- Usually continued perioperatively in vascular surgery patients.
- Generally considered safe in patients having spinal or epidural anaesthesia.
- Can be administered via nasogastric tube, or rectally in the perioperative period.

ADP receptor inhibitors

Mechanism

ADP receptor inhibitors block the P2Y12 subtype of ADP receptors on the platelet surface, thereby preventing ADP-mediated activation of the GIIb/IIIa receptor to which fibrinogen binds to cross-link platelets. Two oral ADP receptor antagonists, clopidogrel and prasugrel, are currently used. Other drugs are in development including cangrelor, a rapidly acting and reversible inhibitor of the P2Y12 receptor which is given by intravenous infusion.

Clopidogrel

Clopidogrel is a thienopyridine drug which on average has a slightly greater inhibitory effect on platelets than aspirin. It is used for the secondary prevention of cardiovascular events, in the treatment of acute myocardial infarction and acute coronary syndromes, and to prevent thrombotic events after the insertion of coronary stents.

Clopidogrel is a pro-drug and is converted in the liver by cytochrome P450 enzymes to an active metabolite which irreversibly inhibits the ADP receptors. Genetic differences result in variable metabolism of clopidogrel. In some patients taking clopidogrel there appears to be little inhibition of platelets and these patients are at increased risk of complications such as coronary stent thrombosis. In other patients there is very marked platelet inhibition and these patients may be at greater risk of excessive bleeding perioperatively if clopidogrel is continued. Point-of-care testing may be used to measure the inhibitory effect of clopidogrel on platelets (see below).

Clinical notes

Clopidogrel is often discontinued before elective surgery because of concern about the risk of bleeding. However, the risk of bleeding in patients having vascular surgery while taking clopidogrel alone may be similar to that in patients taking aspirin alone [5]. The risk of epidural haematoma in patients taking clopidogrel alone and how it compares to the risk in patients taking aspirin alone is not known. However, the American Society for Regional Anaesthesia and Pain Medicine has recommended that clopidogrel be stopped before neuraxial blockade [6]. Since clopidogrel, like aspirin, produces irreversible inhibition of platelets, recovery of normal function depends on production of new platelets and takes 5 to 7 days after stopping the drug.

When patients are taking both aspirin and clopidogrel, the risk of excessive perioperative bleeding is higher than when taking only one of these drugs and it is common practice to stop the clopidogrel 1 week before elective surgery while continuing aspirin therapy. However, randomised trials of giving both aspirin and clopidogrel before carotid endarterectomy [7] and surgery for lower limb ischaemia [8] have reported potential beneficial effects on reducing perioperative thrombotic complications. Spinal or epidural analgesia should not be used in this situation.

Prasugrel

Like clopidogrel, prasugrel is an oral thienopyridine pro-drug which irreversibly inhibits the P2Y12 receptors. However, it produces a greater degree of platelet inhibition than clopidogrel and is associated with a lower incidence of 'non-responsiveness' to the drug.

Dipyridamole

Dipyridamole is used for secondary prevention after transient ischaemic attack or ischaemic stroke, usually in combination with aspirin.

Mechanism

Dipyridamole increases the concentration of cyclic AMP (cAMP) in platelets. High cAMP levels lead to a reduction in intracellular Ca^{2+} levels and this inhibits platelet activation.

Clinical notes

Dipyridamole may cause headache and, particularly in higher doses, tachycardia and vasodilation. It is commonly given in a modified release preparation. The inhibition of platelet function is reversible but the time required after last taking the drug for its effect on platelet function to become insignificant is uncertain. One estimate is that this occurs after 2 days [9].

Glycoprotein IIb/IIIa inhibitors

Glycoprotein IIb/IIIa inhibitors block the binding of fibrinogen to platelets and produce a profound inhibition of platelet aggregation. The currently available agents abciximab, eptifibatide and tirofiban are given intravenously to patients undergoing percutaneous coronary intervention and in acute coronary syndromes.

Anticoagulants and their antagonists

Heparin

'Standard' unfractionated heparin (UFH) is composed of a heterogenous group of polysaccharides produced from animal intestinal mucosa and has an average molecular weight of 15 kDa. It is used for both venous thromboembolism (VTE) prophylaxis (low-dose subcutaneous administration) and for therapeutic anticoagulation (intravenous bolus and infusion) in situations including pulmonary embolism (PE) and acute limb ischaemia. It is also administered as a bolus dose during vascular surgery before arterial cross-clamping to prevent thrombotic complications.

Mechanism

Heparin binds to antithrombin and greatly increases its inhibitory action on thrombin, FXa and other activated coagulation factors. The thrombin inhibition prevents fibrin formation and also leads to reduced activation of platelets, FV and FVIII. Unfractionated heparin has a similar degree of inhibitory activity against thrombin and FXa.

Clinical notes

The effect of intravenous heparin is monitored by measuring APTT (see below). Point of care APTT analysers are available.

The American Society of Regional Anesthesia and Pain Medicine has published advice on spinal and epidural anaesthesia in patients receiving anticoagulants [6].

Heparin-induced thrombocytopaenia (HIT) is an immune complication of heparin administration typically occurring after 5–10 days of treatment, although it can occur earlier with re-exposure.

Low-molecular-weight heparins

Low-molecular-weight heparins (LMWHs) are fragments of standard heparin, produced by depolymerisation processes which yield polysaccharide chains with an average molecular weight of 5000 Da.

Mechanism

The LMWHs exert their effect mainly through inhibition of FXa, with less thrombin inhibition than unfractionated heparin. They differ from each other mainly in their average chain length and molecular weight, and subsequently their ratio of anti-FXa : anti-thrombin activity. Monitoring of the degree

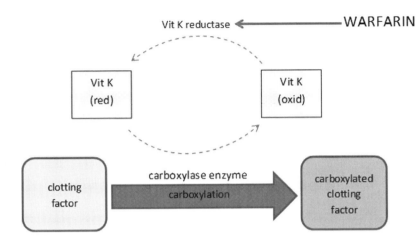

Figure 8.4 Mechanism of action of warfarin.

of inhibition of FXa is possible but is not routinely required.

Fondaparinux

Fondaparinux is a synthetic pentasaccharide adminis-tered subcutaneously for prevention and treatment of deep vein thrombosis (DVT) and PE and in acute coronary syndromes. Its antithrombotic activity is the result of antithrombin-mediated selective inhib-ition of FXa. It does not inactivate thrombin. After discontinuation of fondaparinux, the anticoagulant effect may continue for 2–4 days in patients with normal renal function and for longer in patients with renal impairment.

Oral direct inhibitors of thrombin and factor Xa

Oral drugs which inhibit thrombin or FXa are now available and are used for prophylaxis of DVT and PE after orthopaedic surgery and as an alternative to warfarin in patients with atrial fibrillation.

Rivaroxaban is a direct inhibitor (i.e. it does not act through antithrombin) of FXa.

Dabigatran is a direct thrombin inhibitor.

Protamine

Protamine is used to reverse the effects of unfraction-ated heparin. It is an alkaline substance produced from salmon sperm which combines with the acidic heparin to form a neutral salt. Unlike unfractionated heparin, the anticoagulant effect of LMWHs cannot be fully reversed with protamine. Fondaparinux cannot be reversed with protamine.

Clinical notes

Side-effects of administration include histamine release (more likely if injected quickly) and rarely anaphylaxis. Risk factors for allergic reactions include fish allergies and previous administration of protamine-containing insulins in diabetics.

Vitamin K antagonists e.g. warfarin

Warfarin is an oral anticoagulant, commonly used in the treatment of DVT, PE and atrial fibrillation, and in patients with mechanical heart valves. It is pro-duced from coumarin, a chemical found in various plants including the tonka bean from which it derives its name (coumarou is French for tonka bean plant).

Mechanism

The vitamin-K-dependent coagulation factors II, VII, IX and X contain glutamate residues which must undergo a process of carboxylation in order to perform their normal role in coagulation. This carboxylation process requires a carboxylase enzyme and reduced vitamin K as a co-factor. Vitamin K is oxidised during this process and requires conversion back to the reduced form before it can repeat the process. Warfarin prevents this cyclical conversion of oxidised vitamin K by inhibiting vitamin K reductase (Figure 8.4).

Warfarin does not have an immediate effect because circulating coagulation factors are unaffected and the half-lives of the vitamin-K-dependent coagu-lation factors are between 4 and 72 hours. An anti-coagulant effect may be detected by measurement of the prothrombin time (see below) after about 12 hours but the maximum effect typically occurs several days after starting warfarin. On stopping warfarin it takes several days for coagulation to return to normal.

Clinical notes

Warfarin therapy is monitored buy measuring the prothrombin time (PT) and calculating the international normalised ratio (INR).

Warfarin is typically discontinued 4–5 days before elective surgery with the intention of the INR falling to less than 1.5 by the time of surgery.

The effect of warfarin may be reversed by giving vitamin K or, more rapidly, by giving prothrombin complex concentrate (PCC) which contains factors II, IX and X (three-factor PCC) or factors II, VII, IX and X (four-factor PCC).

Drugs affecting the fibrinolytic system

Fibrinolytics

Fibrinolytics are 'clot dissolvers' and have a role in acute myocardial infarction, pulmonary embolus, ischaemic stroke and catheter-directed thrombolytic therapy for acute limb ischaemia. Examples include recombinant tissue plasminogen activator (rtPa), urokinase and streptokinase.

Mechanism

Fibrinolytics increase the conversion of plasminogen to plasmin. Plasmin causes cleavage of fibrin, resulting in clot breakdown. In addition fibrinolytics increase the breakdown of circulating fibrinogen, FV and FVIII, and cause platelet dysfunction. Systemic fibrinolytic therapy results in a large reduction in fibrinogen concentration and is associated with a high risk of bleeding.

Antifibrinolytics

Antifibrinolytics are used to prevent clot breakdown. There are two main types – lysine analogues (tranexamic acid and epsilon-aminocaproic acid) and serine protease inhibitors (aprotonin).

Tranexamic acid

A synthetic drug derived from the amino acid lysine.

Mechanism

Tranexamic acid prevents the conversion of plasminogen to the fibrin-degrading serine protease plasmin by binding to the lysine binding site on plasminogen. This binding prevents plasminogen from binding to fibrin, a process which is required for the conversion of plasminogen to plasmin.

Aprotonin

Aprotonin is a polypeptide serine protease inhibitor extracted from bovine lung. Its marketing was suspended in 2007 following concerns that morbidity and mortality were higher in patients receiving aprotinin than the lysine analogue antifibrinolytic drugs.

Causes of abnormal haemostasis in vascular surgery

Excessive perioperative bleeding may be 'surgical bleeding' resulting from holes in blood vessels too large to be sealed by the formation of blood clots or may be diffuse microvascular bleeding resulting from an impairment of the ability to form stable clot. Both of these causes of haemorrhage may be present simultaneously and in particular surgical bleeding may lead on to a secondary impairment of haemostasis as a result of the loss of fibrinogen, other coagulation factors and platelets and the development of shock.

Abnormalities of haemostasis may result from congenital deficiencies and abnormalities but these will not be discussed further here. More commonly impaired haemostasis during surgery is the result of one or more of the following acquired abnormalities:

- Low fibrinogen – loss, consumption, dilution
- Impaired fibrin polymerisation – synthetic colloids
- Low platelets – loss, consumption, dilution
- Dysfunctional platelets – antiplatelet drugs, cardiopulmonary bypass
- Low coagulation factors – loss, consumption, dilution; warfarin
- Heparin
- ?Increased activated protein C
- Hyperfibrinolysis
- Hypothermia
- Acidaemia
- Hypocalcaemia.

Fibrinogen, other coagulation factor and platelet deficiencies

Reduced levels of fibrinogen, other coagulation factors and platelets occur in bleeding patients as the result of loss from the circulation, consumption in clot that is formed and dilution as intravenous fluids are given to maintain circulating volume. In bleeding patients, fibrinogen concentration may decrease sufficiently to impair haemostasis before the platelet count or concentrations of other coagulation factors do so [10].

Increased anticoagulant activity – activated protein C

It has been suggested that in shocked trauma patients early coagulopathy is caused by increased conversion of protein C to activated protein C by thrombomodulin–thrombin complexes [11]. Activated protein C exerts an anticoagulant effect by inactivating FVa and FVIIIa and also increases fibrinolysis. The importance of the protein C pathway in impaired haemostasis in vascular surgery patients is not clear.

Hyperfibrinolysis

Excessive fibrinolysis may occur, particularly in shocked patients, leading to rapid breakdown of thrombus.

Drugs and fluids

The effects of antiplatelet and anticoagulant drugs have been discussed above.

The administration of colloids, particularly dextrans and higher-molecular-weight hydroxyethyl starches, impairs haemostasis by mechanisms in addition to purely dilutional effects. These mechanisms include impaired fibrin polymerisation [12], reduced vWF and FVIII and reduced platelet aggregation. Whether modern tetrastarches and gelatin solutions have a clinically significant effect on coagulation is debated. Some authors consider administration of tetrastarch to bleeding patients to be appropriate while others advise against its use in patients with impaired coagulation (see also Chapter 7) [13,14].

Hypothermia, acidaemia and hypocalcaemia

The normal functioning of the coagulation system depends on numerous enzymatic reactions which are both temperature and pH-dependent.

Hypothermia leads to a reduction in platelet adhesion and aggregation through an inhibitory effect on platelet–vWF interaction. It also leads to reduced thrombin generation by impairing TF/FVIIa coupling in the initiation phase.

Acidosis also leads to impaired thrombin generation but in contrast this results mainly from inhibition of the prothrombinase (FXa/FVa) complex during the propagation phase of coagulation.

Calcium is required as a co-factor for the activation of coagulation factors. Hypocalcaemia can occur due to blood loss and subsequent fluid administration and dilution and the administration of citrate-containing blood components. Severe hypocalcaemia should be avoided because of adverse cardiovascular effects as well as potential effects on coagulation. The ionised calcium level should be kept above 0.9 mmol/l [15].

Diagnosis and treatment of impaired haemostasis

There are three approaches to diagnosing and treating abnormalities of haemostasis during vascular surgery:

(1) 'Blind' administration of drugs and blood components in an attempt to improve haemostasis. Sometimes blood components are given in a fixed ratio to the estimated blood loss. The disadvantage of this approach is that treatment is often ineffective because an adequate dose of the correct treatment has not been given while on other occasions blood components are administered unnecessarily, exposing the patient to the risks of transfusion without benefit.

(2) Reliance on the results of laboratory tests to guide treatment. This may be satisfactory in stable patients without much ongoing blood loss and who are not receiving blood components or drugs affecting haemostasis, particularly if the turnaround time from taking a blood sample to receiving results is short. However, when there is significant bleeding during surgery, by the time the results of laboratory tests are received they often do not reflect the current situation and are of little value as a guide to treatment.

(3) Point-of-care testing of coagulation. This has the potential to provide more rapid results than laboratory tests. In addition information can be obtained that is not provided by routine laboratory tests, e.g. on whether excessive fibrinolysis is present and on platelet inhibition resulting from aspirin or ADP antagonist therapy.

Diagnosis

Laboratory testing

Commonly performed tests are a full blood count including platelet count, prothrombin time, activated partial thromboplastin time and fibrinogen concentration. Sometimes the concentration of breakdown products of fibrin lysis – fibrin degradation products (FDPs) or D-Dimers – is also measured.

Prothrombin time

The prothrombin time (PT) is a test which detects deficiencies or inhibitors of factors II, V, VII and X and fibrinogen (the extrinsic and common pathways in the classical model of coagulation). It measures the time in seconds for clot to be formed after the addition of thromboplastin and calcium to the patient's citrated plasma. Thromboplastin is composed of phospholipid, which acts as a platelet substitute, and TF – both are required for activation of the extrinsic pathway.

In patients receiving warfarin therapy, PT is usually reported along with an international normalised ratio (INR). The need for an INR arose due to the variability between laboratories in the sensitivity of the thromboplastin reagent used in the PT test – this variation meant that PT results for identical patient samples could vary in different laboratories. The INR is a mathematical correction of the PT which takes into account the sensitivity of the thromboplastin reagent used.

In patients who have not received warfarin a prolonged PT suggests a low concentration of factors II, V, VII or X, or of fibrinogen. In some assays, the PT may be prolonged by a high concentration of heparin in the sample.

Activated partial thromboplastin time

The activated partial thromboplastin time (APTT) test (also known as partial thromboplastin time or PTT test) assesses the intrinsic and common pathways of the classical model of coagulation. It measures the time in seconds for clot to be formed after the addition of an intrinsic pathway activator (e.g. kaolin), phospholipid and calcium to the patient's citrated plasma. Tissue factor is not required for activation of the intrinsic pathway, hence the term partial thromboplastin. This test can detect deficiencies or inhibitors of factors XII, XI, X, IX, VIII, V and II and fibrinogen. The APTT is prolonged by heparin and

the test is used to monitor the degree of anticoagulation produced by unfractionated heparin.

A prolonged APTT may also result from an inhibitor (autoantibody) such as lupus anticoagulant. Despite the name and the fact that lupus anticoagulant prolongs the APTT, it is associated with an increased risk of thrombosis not of haemorrhage. An APTT mix can be performed to aid diagnosis when an APTT is found to be prolonged. This involves mixing the patient's plasma with normal pooled plasma (1 : 1) – this will correct APTT prolongation due to a deficiency, but not due to an inhibitor.

Fibrinogen

Fibrinogen concentration is usually calculated from a coagulation time test. In the Clauss method a high concentration of thrombin is added to diluted plasma and the time until clot forms is measured – usually optically. A falsely low result can be caused by the presence of high concentrations of heparin. On the other hand, the presence of synthetic colloid fluids may results in a falsely elevated result in some assays.

Point-of-care tests

Point-of-care haemostasis testing allows for rapid diagnosis and appropriate targeted management of coagulation abnormalities during major surgery. Tests can be performed on whole blood samples within or close to the theatre with interpretable results available within minutes.

There are three types of point of care haemostasis analyser:

(1) Coagulation time analysers, e.g. PT/APTT/ACT analysers
(2) Viscoelastic clot strength analysers – thromboelastography/thromboelastometry
(3) Platelet function analysers.

Coagulation time analysers

Prothrombin time and APTT can be rapidly determined by adding a drop of whole blood to a test cuvette inserted into small portable analysers. These analysers are primarily intended for monitoring warfarin or heparin therapy and are excellent for this purpose with the results usually correlating well with laboratory PT and APTT results. In bleeding patients where other abnormalities such as anaemia and thrombocytopaenia may be present the correlation

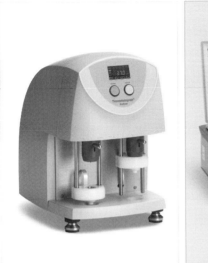
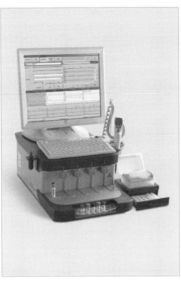

Figure 8.5 TEG®5000 Thromboelastograph® Analyser (Haemonetics, Braintree, MA, USA) and ROTEM® Delta Analyser (Tem International GmbH, Munich, Germany).

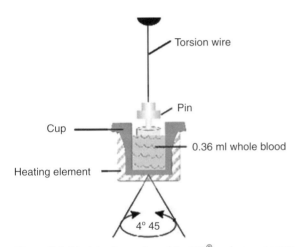

Figure 8.6 Principle of operation of the TEG® analyser – see text.

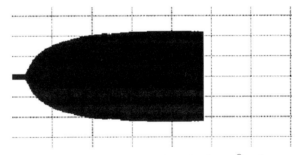

Figure 8.7 Example of a trace produced by the TEG® analyser: time in seconds on the *x*-axis, clot strength in millimetres on the *y*-axis.

between point of care and laboratory tests may be poorer.

The activated clotting time (ACT) test is a point-of-care test for monitoring treatment with high concentrations of unfractionated heparin. An activator (usually celite or kaolin) is added to a whole blood sample and the time taken for clot to form is measured.

Thromboelastography/thromboelastometry: principles

Two analysers, TEG® and ROTEM® (Figure 8.5), are available which measure the elasticity or strength of blood clot as it forms in a whole blood sample. The manufacturer of the TEG® analyser uses the term

thromboelastography and that of the ROTEM® analyser uses thromboelastometry but for convenience we will use thromboelastometry here to refer to both analysers.

In the original version of the TEG® analyser blood is placed into a small cup which is heated to 37 °C and rotated slowly backwards and forwards through about 4° (Figure 8.6). A pin is suspended in the blood sample by a torsion wire. A light source is deflected by a small mirror attached to the torsion wire and shines onto light-sensitive paper moving on a chart recorder. Initially there is no clot and, although the cup rotates, the pin and wire remain stationary and the light produces a straight line on the chart recorder (Figure 8.7). However, when clot starts to form, fibrin strands and platelet aggregates form between the cup and the pin, transmitting some of the cup's movement to the pin which then also starts to rotate

Table 8.1 ROTEM® variables and typical causes of abnormal traces seen in vascular surgery

Parameter	Definition	Abnormalities
Clotting time (**CT**)	Time in seconds from start of test until detection of clot	Prolonged CT can be caused by: Coagulation factor deficiency Heparin effect Severe fibrinogen deficiency
Maximum clot firmness (**MCF**)	Maximum width of trace	Reduced MCF and A10 can be caused by: Low fibrinogen or impaired fibrin polymerisation
A10	Width of the trace 10 minutes after clot is first detected	Low platelets Low fibrinogen and platelets
Maximum lysis (**ML**)	Percentage reduction in width of trace from MCF	Increased ML can be caused by: Hyperfibrinolysis

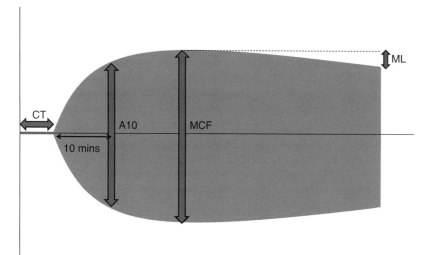

Figure 8.8 ROTEM® variables: time in seconds on the *x*-axis, clot strength in millimetres on the *y*-axis.

backwards and forwards, causing the light beam to move up and down on the paper. Initially, when the clot is weak, the amount of movement of the pin and deflection of the light beam is slight and the amplitude of the trace on the paper is small. As the clot becomes stronger, the pin rotates more and the amplitude of the trace increases. The trace that is produced has time in seconds on the *x*-axis and clot strength on the *y*-axis. The modern version of the TEG® analyser uses a computer to display the trace rather than a chart recorder.

The ROTEM® analyser was developed with the intention of producing a more robust analyser which was less sensitive to movement and vibration. It is actually the pin that rotates in the ROTEM® rather than the cup but a similar trace of clot strength in millimetres against time in seconds is produced on a computer display.

A number of different variables can be determined from the thromboelastometry trace and the situation is complicated somewhat by different terms being used on the two analysers. However, there are three important pieces of information to derive from the thromboelastometry trace (Figure 8.8 and Table 8.1).

(1) *The strength of the clot.* This is indicated by the maximum width of the trace in millimetres (maximum clot firmness or MCF in ROTEM® and maximum amplitude or MA in TEG®). A measure of clot strength can be obtained more rapidly by measuring the width of the trace 10 minutes after clot is first detected and this is known as the amplitude at 10 minutes or A10. Clot strength is reduced by thrombocytopaenia or a low fibrinogen concentration or a combination of the two. The effect of drugs such as aspirin or clopidogrel is not

Table 8.2 ROTEM® tests

Test	Description	Normal range
Extem	Assessment of (extrinsic) clotting factors, fibrinogen, and platelets, and detection of excessive fibrinolysis	CT 38–79 s, A10 43–65 mm, ML <15%
Intem	Assessment of (intrinsic) clotting factors, fibrinogen and platelets, and detection of excessive fibrinolysis	CT 100–240 s, A10 44–66 mm, ML <15%
Fibtem	Assessment of fibrinogen component of clot. (Fibtem test = Extem test with addition of platelet inhibitor – cytochalasin D) Compare with Extem to assess platelet component of clot	A10 7–23 mm
Heptem	Assesses whether heparin effect present (Heptem test = Intem test with addition of heparinase)	Compare Heptem CT with Intem CT
Aptem	Confirms the presence of excessive fibrinolysis (Aptem test = Extem test with addition of aprotinin)	Compare Aptem with Extem

seen on standard thromboelastometry tests because the thrombin that forms when blood clots is a very powerful stimulus to platelet aggregation. Tests for the effect of these drugs on platelet function have to be performed on anticoagulated samples in which the production of thrombin is prevented.

(2) *The time it takes for detectable clot to form.* This is indicated by the length of the straight line at the start of the trace (clotting time or CT in ROTEM® and Reaktionszeit or R-time in TEG®) and is measured in seconds. It is prolonged by low concentrations of coagulation factors including fibrinogen and in the presence of heparin.

(3) *Whether the clot remains strong or breaks down.* A small decrease in the width of the trace after it reaches its maximum occurs as a result of clot retraction. However the percentage reduction from the maximum width (maximum lysis or ML in ROTEM®) does not normally exceed 15%.

Thromboelastometry analysers may be used with samples of venous or arterial blood. A blood sample to which no anticoagulant has been added may be placed into the analyser immediately or alternatively citrate may be added to the sample as anticoagulant and the effect of the citrate reversed by adding calcium when the sample is put in the analyser. The TEG® analyser has two channels (two cups and pins) allowing two different tests to be performed simultaneously while the ROTEM® analyser has four channels.

Different tests are performed by adding different activators or inhibitors of coagulation to determine for example:

- if reduced clot strength is the result of reduced platelets or fibrinogen or both
- if a prolonged CT the result of heparin or of factor deficiency
- if excessive clot breakdown is present and can be reversed by an antifibrinolytic drug.

The tests usually performed on the ROTEM® are listed in Table 8.2. An example of normal results is shown in Figure 8.9. Four tests have been performed simultaneously on a blood sample.

The Fibtem trace is narrower than the others because platelet aggregation has been prevented in this test, resulting in a clot containing only fibrin rather than fibrin and platelets. Comparison with the Extem enables the relative contributions of fibrin and platelets to clot strength to be assessed. For example Figure 8.10 shows the Extem and Fibtem results from a patient with thrombocytopaenia. The A10 amplitude is reduced in the Extem indicating a deficiency of either platelets or fibrin in the clot. The A10 amplitude is normal in the Fibtem trace indicating a normal fibrin component of the clot. Therefore the deficiency is of platelets. Figure 8.11 on the other hand also has a reduced A10 amplitude in the Extem but in this case the A10 is also very low in the Fibtem indicating a very weak fibrin clot. This is usually the result of a very low fibrinogen concentration. The ROTEM® results can thus be used to determine what specific treatment is appropriate. Figure 8.12 shows how we use ROTEM® for the diagnosis and treatment of impaired haemostasis.

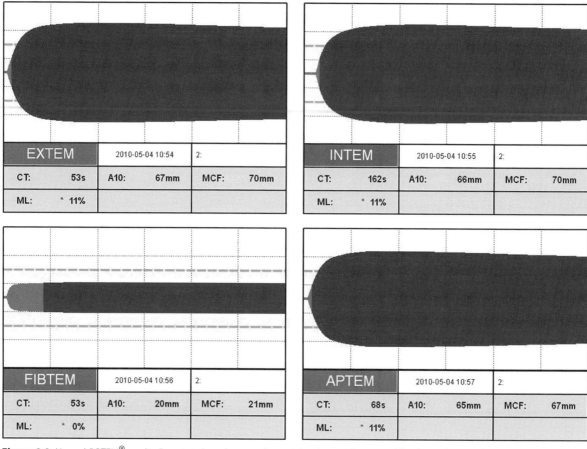

Figure 8.9 Normal ROTEM® results. Four tests have been performed simultaneously on one blood sample. See plate section for colour version.

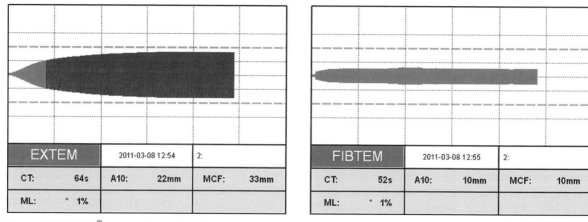

Figure 8.10 ROTEM® traces indicating thrombocytopaenia – see text. See plate section for colour version.

An alternative approach to distinguishing between reduced clot strength caused by thrombocytopaenia and that caused by low fibrinogen is often used on the TEG® analyser. This involves performing only one test and looking at the speed of development of clot strength by measuring how long it takes from clot first being detected until the trace width reaches 20 mm (Koagulationszeit or K-time in the TEG®, clot

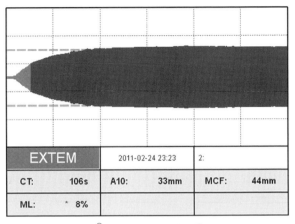

EXTEM	2011-02-24 23:23	2:			
CT:	106s	A10:	33mm	MCF:	44mm
ML:	* 8%				

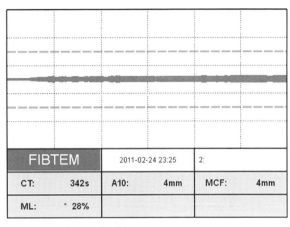

FIBTEM	2011-02-24 23:25	2:			
CT:	342s	A10:	4mm	MCF:	4mm
ML:	* 28%				

Figure 8.11 ROTEM® traces indicating low fibrinogen concentration – see text. See plate section for colour version.

formation time or CFT in the ROTEM®) or measuring the angle made by a line drawn at a tangent to the first part of the curve (α angle). It is then assumed that abnormalities of the K-time and α angle are likely to be caused by a reduced fibrinogen concentration but that reduced amplitude of the trace is likely to be caused by thrombocytopaenia. However, thrombocytopaenia and a low fibrinogen can give similar values for these variables and treatment algorithms based on this approach may result in the transfusion of platelets when the main problem is a reduced fibrinogen concentration [16].

Figure 8.13 shows ROTEM® traces from a patient with hyperfibrinolysis – excessive clot breakdown. Clot forms but then dissolves, except in the Aptem test in which aprotinin is added to the sample being tested to prevent fibrinolysis. Hyperfibrinolysis is seen in some patients with ruptured aortic aneurysms and can be treated with intravenous tranexamic acid or epsilon-aminocaproic acid.

Value and limitations of thromboelastometry

We have found thromboelastometry monitoring during major vascular surgery to be invaluable in permitting rapid diagnosis and targeted appropriate treatment of impaired haemostasis. It enables us to return patients who have had thoracoabdominal aortic aneurysm repair involving massive haemorrhage to the intensive care unit with haemostasis restored to normal so that little or no administration of blood or blood components is usually required after surgery. However, it is important to be aware that thromboelastometry does not detect all disorders of haemostasis. In particular:

(1) Standard thromboelastometry tests do not detect the effect of antiplatelet drugs such as aspirin or clopidogrel. In a test of haemostasis in which the blood sample clots, a large amount of thrombin is produced and acts as a very powerful stimulus to platelet aggregation.

The effect of antiplatelet drugs must be assessed in anticoagulated samples where the formation of thrombin is prevented. Tests known as platelet mapping for the effect of aspirin and clopidogrel may be performed on anticoagulated samples on the TEG® analyser. Alternatively a point-of-care platelet function analyser may be used (see below).

(2) Standard thromboelastometry tests are not very sensitive tests for the effect of some anticoagulants, e.g. warfarin, LMWH.

(3) Thromboelastometry does not detect vWF deficiency.

Platelet function analysers

In the laboratory, platelet function is usually assessed by the technique of optical or light transmittance aggregometry first described by Born. An anticoagulated blood sample is centrifuged to produce platelet-rich plasma (PRP) which is then placed in a cuvette at 37 °C between a light source and a photocell. When an agonist is added to the cuvette the platelets aggregate, the plasma becomes clearer and absorbs less light, and this is detected by the photocell. The preparation of PRP and concentration of agonists used vary between laboratories so that it can be difficult to compare results from different laboratories.

DIAGNOSIS

1. Clot firmness
- in the presence of heparin use the HEPTEM result
- if there is hyperfibrinolysis (ML > 15 %) use the APTEM result

CLOT FIRMNESS		A10 in EXTEM / INTEM / HEPTEM / APTEM		
		< 22 mm	22-38 mm	≥ 39 mm
A10 in FIBTEM	< 5 mm	Low fibrinogen Low platelets	Low fibrinogen (†platelets - see below)	Low fibrinogen
	5-7 mm	Low platelets Low fibrinogen	Low platelets Low fibrinogen	Clot firmness appears satisfactory. See Sections 2, 3 & blue box below. (If bleeding isn't controlled consider: -raising fibrinogen (FIBTEM A10≥10mm) -in patients on aspirin* or clopidogrel* giving platelets and/or desmopressin).
	≥ 8 mm	Low platelets	Low platelets	

†Typically fibrinogen < 1.5 g/l & platelets 50-100. Also consider giving platelets if ongoing bleeding

2. Clotting time
- in the presence of heparin run a HEPTEM test

Causes of a prolonged CT	
Fibtem A10 < 5 mm	= Low fibrinogen
CT prolonged in Intem but normal in Heptem	= Heparin effect
Fibtem A10 ≥ 5 mm and no heparin effect	= Low coagulation factors

When to treat CT		
CT in Intem / Heptem > 300	or	CT in Extem / Aptem > 100s
CT in Intem / Heptem 240 - 300 s	or	CT in Extem / Aptem 80 - 100s
CT in Intem / Heptem < 240 s	or	CT in Extem / Aptem <80 s

3. Hyperfibrinolysis

Lysis of clot within 20 mins	Fulminant lysis
Lysis of clot within 20 – 40 mins	Early lysis
Lysis of clot after more than 40 mins	Late lysis - ?treat

Repeat Rotem tests including Aptem after treatment (or if no treatment is given)

TREATMENT

Treat	Treat if bleeding / high risk of bleeding	See below*

Low fibrinogen – FFP or fibrinogen concentrate or cryoprecipitate
Low platelets – platelets
Low coagulation factors – FFP or PCC   Heparin – protamine (if reversal appropriate)
Hyperfibrinolysis – tranexamic acid (1 g – 2 g bolus)

* IMPORTANT
Rotem® does not detect the effect of aspirin, clopidogrel or Reopro® on platelets
Rotem® is not a sensitive test for some anticoagulants e.g. warfarin, LMWH
Rotem® does not detect von Willebrand factor deficiency

Figure 8.12 Example of a guideline which uses the ROTEM® results to diagnose and treat impaired haemostasis during surgery. See plate section for colour version.

Point-of-care platelet function analysers use anti-coagulated whole blood samples. A number of different methods are used to detect platelet aggregation in response to the addition of different agonists:

(1) Light transmittance aggregometry – Verify Now®
(2) Platelet count determined by a cell counter – Plateletworks®
(3) Impedance aggregometry – Multiplate®. Also TEMplate® (add-on to the ROTEM® analyser)
(4) Thromboelastography – additional Platelet Mapping® tests – TEG®
(5) Time taken for platelets to block an aperture in a membrane – PFA-100®.

In impedance aggregometry the blood sample is placed in a cuvette in which an electrical current is passed between two electrodes. As platelets aggregate they stick to the electrodes and increase the electrical resistance or impedance between them. Aggregation is measured from the area under the curve of impedance against time. Figure 8.14 shows the results of tests using the Multiplate® analyser on a blood sample from a patient taking aspirin. The aggregation

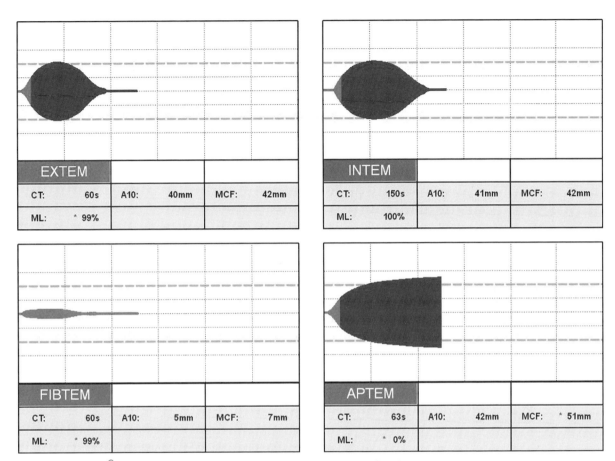

EXTEM					
CT:	60s	A10:	40mm	MCF:	42mm
ML:	* 99%				

INTEM					
CT:	150s	A10:	41mm	MCF:	42mm
ML:	100%				

FIBTEM					
CT:	60s	A10:	5mm	MCF:	7mm
ML:	* 99%				

APTEM					
CT:	63s	A10:	42mm	MCF:	* 51mm
ML:	* 0%				

Figure 8.13 ROTEM® traces showing hyperfibrinolysis – see text. See plate section for colour version.

response to thrombin receptor agonist peptide (TRAP) which mimics the effect of thrombin and causes maximal platelet aggregation is normal as is the response to ADP. However, the aggregation response to arachidonic acid in the 'ASPItest' is markedly reduced, indicating that the patient's platelets are inhibited by aspirin. The degree of platelet inhibition produced by aspirin and in particular by clopidogrel varies markedly between patients. In some patients there appears to be little inhibition and these patients are at increased risk of complications such as coronary stent thrombosis. In other patients there is very marked platelet inhibition and these patients may be at greater risk of excessive bleeding perioperatively.

Treatment of impaired haemostasis

Treatment of impaired haemostasis in vascular surgery patients may consist of general measures such as correcting hypothermia and acidaemia and specific treatments with drugs or blood components. Treatment is best guided by point-of-care testing of haemostasis in combination with other point-of-care tests including haemoglobin, acid–base status and calcium. If point-of-care testing is not available, treatment is guided either by laboratory results or by the anaesthetist's best judgement of the abnormalities likely to be present.

A low fibrinogen concentration is often the first abnormality requiring treatment in a bleeding patient. Newer guidelines on the management of bleeding surgical and trauma patients have recommended maintaining a fibrinogen concentration above 1.5 g/l rather than 1.0 g/l as was previously recommended [15,17]. Fibrinogen may be given in the form of purified freeze-dried fibrinogen concentrate, cryoprecipitate or fresh frozen plasma (FFP) (see also Chapter 9).

Platelet transfusion may be required either because haemostasis is impaired by severe thrombocytopaenia,

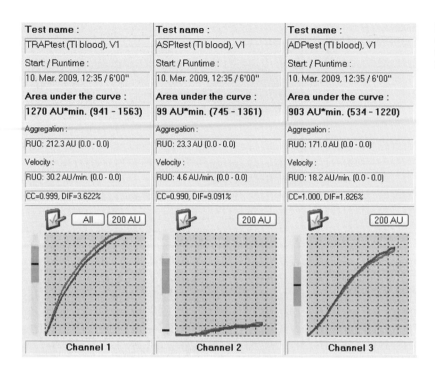

Test name :	Test name :	Test name :
TRAPtest (TI blood), V1	ASPItest (TI blood), V1	ADPtest (TI blood), V1
Start: / Runtime :	**Start: / Runtime :**	**Start: / Runtime :**
10. Mar. 2009, 12:35 / 6'00"	10. Mar. 2009, 12:35 / 6'00"	10. Mar. 2009, 12:35 / 6'00"
Area under the curve :	**Area under the curve :**	**Area under the curve :**
1270 AU*min. (941 – 1563)	99 AU*min. (745 – 1361)	903 AU*min. (534 – 1220)
Aggregation :	Aggregation :	Aggregation :
RUO: 212.3 AU (0.0 - 0.0)	RUO: 23.3 AU (0.0 - 0.0)	RUO: 171.0 AU (0.0 - 0.0)
Velocity :	Velocity :	Velocity :
RUO: 30.2 AU/min. (0.0 - 0.0)	RUO: 4.6 AU/min. (0.0 - 0.0)	RUO: 18.2 AU/min. (0.0 - 0.0)
CC=0.999, DIF=3.622%	CC=0.990, DIF=9.091%	CC=1.000, DIF=1.826%
All 200 AU	200 AU	200 AU
Channel 1	Channel 2	Channel 3

Figure 8.14 Multiplate® impedance aggregometry results in a patient taking aspirin – see text. See plate section for colour version.

e.g. a platelet count of less than $50 \times 10^9/l$ or because of the effect of antiplatelet drugs – particularly the combination of both aspirin and clopidogrel. The use of intravenous desmopressin to improve platelet function in patients taking aspirin and/or clopidogrel has been reported.

A PT that is prolonged to more than 1.5 times normal despite a normal fibrinogen concentration (and in the absence of an anticoagulant drug) suggests that the concentration of other coagulation factors may be too low for satisfactory haemostasis. Coagulation factors may be administered using FFP or PCC.

Excessive fibrinolysis is usually treated with intravenous tranexamic acid or epsilon-aminocaproic acid.

Reversal of the effect of anticoagulants is discussed above. When a moderate dose of intravenous heparin, e.g. 70 units/kg, is given during vascular surgery it may not be necessary to reverse the effect of the heparin unless there appears to be excessive microvascular bleeding after arterial clamps have been removed. In that case point of care measurement of APTT may be useful in confirming that marked anticoagulation by heparin is still present. If that is the case intravenous protamine (e.g. 5 mg per 1000 units of heparin administered) may be given.

Thrombosis

The benefits of improving haemostasis in vascular surgery patients have to be balanced against the risks of thrombotic complications. Thus it is common to continue antiplatelet drugs, particularly aspirin, perioperatively and not to routinely reverse the effect of moderate doses of intravenous heparin given during surgery even although these drugs increase bleeding. Vascular surgical patients are a high-risk population for thrombotic events. Patients with critical limb ischaemia may have an elevated fibrinogen concentration and activated platelets before surgery. Postoperatively a raised fibrinogen concentration and prothrombotic state commonly occurs. Therefore thrombotic complications are common in the perioperative period and lead to an increase in morbidity and mortality. The more common thrombotic events include coronary artery thrombosis leading to myocardial infarction, venous thromboembolism and arterial graft occlusion. Cardiac complications are discussed in Chapter 4.

Venous thromboembolism

Venous thromboembolism (VTE) refers to a spectrum of disease ranging from asymptomatic thrombosis in the deep veins of the leg to fatal PE.

Potentially preventable hospital-acquired VTE is estimated to cause 25 000 deaths annually in the UK. Asymptomatic DVT has been reported in approximately 20% of patients undergoing abdominal aortic surgery without VTE prophylaxis. The vascular surgical population contains many elderly, immobile patients who are at particular risk.

Pathophysiology

Whereas arterial thrombosis is often precipitated by endothelial injury, venous thrombosis is triggered by one or more prothrombotic factors known as Virchow's triad – alterations in the blood vessel wall, alteration to blood flow and alterations in the composition of blood. Alterations in the blood vessel wall include the endothelial release of prothrombotic granules known as Weibel–Palade bodies during periods of inflammation. These granules contain substances including vWF which can bind to the endothelium and promote clot formation. Alteration to blood flow includes the venous stasis that occurs in the perioperative period. Generalised immobility during hospitalisation, immobility during surgery and vascular clamping intraoperatively can all contribute to a reduction in venous blood flow which can result in thrombosis through a variety of mechanisms – stasis allows the accumulation and interaction of prothrombotic substances, causes endothelial activation and leads to haemoglobin desaturation which leads to activation of leukocytes and platelets. Alterations in the composition of blood usually refer to an acquired hypercoagulability. This can occur during acute or chronic illness, or as a result of the inflammatory responses known to occur in the perioperative period.

Prevention

Simple conservative measures including early mobilisation and hydration are integral to good care and VTE risk reduction. Compression stockings are contraindicated in patients with severe lower limb arterio-occlusive disease but may be considered in appropriate vascular patients after discussion with the surgical team. Pharmacological VTE prophylaxis should be considered in all vascular patients (and in all hospital patients) – all units should have a simple system of risk stratification to enable clear identification at the time of hospital admission of those requiring prophylaxis. Usually LMWH is prescribed to vascular patients requiring pharmacological prophylaxis. Alternatively UFH or fondaparinux are suitable where contraindications exist to treatment with LMWH (UFH in renal impairment, fondaparinux in HIT). There is some limited evidence that regional anaesthesia reduces the risk of VTE when compared with general anaesthesia. The administration of a heparin bolus intraoperatively immediately before vascular clamping may also reduce the risk of VTE.

Treatment

Depending on local facilities, the diagnosis of VTE is usually confirmed by lower limb Doppler ultrasound examination for DVT and by computed tomography pulmonary angiography (CTPA) for PE. Unless contraindicated, immediate anticoagulation is required with a parenteral anticoagulant – typically therapeutic dose LMWH, or intravenous UFH (more easily reversible) if there are concerns regarding bleeding risk. This treatment should be commenced before radiological confirmation if there is a high clinical suspicion of VTE and there are no prohibitive contraindications, especially if there is likely to be a delay in organising the necessary diagnostic imaging. Ultimately patients will require medium- or long-term anticoagulation, usually with warfarin. If the enteric route is available, this may be commenced immediately after diagnosis (concurrently with parenteral anticoagulant therapy) and requires careful INR monitoring – parenteral therapy can be discontinued once a therapeutic INR has been achieved.

Graft occlusion

Many vascular operations involve the use of vein or prosthetic grafts. Unfortunately, a significant proportion of grafts fail, often leading to repeat procedures or amputation. The risk of occlusion of arterial grafts is higher in long narrow grafts than in shorter wider grafts. Thus lower limb bypass grafts are more likely to become occluded than aortic grafts. Autologous vein grafts have a lower risk of occlusion than synthetic grafts. Grafts may fail in the early postoperative period or later. The failure rate for lower limb grafts inserted to treat critical limb ischaemia or claudication has been variably reported to be between 20% and 90% at 5 years.

Pathophysiology

Graft occlusion can occur by a number of mechanisms – thrombosis, neointimal hyperplasia and progression of the underlying atherosclerotic disease.

Thrombosis can occur at any point along the graft but is most likely at anastomoses where a prothrombotic combination of endothelial injury and suturing exists. The risk of thrombosis is increased by low flow through the graft – which may be the result of narrowed or occluded arteries proximal or distal to the graft, low blood pressure or low cardiac output – and by the generalised prothrombotic state that exists after surgery as a result of the stress response. Neointimal hyperplasia refers to the exaggerated endothelialisation that can occur on the inner surface of grafts – endothelialisation is an important biological process to provide a non-thrombogenic surface, but if excessive can lead to graft narrowing or complete occlusion. This hyperplasia is more likely when there is a significant mismatch between the compliance of the native artery and the graft – this mismatch causes turbulent flow and can lead to anastamotic occlusion.

Prevention

Attempts to prevent graft occlusion have focussed on two main areas – the development of better synthetic grafts, and antithrombotic or antiplatelet drugs. Important features of a synthetic graft include manufacture using a non-thrombogenic material, having similar compliance to native vessels, suturability, tensile strength and resistance to infection. Currently most synthetic grafts used in vascular surgery are made from Dacron (polyethylene terephthalate) or PTFE (polytetrafluorethylene). Numerous novel grafts have been produced in an attempt to reduce thrombogenicity and neointimal hyperplasia – examples include

Dacron or PTFE grafts impregnated with carbon, grafts coated with anticoagulants such as heparin or hirudin, grafts seeded with endothelial cells (providing a biologically active surface which will release anticoagulant substances) and grafts incorporating substances capable of acting as nitric oxide donors. Efforts to date have yielded mixed results and there is much ongoing research. Additional measures to prevent graft occlusion have included the use of vein cuffs at the distal anastamosis to reduce compliance mismatch and hyperplasia.

A *Cochrane Review* of the effectiveness of antithrombotic drugs in preventing graft occlusion after infrainguinal arterial bypass surgery concluded that patients with vein grafts are more likely to benefit from warfarin than antiplatelet drugs and that patients with a prosthetic graft benefit from antiplatelet drugs [18].

Treatment

Acute graft occlusion is most commonly due to thrombosis and attempts can be made to treat with catheter-guided thrombolysis, surgical thrombectomy, or by redoing bypass graft surgery. In addition systemic anticoagulation may be undertaken preoperatively in an attempt to minimise the degree of thrombosis/occlusion, and postoperatively to reduce the risk of recurrent thrombosis. Management of chronic graft occlusion may include repeat attempts at revascularisation, or amputation where this is not feasible or is unsuccessful and there is severe pain, tissue loss or gangrene.

References

1. Furie B, Furie BC. Mechanisms of thrombus formation. *N Engl J Med* 2008;**359**:938–49.

2. Furie B. Pathogenesis of thrombosis. *Hematol Am Soc Hematol Educ Program* 2009: 255–8.

3. Hoffman M, Monroe DM, 3rd. A cell-based model of hemostasis. *Thromb Haemost* 2001;**85**:958–65.

4. Hoffman M, Monroe DM. Coagulation 2006: a modern view of Hemostasis. *Hematol Oncol Clin N Am* 2007;**21**:1–11.

5. Stone DH, Goodney PP, Schanzer A, *et al*. Clopidogrel is not associated with major bleeding complications during peripheral arterial surgery. *J Vasc Surg* 2011;**54**:779–84.

6. Horlocker TT, Wedel DJ, Rowlingson JC, *et al*. Regional anesthesia in the patient receiving antithrombotic or thrombolytic therapy: American Society of Regional Anesthesia and Pain Medicine Evidence-Based Guidelines (3 edn). *Reg Anesth Pain Med* 2010;**35**:64–101.

7. Payne DA, Jones CI, Hayes PD, *et al*. Beneficial effects of clopidogrel combined with aspirin in reducing cerebral emboli in patients undergoing carotid endarterectomy. *Circulation* 2004;**109**:1476–81.

8. Burdess A, Nimmo AF, Garden OJ, *et al*. Randomized controlled trial of dual antiplatelet therapy in patients undergoing surgery for critical limb ischemia. *Ann Surg* 2010;**252**:37–42.

9. Hall R, Mazer CD. Antiplatelet drugs: a review of their pharmacology and management in the perioperative period. *Anesth Analg* 2011;**112**:292–318.

10. Hiippala ST, Myllyla GJ, Vahtera EM. Hemostatic factors and replacement of major blood loss with plasma-poor red cell concentrates. *Anesthes Analg* 1995;**81**:360–5.

11. Brohi K, Cohen MJ, Ganter MT, *et al*. Acute coagulopathy of trauma: hypoperfusion induces systemic anticoagulation and hyperfibrinolysis. *J Trauma* 2008;**64**:1211–17.

12. Mittermayr M, Streif W, Haas T, *et al*. Hemostatic changes after crystalloid or colloid fluid administration during major orthopedic surgery: the role of fibrinogen administration. *Anesth Analg* 2007;**105**:905–17.

13. Kozek-Langenecker SA. Influence of fluid therapy on the haemostatic system of intensive care patients. *Best Pract Res Clin Anaesthesiol* 2009;**23**:225–36.

14. Hartog CS, Reuter D, Loesche W, Hofmann M, Reinhart K. Influence of hydroxyethyl starch (HES) 130/0.4 on hemostasis as measured by viscoelastic device analysis: a systematic review. *Intens Care Med* 2011;**37**:1725–37.

15. Rossaint R, Bouillon B, Cerny V, *et al*. Task Force for Advanced Bleeding Care in Trauma. Management of bleeding following major trauma: an updated European guideline. *Crit Care* 2010;**14**:R52.

16. Larsen OH, Fenger-Eriksen C, Christiansen K, Ingerslev J, Sørensen B. Diagnostic performance and therapeutic consequence of thromboelastometry activated by kaolin versus a panel of specific reagents. *Anesthesiology* 2011;**115**:294–302.

17. Association of Anaesthetists of Great Britain and Ireland. Blood transfusion and the anaesthetist: management of massive haemorrhage. *Anaesthesia* 2010;**65**:1153–61.

18. Geraghty AJ, Welch K. Antithrombotic agents for preventing thrombosis after infrainguinal arterial bypass surgery. *Cochrane Database Syst Rev* 2011;**CD000536**.

Transfusion and blood conservation

Alastair F. Nimmo and Danny McGee

Introduction

Transfusion of allogeneic (donor) blood components – red cells, fresh frozen plasma (FFP), cryoprecipitate and platelets to avoid or correct severe anaemia and impaired haemostasis may be life-saving in acutely bleeding patients. However, many blood transfusions are given to patients who are not bleeding or are no longer severely anaemic and a number of observational studies have found blood transfusion to be an independent risk factor for increased mortality and morbidity, suggesting that some transfusions may be inappropriate and harmful. Furthermore, allogeneic blood components are expensive and their availability is limited. Recruitment and retention of blood donors, and ensuring that donated blood is safe for use, has become increasingly challenging in recent years. Restrictions on who may donate blood aimed at reducing the risk of transmission of HIV and variant Creutzfeldt–Jakob disease (vCJD) have seen a reduction in the number of donors, while additional testing and leucodepletion have resulted in a rise in the cost of producing each unit.

Blood component therapy

The separation or fractionation of blood into its components – red cells, platelets and plasma – became common practice in the UK in the 1980s. Whole blood is now rarely transfused in developed countries although fresh warm whole blood transfusion has been used in recent years by the US military in some patients with life-threatening injuries [1]. When whole blood is stored refrigerated there is a loss of platelet function and decline in the concentration of some coagulation factors.

Blood components are obtained either from a donation of whole blood or by apheresis. Selection of blood donors and testing a sample of the donated blood reduces the risk of transmission of infections. A whole blood donation of 450–500 ml is collected into a bag containing citrate phosphate dextrose (CPD) anticoagulant solution and may then be passed through a leucodepletion filter to remove most of the white blood cells. The blood bag is centrifuged to separate the red cells, plasma and platelets, and the plasma and platelets are then transferred into 'satellite bags'. Apheresis involves blood from a donor being centrifuged to separate the required component, e.g. platelet concentrate, which is then removed, and the remaining blood is returned to the donor.

An additive solution such as SAGM (saline, adenine, glucose and mannitol) is added to the red cell concentrate (RCC) which may then be kept refrigerated at $4\,^{\circ}C$ for up to 35 or 42 days before transfusion. Plasma is stored frozen and may be kept at $-30\,^{\circ}C$ for up to 2 years before use. The number of platelets obtained from a single whole-blood donation is too small to have a therapeutic effect in an adult patient so the platelets from four or five donors are usually pooled, i.e. transferred into one storage bag. The collection of platelets by apheresis results in a more concentrated product, such that a single apheresis platelet donation is equivalent to the platelets in a pooled product from four or five donors. Platelets are kept at room temperature on an agitator for up to 5 days before transfusion. Table 9.1 shows typical blood components specifications in the UK [2,3]. The *Handbook of Transfusion Medicine* published by the United Kingdom Blood Services and available online contains useful clinical information about blood transfusion [2].

Red cell concentrate transfusion

Anaemia before or after surgery is associated with an increased risk of death and complications. In a retro-

Core Topics in Vascular Anaesthesia, ed. Carl Moores and Alastair F. Nimmo. Published by Cambridge University Press.
© Cambridge University Press 2012.

Table 9.1 Blood components supplied by the United Kingdom Blood Services

	Red cells	Fresh frozen plasma (FFP)	Cryoprecipitate	Platelets
Number of donors per adult dose	1 (1 unit of red cells)	4 (4 units of FFP)	10	4 (pooled) 1 (apheresis)
Storage	Refrigerated (2–6 °C)	Frozen (−30 °C)	Frozen (−30 °C)	'Room temperature.' (20–24 °C)
Shelf life	35 days	2 years	2 years	5–7 days
Typical volume	280 ml	270 ml	330 ml	300 ml (pooled) 200 ml (apheresis)
Typical content	Hb 55 g/pack Haematocrit 57%	Fibrinogen – variable; typically around 3 g in 4 units; FVIII > 0.7 iU/ml; other factors variable	Fibrinogen 4 g	300×10^9 platelets
Administration	Within 4 hours once removed from controlled-temperature storage	Within 4 hours of issue. May be stored at 4 °C for up to 24 hours after thawing	Within 4 hours once thawed	Do not refrigerate

spective study of adults who refused perioperative blood transfusions for religious reasons, Carson found the risk of death increased progressively with preoperative haemoglobin concentrations below 10 g/dl and more dramatically so in patients with cardiovascular disease than in patients without [4]. However, it does not necessarily follow that giving a transfusion to treat the anaemia is beneficial because the harmful effects of the transfusion may outweigh the benefit of a higher haemoglobin concentration.

Risks of transfusion

Some of the risks of red cell transfusion such as transfusion of an incompatible unit (for example the wrong ABO blood group), transmission of bacterial and known viral infections and specific immunological reactions (such as haemolytic transfusion reactions) can be quantified, and are low in developed countries. For example the United Kingdom Serious Hazards of Transfusion (SHOT) haemovigilance scheme report for 2010 contained no confirmed cases of transfusion-transmitted infection. However, two major concerns about the safety of blood transfusions remain.

The first is the transmission of variant Creutzfeldt–Jakob disease (vCJD) by transfusion. This applies particularly to the United Kingdom and several other European countries where an as yet unquantifiable number of blood donors are thought to be carriers of the prions responsible for the disease as a result of eating infected beef products in the 1980s. Animal experiments have shown that vCJD can be transmitted by red cell, platelet or plasma transfusion and that the risk is not eliminated by leucodepletion. A small number of human cases of vCJD resulting from a blood transfusion have been reported but it is difficult to assess the magnitude of the risk because in some cases there may be an interval of many years between infection and symptoms becoming apparent.

The second concern is that a number of observational studies have concluded that red cell transfusion is an independent risk factor for death and complications. For example a study by Koch in cardiac surgery patients concluded that transfusion of red cells was associated with a dose-dependent, risk-adjusted increase in the occurrence of every postoperative morbidity and mortality outcome after isolated coronary artery bypass graft (CABG) [5]. Another study in cardiac surgery by Murphy found similar associations [6]. The adjusted odds ratio for transfused versus non-transfused patients was 3.38 for infections and 3.35 for ischaemic complications. Death within 30 days of surgery was six times commoner in patients who were transfused. No difference was apparent when the periods before and after the introduction of universal leucodepletion of red cells were compared. An association between red cell transfusion and adverse outcomes has also been reported in vascular surgery patients undergoing lower limb revascularisation [7]. Studies such as these have attempted to correct for the influence of factors other than transfusion on death and complications. However, with observational studies there always remains the possibility that there are residual confounding factors and that the association of red cell transfusion with a large increase in mortality and morbidity may not necessarily mean that the transfusions caused the deaths and complications. There is uncertainty about the haemoglobin level at which the benefits of a red cell transfusion outweigh the risks. Randomised trials are required to answer this question.

Transfusion thresholds

There have been remarkably few randomised trials of blood transfusion. One exception, the Transfusion Requirements in Critical Care (TRICC) trial included 833 patients with a haemoglobin (Hb) of <90 g/l within 72 hours of admission to the intensive care unit who were considered to be volume resuscitated [8]. They were randomised to either a restrictive or liberal transfusion strategy. The restrictive strategy involved transfusing one unit of red cells when the Hb concentration decreased below 70 g/l and then maintaining the concentrations between 70 and 90 g/l. In the liberal red blood cell group, the Hb concentration was maintained between 100 and 120 g/l and a unit of red cells was given when the Hb concentration fell below 100 g/l. There was a trend to reduced 30-day mortality in the restrictive transfusion group. This was statistically significant in patients who were less acutely ill and in patients under 55 years of age.

A subsequent subgroup analysis of the 357 patients in the TRICC trial who had cardiovascular disease found no difference in outcome between the restrictive and liberal transfusion strategies [9]. A non-significant ($p = 0.3$) decrease in overall survival rate in the restrictive group was noted in the patient group with confirmed ischaemic heart disease, severe peripheral vascular disease, or severe comorbid cardiac disease. The authors concluded that 'a restrictive red blood cell transfusion strategy generally appears to be safe in most critically ill patients with cardiovascular disease,

with the possible exception of patients with acute myocardial infarcts and unstable angina'.

A clinical practice guideline on perioperative blood transfusion and blood conservation in cardiac surgery from the Society of Thoracic Surgeons and the Society of Cardiovascular Anesthesiologists suggests 'Transfusion is reasonable in most postoperative patients whose hemoglobin is less than 7 g/dl, but no high-level evidence supports this recommendation' [10]. It is not clear whether a similar policy is appropriate in vascular surgery patients with coronary artery disease who have not undergone coronary revascularisation and many anaesthetists would maintain a higher Hb concentration, e.g. ≥80 g/l, in such patients.

It should not be forgotten that there is a significant danger of undertransfusing patients who are actively bleeding. In such patients we would recommend aiming to maintain a Hb concentration greater than 7 g/l because when Hb concentration is measured in bleeding patients it is common for it to be found to be considerably lower (or higher) than intended.

'Age' of blood

Some but not all observational studies have found that transfusion of red cells which have been stored for longer after donation is associated with a higher rate of death and complications in cardiac surgery and intensive care patients than transfusion of red cells stored for a shorter period [11,12]. Randomised trials are being undertaken in an attempt to establish whether it is indeed the 'age' of the red cells that causes the increase in mortality and morbidity or if this is the result of other differences between the groups in the observational studies.

Blood conservation

It is desirable to avoid or reduce perioperative red cell transfusions both because of the potential for harm to the patient and because donor blood is a scarce and expensive resource. Many hospitals have developed a blood conservation strategy involving a number of blood conservation techniques that often begins before the patient enters the operating theatre. Methods that may be used to avoid or reduce red cell transfusion are shown in Table 9.2.

Table 9.2 Blood conservation methods that may be used to avoid or reduce red cell transfusion

Diagnosis and treatment of preoperative anaemia

Stopping anticoagulant/ antiplatelet drugs in advance of surgery

Choice of procedure

Preoperative donation

Normovolaemic haemodilution

Surgical technique

Topical haemostatic agents, e.g. sealants or glues

Restrictive transfusion strategy

Intraoperative red cell salvage

Point-of-care testing of coagulation

Antifibrinolytic drug therapy

Preoperative management

Patients at greatest risk of requiring an allogeneic transfusion during vascular surgery include those presenting for surgery with a low Hb level resulting in a low tolerance for blood loss, and patients with impaired coagulation increasing their risk of bleeding during surgery.

Assessing the patient several weeks before their date of surgery offers the first opportunity to minimise the requirement for allogeneic transfusion, although this may not be possible if the vascular surgery needs to be undertaken urgently, e.g. repair of a large or symptomatic aortic aneurysm. A detailed medical history should be taken with particular attention given to bleeding disorders, previous surgical challenges and transfusion requirements. Anaemia should be investigated and treated if time permits. Occasionally treatment of the condition causing the anaemia will be a higher priority than the planned vascular surgery. Erythropoietin and intravenous or oral iron have been used to increase red cell mass and Hb concentration before surgery but their role in vascular surgery patients is not clear.

Antiplatelet drugs and anticoagulants will increase bleeding during surgery. Anticoagulants are usually stopped before surgery but in the case of antiplatelet drugs the risk of increased bleeding has to be weighed against the risk of thrombotic complications, particularly cardiac complications, if the drugs are stopped.

It is common to continue aspirin perioperatively in vascular surgery (see Chapters 4 and 8).

Autologous transfusion techniques

Autologous blood is blood derived from the same individual. Preoperative autologous blood donation (PABD) requires the patient to donate their own blood before the date of surgery. The patient may donate several times before surgery with the blood being stored and then made available for transfusion on the day of surgery if required. This technique requires a significant investment of time and money for the patient and the blood establishment. As a consequence of PABD, the patient may present on the day of surgery with a lower Hb and therefore although in theory this technique may reduce the transfusion of allogeneic blood, in practice it may increase the patient's requirement for any form of transfusion. Furthermore, because the predonated units are stored in the blood bank this technique does not reduce one of the significant risks associated with donor transfusion, namely receiving an incorrect blood component. This technique is only suitable for elective surgery; should the surgery be postponed or rescheduled then some or all of the predonated blood may be wasted. In the UK, PABD is not currently routine practice but may be considered in cases where patients have unusual antibodies making sourcing compatible donor blood problematic.

Acute normovolaemic haemodilution (ANH) takes place on the day of surgery usually in the anaesthetic room with the patient anaesthetised. A volume of blood (for example 1 litre) is withdrawn into a blood bag containing anticoagulant which is kept beside the patient at room temperature. The patient's circulating volume is maintained by the simultaneous intravenous infusion of colloid (or crystalloid) fluid. The deliberate haemodilution of the patient means that bleeding during surgery results in fewer red cells, platelets and clotting factors being lost, with a readily available volume of undiluted autologous whole blood available for reinfusion if required. The efficacy of ANH has been compared with no ANH in randomised study in patients undergoing open abdominal aortic aneurysm (AAA) repair under combined general and epidural anaesthesia (with intraoperative cell salvage also used in all patients) [13]. No reduction in blood transfusion was found in the ANH group and it was suggested that large volumes of intravenous fluids

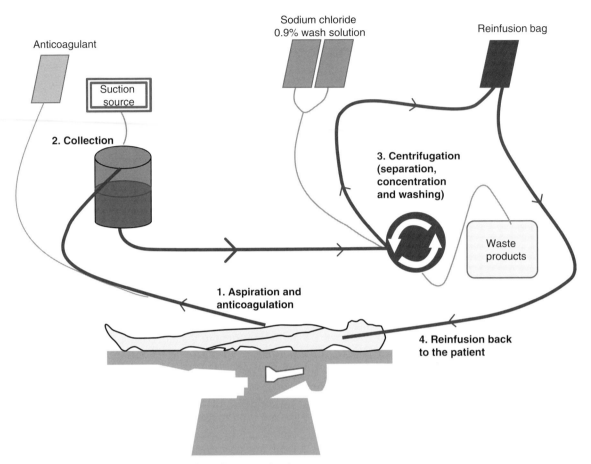

Figure 9.1 Principles of autologous blood transfusion. For details see text.

infused in the control group in response to the effects of anaesthesia and aortic clamp release were producing 'hypervolaemic haemodilution' so that additional haemodilution was not beneficial.

Intraoperative cell salvage (ICS) is a technique that collects and anticoagulates blood shed from the surgical field. The blood is aspirated into a collection reservoir and filtered to remove gross debris. Depending on the specific ICS machine used, the salvaged blood will either be processed in batches to produce between 100–250 ml of concentrated red cells on each occasion or will be processed continuously. During batch processing, once a predetermined volume of anticoagulated blood has been collected, the ICS machine will draw the reservoir contents into a centrifuge where the red cell component is retained and concentrated, while the other components – plasma, platelets and anticoagulant – are removed. The concentrated red cells are then washed using a 0.9% sodium chloride

solution. At the end of the washing process the centrifuge contains red cells in 0.9% sodium chloride and this is pumped into a bag for reinfusion (Figure 9.1). The haematocrit of the product depends on the ICS machine but is typically between 50% and 70%. Of the three autologous techniques, ICS is the most commonly used and is suitable for both elective and emergency vascular surgery.

Other intraoperative techniques

Both the choice of procedure (e.g. open versus endovascular aortic aneurysm repair) and surgical technique affect the amount of blood lost and the options available to reduce this. Topical haemostatic sealants or glues may be applied for example to vascular anastomoses.

The Hb concentration may fall in the absence of significant bleeding if a large volume of intravenous fluid is given. This may occur when fluid is given to treat hypotension after inducing general anaesthesia or establishing spinal or epidural analgesia and may be more common in patients taking drugs that can lead to marked falls in blood pressure with anaesthesia, such as angiotensin-converting enzyme (ACE) inhibitors and angiotensin receptor blockers. In this situation the Hb falls although there has been little or no change in the red cell mass in the patient's circulation and the anaesthetist should consider carefully whether or not a red cell transfusion is necessary.

Impaired haemostasis during surgery can result in diffuse excessive bleeding. Blood loss and the need for red cell transfusion may be reduced by rapid appropriate treatment guided by point-of-care testing of haemostasis (see Chapter 8).

The antifibrinolytic drugs tranexamic acid and epsilon-aminocaproic acid are used to reduce bleeding in cardiac and orthopaedic surgery and in trauma patients. They have not been widely used in vascular surgery and it is not clear whether any benefit that might result from reduced bleeding and transfusion outweighs a possible risk of increased thrombotic complications.

Plasma, cryoprecipitate and platelet transfusion

Red cell concentrate transfusions, whether allogeneic or autologous, do not contain therapeutic amounts of fibrinogen, other coagulation factors or platelets. When major surgical blood loss is replaced with red cell concentrates and colloid plasma substitutes, the fibrinogen concentration typically falls to a level that impairs haemostasis before the platelet count or concentrations of other coagulation factors do [14]. Point-of-care testing is a useful guide to the need for replacement of fibrinogen, platelets and coagulation factors in bleeding patients. When laboratory tests are used as a guide to the need for replacement there are varying guidelines on when treatment is required. Recent guidelines on the management of bleeding following major trauma recommend that a fibrinogen concentration of at least 1.5 g/l should be maintained and a platelet count of at least 50×10^9/l (and perhaps higher in some situations) [15]. These are similar values to those we have found to be associated with satisfactory haemostasis during thoracoabdominal aortic aneurysm repair. The Association of Anaesthetists of Great Britain and Ireland's guideline on the management of massive haemorrhage suggests maintaining a fibrinogen concentration above 1.5 g/l and a platelet count at least 75×10^9/l [16].

Fibrinogen may be given in FFP, in cryoprecipitate or as fibrinogen concentrate. A prothrombin time (PT) or activated partial thromboplastin time (APTT) that is prolonged to over 1.5 times normal (in the absence of an anticoagulant) suggests a low concentration of fibrinogen and/or other coagulation factors (see also Chapter 8). Coagulation factors may be given in FFP which also contains fibrinogen or in prothrombin complex concentrate (PCC) which does not. The benefits and risks of giving PCC rather than FFP in bleeding patients are uncertain.

Fresh frozen plasma

A pack of FFP contains the plasma from one whole-blood donation. In the UK the mean volume of plasma in a pack is 220 ml plus 50 ml of anticoagulant. The plasma contains fibrinogen, the other coagulation factors, and the naturally occurring anticoagulants protein C, protein S and antithrombin in similar concentrations to those normally present in plasma. It is stored frozen at $-30\,^\circ$C and then thawed before use. Once thawed the unit should be transfused within 4 hours if stored at ambient temperature or may be stored at $4\,^\circ$C and used within 24 hours. Some hospitals hold a stock of thawed plasma at $4\,^\circ$C so that it can be issued in an emergency without the delay that thawing entails. The standard adult dose is 15 ml/kg, i.e. four units for a 70-kg patient. The FFP should be ABO compatible with the recipient to avoid the risk of haemolysis in the recipient caused by anti-A or anti-B antibodies in the donor plasma but does not need to be matched for RhD (Rhesus) group. Therefore, group O FFP must only be given to group O recipients. Conversely, group AB FFP (lacking naturally occurring anti-A and anti-B antibodies) can be given to recipients irrespective of their ABO group but is in short supply in many countries where only a small proportion of the population is group AB.

The use of FFP is indicated for the treatment of bleeding patients who have impaired haemostasis as the result of low concentrations of fibrinogen and/or other clotting factors resulting from consumption, loss or dilution. Some observational studies in patients who have suffered severe trauma have found that transfusion of an increased ratio of FFP to red cells is associated with decreased mortality. Such observational studies are subject to confounding factors, such as 'survivor bias'. The most severely injured patients who die soon after admission may receive red cells but little or no FFP because FFP is not available as quickly as red cells whereas less severely injured patients survive and receive more FFP. Nevertheless, when massive injury or haemorrhage is associated with coagulopathy, early and aggressive correction of haemostasis, for example with plasma and platelets, is likely to be beneficial.

There is little evidence to support the use of FFP in other situations such as attempting to correct an isolated prolongation of PT in patients who are not bleeding [17,18]; and FFP is no longer recommended for the emergency reversal of warfarin (see Chapter 8).

Transfusion of FFP carries risks including the transmission of viral infections and vCJD, immunological reactions including transfusion-associated lung injury (TRALI), and circulatory overload. The risk of transmission of viruses can be reduced by treatment with light-activated methylene blue or with a solvent detergent process. However, these processes may reduce the amount of fibrinogen and coagulation factors and do not prevent transmission of prions. The FFP given to adults in the UK is not virus-inactivated and in addition there are major concerns regarding the possibility of prion transmission. These concerns are such that in the UK children receive only imported FFP from non-European blood donors. An alternative to giving units of FFP, each of which has been obtained from a single blood donor, is to give a pooled plasma product which has been obtained by combining plasma from multiple donors of the same ABO blood group and then subjected to a pathogen reduction process such as solvent detergent treatment.

Cryoprecipitate

Cryoprecipitate is produced by controlled thawing of frozen plasma to precipitate high molecular weight proteins, including fibrinogen, factor VIII, von Willebrand factor and factor XIII. The cryoprecipitate is then frozen again for storage and must be thawed before use. Cryoprecipitate prepared from a single donor unit contains 300−600 mg of fibrinogen in a volume of 20−50 ml. In the past cryoprecipitate was given as a source of factor VIII to patients with haemophilia but factor VIII concentrates are now used for this purpose. Cryoprecipitate is now used as a source of fibrinogen to raise the fibrinogen concentration in bleeding patients. The standard adult dose is the cryoprecipitate from 10 donors, often administered as two bags, each of which contains cryoprecipitate pooled from five donors. This dose will typically raise the plasma fibrinogen level by about 1 g/l. Cryoprecipitate should be ABO 'plasma compatible' (see under FFP above).

As plasma from 10 donors is required to provide one standard adult dose of cryoprecipitate, this may increase the risk of viral or prion infection being transmitted to the recipient. Cryoprecipitate given to adults in the UK does not routinely undergo pathogen reduction treatment. However, cryoprecipitate given to children is made from methylene-blue-treated plasma imported from outside Europe in order to reduce the risk of pathogen transmission. The methylene blue treatment reduces the fibrinogen in the cryoprecipitate.

In most European Union countries cryoprecipitate is no longer used and in several of these countries fibrinogen concentrate is used instead [19]. Fibrinogen concentrate is derived from pooled plasma sourced from countries where there is a low risk of vCJD being present in donors. It is subjected to purification and pathogen reduction steps before being freeze-dried to produce a white powder which may be stored at room temperature. The concentrate is dissolved in sterile water before administration.

Platelet concentrate

A standard adult dose of platelet concentrate contains around 300×10^9 platelets in 250 ml of plasma (which maintains platelet function during storage) and is obtained from four or five whole-blood donors or one apheresis donor. Platelets that are refrigerated have reduced survival in the circulation after administration. Therefore platelet concentrates are stored at 20−24 °C. This increases the risk of transmission of bacterial infections and limits the maximum period of storage before use – typically to 5 days, though this may be extended to 7 days in conjunction with preissue bacterial testing. The limited storage life of platelets causes logistic problems for blood transfusion services trying to maintain sufficient stock to cope with emergency requests and leads inevitably to overcollection and unavoidable wastage of unused platelet concentrates. Platelet quality and survival in the circulation after transfusion is improved by storing them on an agitator which produces gentle continuous movement.

Platelet concentrates of the same ABO and RhD group as the recipient should be given where possible [20].

Practical aspects of blood component transfusion

Transfusions of blood components should be given through a blood administration set which contains an integral screen filter (170–200 μm pore size). Platelet transfusions may be given either through a standard blood administration set or a platelet infusion set but should not be given through an administration set which has previously been used for red cell transfusion. Blood components should not be mixed with intravenous fluids containing calcium because the calcium may interact with the citrate anticoagulant and result in clot formation within the administration line before the blood component enters the circulation.

Large and rapid transfusions of blood components may cause hypothermia, hypocalcaemia and hyperkalaemia. A fluid warmer should be used. Hypocalcaemia results from administration of citrate present in blood components which exerts its anticoagulant activity by binding ionised calcium. Point-of-care measurement of ionised calcium is desirable and the ionised calcium concentration should be kept above 0.9 mmol/l to avoid cardiovascular effects as well as effects on haemostasis [15]. The concentration of potassium in the supernatant fluid in allogeneic red cell concentrate rises during storage, reaching around 35 mmol/l after 35 days in the case of red cells in CPD anticoagulant and SAGM additive solution [21]. This may result in hyperkalaemia after rapid transfusion of stored red cells. The hyperkalaemia is usually short-lived but if severe can result in cardiac arrest. Point-of-care measurement of potassium, e.g. using a blood gas analyser, is desirable.

When a blood component is administered it is essential that the patient's name, date of birth and identification number are checked against an identification band attached to the patient. Performing these checks against case notes, charts or information on a computer screen is not acceptable because the notes, charts or computer record may be those of a different patient and this may result in an incompatible blood component being transfused and a serious or fatal transfusion reaction.

References

1. Spinella PC. Warm fresh whole blood transfusion for severe haemorrhage: US military and potential civilian applications. *Crit Care Med* 2008;**36**:S340–5.

2. United Kingdom Blood Services. *Handbook of Transfusion Medicine*, 4th edn. London: The Stationery office, 2007. Available at www.transfusionguidelines.org/docs/pdfs/htm_edition-4_all-pages.pdf

3. Specification SPN223/3. *NHSBT Portfolio of Blood Components and Guidance for their Clinical Use.* Available at http://hospital.blood.co.uk/library/pdf/components/SPN223_version3.pdf

4. Carson JL, Duff A, Poses RM, *et al.* Effect of anaemia and cardiovascular disease on surgical mortality and morbidity. *Lancet* 1996;**348**:1055–60.

5. Koch CG, Liang L, Duncan AI, *et al.* Morbidity and mortality risk associated with red blood cell and blood-component transfusion in isolated coronary artery bypass grafting. *Crit Care Med* 2006;**34**:1608–16.

6. Murphy GJ, Reeves BC, Rogers CA, *et al.* Increased mortality, postoperative morbidity, and cost after red blood cell transfusion in patients having cardiac surgery. *Circulation* 2007;**116**:2544–52.

7. O'Keeffe SD, Davenport DL, Minion DJ, *et al.* Blood transfusion is associated with increased morbidity and mortality after lower extremity revascularization. *J Vasc Surg* 2010;**51**:616–21.

8. Hebert PC, Wells G, Blajchman MA, *et al.* A multicenter, randomized, controlled clinical trial of transfusion requirements in critical care. *N Engl J Med* 1999;**340**:409–17.

9. Hebert PC, Yetisir E, Martin C, *et al.* Is a low transfusion threshold safe in critically ill patients with cardiovascular diseases? *Crit Care Med* 2001;**29**:227–34.

10. Ferraris VA, Brown JR, *et al.* 2011 Update to The Society of Thoracic Surgeons and the Society of Cardiovascular Anesthesiologists Blood Conservation Clinical Practice Guidelines. *Ann Thorac Surg* 2011;**91**:944–82.

11. Koch CG, Li L, Sessler DI, *et al.* Duration of red-cell storage and complications after cardiac surgery. *N Engl J Med* 2008;**358**:1229–39.

12. Pettilä V, Westbrook AJ, Nichol AD, *et al.* Age of red blood cells and mortality in the critically ill. *Crit Care* 2011;**15**:R116.

13. Wolowczyk L, Nevin M, Smith FC, Baird RN, Lamont PM. Haemodilutional effect of standard fluid management limits the effectiveness of acute normovolaemic haemodilution in AAA surgery: results of a pilot trial. *Eur J Vasc Endovasc Surg* 2003;**26**:405–11.

14. Hiippala ST, Myllyla GJ, Vahtera EM. Hemostatic factors and replacement of major blood loss with plasma-poor red cell concentrates. *Anesth Analg.* 1995;**81**:360–5.

15. Rossaint R, Bouillon B, Cerny V, *et al.* Management of bleeding following major trauma: an updated European guideline. *Crit Care* 2010;**14**:R52.

16. Association of Anaesthetists of Great Britain and Ireland. Blood transfusion and the anaesthetist: management of massive haemorrhage. *Anaesthesia* 2010;**65**:1153–61.

17. Murad MH, Stubbs JR, Gandhi MJ, *et al.* The effect of plasma transfusion on morbidity and mortality: a systematic review and meta-analysis. *Transfusion* 2010;**50**:1370–83.

18. Stanworth SJ, Grant-Casey J, Lowe D, *et al.* The use of fresh-frozen plasma in England: high levels of inappropriate use in adults and children. *Transfusion* 2011;**51**:62–70.

19. Sørensen B, Bevan D. A critical evaluation of cryoprecipitate for replacement of fibrinogen. *Br J Haematol* 2010;**149**: 834–43.

20. Lozano M, Cid J. The clinical implications of platelet transfusions associated with ABO or Rh(D) incompatibility. *Transfus Med Rev* 2003;**17**:57–68.

21. Vraets A, Lin Y, Callum JL. Transfusion-associated hyperkalemia. *Transfus Med Rev* 2011;**25**:184–96.

Anaesthesia for elective abdominal aortic aneurysm surgery

Richard Telford

Epidemiology of abdominal aortic aneurysms and risk of rupture

Abdominal aortic aneurysm (AAA) is a dilatation of the aorta as it passes through the abdomen. The abdominal aorta is aneurysmal when its diameter is greater than 3.0 cm. The prevalence of AAAs is rising, and is around 10% in men and 3% in women aged more than 65. Abdominal aortic aneurysms are usually asymptomatic. Chronic cigarette smoking is the single most important risk factor in both the development and progression of AAA. The prevalence of AAAs in chronic smokers is more than four times that in lifelong non-smokers, and the average rate of increase in aneurysm size in smokers is 2.8 mm per year versus 2.5 mm per year in non-smokers. The most common cause of AAA is atherosclerosis; rare causes include Marfan syndrome, salmonella, brucellosis, tuberculosis and Takayasu disease.

Abdominal aortic aneurysms account for more than 6000 deaths per year in England and Wales. This is around 2% of all deaths of men aged greater than 65. Most deaths occur as a result of rupture of the aneurysm, which is a surgical emergency. The mortality after rupture is high – approximately 80% of those who reach hospital and 50% of those undergoing emergency surgery for ruptured aortic aneurysm will die. These deaths are potentially preventable because elective repair of the abdominal aorta can be performed with an operative mortality of less than 7%.

The risk of rupture is related to the size of the aneurysm. Small aneurysms of less than 5 cm in diameter rarely rupture (<2%). There is no survival benefit from early surgical intervention. Patients with small aneurysms greater than 3 cm and less than 5.4 cm in diameter should undergo regular ultrasound scanning to monitor the aneurysm size. The estimated annual rupture rate of aneurysms larger than 6 cm in diameter is 9%, rising to more that 25% for aneurysms larger than 8 cm in diameter. The 5-year survival of patients if aneurysms greater than 5 cm are not operated on is around 20%. Current guidelines are to offer operative intervention when the aneurysm exceeds 5.5 cm, provided the patient is deemed fit enough for surgery.

Screening for aortic aneurysms

Since most aneurysms are asymptomatic the key to reducing mortality from rupture is early diagnosis. The NHS Abdominal Aortic Aneurysm Screening Programme (NAAASP) has been introduced in England and Wales, with the aim of reducing deaths from aneurysm rupture. The first three phases of NAAASP have been rolled out, with the remainder of England expected to be covered by April 2013. The Scottish AAA screening programme is due to be rolled out from autumn 2012. The aim is for nationwide coverage by 2013. The key evidence underpinning this policy is the multicentre aneurysm screening study (MASS), funded by the Medical Research Council [1]. More than 67 000 men aged 65–74 were recruited from four centres in the UK and were randomised to either receive or not receive an invitation to screening. The results after 4 years' follow-up showed a 42% relative risk reduction in mortality related to AAA (absolute risk reduction from 0.33% to 0.19%). All men will automatically be invited for screening in the year they turn 65. Men who are older than 65, and who have not previously been screened or treated for an AAA, will be able to opt-in through self-referral direct to the screening programme. Men who are found to have aortic diameters of less than

Core Topics in Vascular Anaesthesia, ed. Carl Moores and Alastair F. Nimmo. Published by Cambridge University Press.
© Cambridge University Press 2012.

3 cm will be discharged (96%). Those with aortic diameters between 3 and 5.4 cm will be enrolled in a surveillance programme (3.5%). Those with aortic diameters greater than 5.5 cm will be referred to a vascular surgeon (0.5%).

Surgical techniques

The abdominal aorta is a retroperitoneal structure. The majority of open AAA repairs are performed via either long midline or subumbilical transverse incision [2]. A midline incision is quicker to perform, but may be associated with a higher incidence of incisional hernia when compared to a transverse incision. A left retroperitoneal approach is sometimes advocated if the patients have severe respiratory disease. The peritoneum is not opened; there is less postoperative ileus and reduced postoperative atelectasis. The main disadvantage of this approach is that access to the right iliac artery can be difficult, particularly if there is a large iliac aneurysm. Whichever surgical approach is chosen the neck of the aneurysm needs to be identified to apply an aortic cross clamp. The inferior mesenteric artery (IMA), which takes its origin from the front of the aneurysm, is usually sacrificed. Rarely the IMA may be reimplanted into the aortic prosthesis with a Carroll patch if there are concerns about the adequacy of collateral circulation to the descending colon, sigmoid colon and rectum.

The aortic graft is made of woven Dacron. The upper anastomosis is end to end. The distal anastomoses may be to the aortic bifurcation (a 'tube' graft) or to the iliac or femoral arteries (a bifurcated or 'trouser' graft). The site of the distal anastomosis(es) is dependent whether the iliac arteries are involved in the aneurysm. Wherever possible femoral anastomoses should be avoided because of the increased risk of infection associated with groin incisions.

Preoperative assessment and risk management

Surgery for AAA is a high-risk procedure. The 30-day mortality in the UK is approximately 7% [3]. Abdominal vascular surgery is a major physiological insult which provokes an increase in oxygen consumption of 40%. Patients presenting for abdominal vascular surgery are elderly and frequently unfit with a high incidence of comorbidities which may mean they lack the physiological reserve to meet this increased demand. Major morbidity or even mortality may ensue.

Meticulous preassessment is essential to assess the risk–benefit ratio of the proposed intervention and to enable informed consent to be obtained. There is little point performing a prophylactic operation designed to increase life expectancy if the patient succumbs to the complications of the procedure.

Comorbidities may include:

- coronary artery disease, often with impaired ventricular function
- hypertension
- pulmonary disease (often related to smoking)
- renal impairment
- diabetes mellitus.

Careful preassessment is required to identify high-risk patients and to optimise medical management of their comorbidities. Ideally this should be performed by a consultant vascular anaesthetist as soon as possible after the patient is listed for surgery [4,5].

The ability to exercise is an excellent indicator of cardiovascular and respiratory fitness. Patients who cannot climb a flight of stairs or walk on level ground at 6 km/hour frequently have adverse outcomes.

Other major cardiac risk factors include:

- recent myocardial infarction (<1 month)
- unstable or severe angina
- decompensated heart failure
- significant arrhythmias (high-grade atrial ventricular block, symptomatic arrhythmias or supraventricular arrhythmias with uncontrolled ventricular rate)
- severe valvular heart disease (aortic, mitral stenosis)
- recent percutaneous coronary intervention (balloon angioplasty <4 weeks, bare metal stent insertion <6 weeks or drug eluting stent insertion <1 year).

Pharmacological stress tests (dipyridamole–thallium scintography and dobutamine stress echocardiography) may be used. They have a low positive predictive value (20–30%) but a reassuringly a high negative predictive value (95–100%) for perioperative cardiovascular complications. Patients with positive stress tests should have coronary angiography. Heart murmurs should be investigated with transthoracic echocardiography.

Cardiopulmonary exercise (CPET) testing can help identify high-risk patients [6]. It is performed on a cycle ergometer with simultaneous respiratory gas analysis and ECG recording. An anaerobic threshold of less than 11 ml/kg per minute, particularly if associated with ECG evidence of ischaemia, is associated with high perioperative mortality.

Lifestyle advice should be given to the patient at the time of preassessment. Cessation of smoking and structured exercise programmes may improve cardio-respiratory fitness.

All patients presenting for abdominal vascular surgery should receive antiplatelet medication to protect against the thromboembolic complications of cardiovascular disease (aspirin 75–150 mg once daily or clopidogrel 75 mg once daily if aspirin-intolerant) Statins should be prescribed because they improve both short- and long-term outcomes following non-cardiac surgery regardless of the baseline low-density lipoprotein concentration [7]. Statin therapy improves endothelial function, reduces vascular inflammation and stabilises atherosclerotic plaques.

Acute beta-blockade for all patients presenting for vascular surgery is associated with increased peri-operative mortality and increased risk of stroke [8]. However some extremely high-risk patients who demonstrate inducible ischaemia on pharmacological stress testing have improved outcomes if they receive carefully titrated beta-blockade (low dose bisoprolol titrated to a resting heart rate of 50–80 beats per minute).

Modern medical treatment of coronary artery disease with aspirin and statins has negated the benefits of coronary revascularisation before non-cardiac surgery. Two well-conducted trials have shown no significant difference in perioperative death or myocardial infarction (MI), or longer-term mortality [9]. Preoperative coronary artery bypass grafting (CABG) should be performed prior to open AAA surgery only if indicated on prognostic grounds (significant (>50%) left main stem stenosis, severe (>70%) two or three vessel disease (including the proximal LAD) and/or left ventricular systolic dysfunction.). If CABG is performed AAA surgery should be deferred for 3 months if possible.

Percutaneous coronary intervention (PCI) is very rarely indicated prior to AAA surgery [10]. Major surgery following recent PCI is associated with increased 30-day mortality and increased risk of non-fatal myocardial infarction. Percutaneous coronary intervention traumatises the vessel wall rendering the endoluminal surface thrombogenic until the vessel wall has healed or the stent has re-endothelialised. Antiplatelet therapy is necessary to prevent local coronary thrombosis after PCI – aspirin for life and clopidogrel for 3 weeks after balloon angioplasty, 6 weeks after bare metal stent insertion and for 12 months after drug-eluting stent insertion. Interference with dual antiplatelet medication perioperatively because of bleeding concerns is associated with a very high cardiac complication rate. If surgery for AAA is deemed essential within the above timeframes it has been suggested that clopidogrel should be stopped 7 days prior to surgery and bridging therapy instituted with a short-acting platelet glycoprotein IIa/IIIb inhibitor (tirofiban or epfifibatid) stopping this 6 hours prior to surgery.

Anaesthetic management

Patients should receive their regular medications on the day of surgery with the possible exception of angiotensin-converting enzyme (ACE) inhibitors and angiotensin II receptor blockers which should be discontinued 24–48 hours prior to surgery. The aim of anaesthesia is to have a normovolaemic, haemodynamically stable, normothermic, pain-free patient on completion of surgery. Most vascular anaesthetists in the UK use a balanced general anaesthetic technique (high-dose opioid, oxygen, air, low-dose volatile agent) with a thoracic epidural to provide postoperative pain relief [3]. There is some evidence that volatile anaesthetics and opioids improve tolerance of myocardial ischaemia by their effects on mitochondrial and sarcolemmal ATP-regulated potassium channels. The mechanism may be similar to ischaemic preconditioning. An effective epidural helps ameliorate the stress response to surgery, reducing cardiovascular demands. Epidurals provide high-quality dynamic postoperative analgesia, facilitating early extubation and reducing the incidence of pulmonary complications. There is no evidence that epidurals reduce mortality [11]. Epidurals can safely be inserted in patients taking aspirin. The situation with clopidogrel is less clear. If an epidural is inserted in a patient taking clopidogrel, careful documentation of the risk–benefit ratio is essential. Patients should be monitored closely for the symptoms and signs of epidural haematoma (back pain, bladder dysfunction, leg weakness).

Systemic heparinisation is required prior to aortic cross-clamping. Administration of heparin has been shown to reduce thrombotic and embolic events. One paper suggested an increase in perioperative mortality from myocardial infarction if heparin was not used. Additional heparin may be required in the presence of prolonged clamp times. Heparin can be reversed by protamine if bleeding is thought to be due to excessive heparinisation. However, protamine should be used with caution as it may lead to myocardial depression, anaphylaxis and pulmonary hypertension.

Physiology of aortic clamping and declamping

Aortic cross-clamping is necessary in open infrarenal AAA surgery. Usually the aortic cross-clamp is placed below the origin of the renal arteries but occasionally a juxtarenal or suprarenal cross-clamp may be required. The physiological response to cross-clamping is complex and depends on myocardial function, the amount of collateral circulation present, the volume status of the patient and the function of the sympathetic nervous system. Arterial hypertension is the most common occurrence due to an increase in systemic vascular resistance of around 30%. Blood pressure typically rises by 7–10%. Cardiac filling pressures also increase for two reasons. Firstly, blood volume is shifted to the central veins because of reduced venous capacitance in organs distal to the clamp. Secondly, a diseased coronary system may be unable to respond to increases in cardiac workload, resulting in cardiac failure. This may be exacerbated by the administration of too much fluid before cross-clamping. Studies show reductions of cardiac output of between 9% and 33% after infrarenal cross-clamping. However, some patients with good cardiac performance may increase cardiac output. Vasodilators (e.g. glyceryl trinitrate) are effective in treating hypertension and cardiac failure, but theoretically risk exacerbating organ ischaemia by reducing perfusion pressure in the collateral circulation.

Release of the aortic cross-clamp may result in a dramatic reduction in blood pressure. This is multifactorial. There is a sudden decrease in systemic vascular resistance due to the removal of the cross-clamp and the release of vasoactive cytokines and metabolites as the ischaemic tissues of the lower part of the body are reperfused. Ischaemic metabolites and the ensuing metabolic acidosis may exacerbate myocardial depression. There may be central hypovolaemia due to sequestration of blood in the reperfused organs. The severity of hypotension is proportional to cross-clamp time. Ensuring adequate cardiovascular filling prior to cross-clamp release and a gradual release of the cross-clamp helps to minimise declamping hypotension. Vasodilators, if used, should be gradually reduced or discontinued before cross-clamp release. Vasopressors may be required after cross-clamp release, but have the potential disadvantage of preferential vasoconstriction of the vasculature above the clamp. Reclamping may be required if the hypotension is severe and refractory to treatment.

Intraoperative monitoring

In addition to standard monitoring, direct measurement of arterial and central venous pressure, temperature and urine output is mandatory. A five-lead ECG will aid detection of ST segment changes.

In the UK anaesthetists rarely measure cardiac output during elective AAA surgery. In the 2005 NCEPOD report cardiac output was measured in 7% of AAA repairs, with a pulmonary artery flotation catheter (PAFC) being used in 2% of cases. Interestingly inotropes and vasopressors were administered to 70% of these patients. The NCEPOD report authors questioned whether greater use of cardiac output monitoring and computation of the derived haemodynamic variables might lead to more rational use of inotropes and vasopressors and contribute to improved outcome. There is some evidence from other forms of major abdominal surgery that haemodynamic management to achieve an optimal value of stroke volume may reduce postoperative complication rates and shorten hospital stay.

The PAFC remains the gold standard monitor of the cardiovascular system and should be considered in patients with impaired ventricular function. Randomised trials support its use in the high-risk surgical patient.

Oesophageal Doppler monitoring can give an indication of myocardial contractility (peak velocity, PV) and cardiac filling (flow time corrected for heart rate, FTC). A Doppler probe is positioned in the oesophagus to insolate the descending thoracic aorta. A derived cardiac output is calculated via the equipment software. Although there are published data to support its use in other forms of abdominal surgery there are no published data in open aortic surgery. Readings obtained are of limited value during the period of aortic cross-clamping. However the haemodynamic variables obtained before and after aortic cross-clamping and release may provide useful information to help optimise the circulation.

Pulse contour analysis cardiac output monitoring (LiDCO™ and PiCCO™) is not popular in the operating theatre. Muscle relaxants interfere with the calibration of LiDCO™, whereas PiCCO™ necessitates cannulation of the brachial artery. The recently developed LiDCOrapid™ which uses a patented, clinically validated PulseCO algorithm to derive haemodynamic variables from a radial arterial line trace without the need for prior calibration may prove a useful monitor of the cardiovascular system. The values obtained will not be influenced by aortic cross-clamping.

The UK National Institute for Clinical Excellence (NICE) has emphasised the importance of avoiding hypothermia in surgical patients [12]. Perioperative hypothermia is common in open AAA surgery because the abdomen may be open for a considerable time, there is a period of reduced perfusion of the lower body and fluid losses may be significant. Perioperative hypothermia is associated with myocardial ischaemia and dysrhythmias [13]. It contributes to a coagulopathy and increases wound infections. Shivering can increase oxygen consumption up to sixfold, placing excessive demands on the cardiovascular system. Forced air warming devices, fluid warmers and increased ambient theatre temperatures are important to minimise heat loss. The legs should not be actively warmed when the aorta is cross-clamped. It is important to institute heat conservation measures starting in the anaesthetic room. One group has suggested that insertion of central neuraxial blocks and invasive monitoring lines prior to induction of general anaesthesia may be beneficial as in their study the majority of heat loss occurred in the anaesthetic room.

Blood loss during elective AAA surgery is highly variable. In the 2005 NCEPOD report 7% of elective AAA repairs had a measured blood loss >5 litres [3]. Adequate wide-bore intravenous access is important. A valid group and save sample must be performed. In the absence of antibodies the blood transfusion laboratory will be able to issue type-specific blood and perform a full retrospective cross-match. The vascular anaesthetist needs to be familiar with local protocols for the management of massive blood transfusion [14]. Significant bleeding can occur when opening the aortic aneurysm because of 'backbleeding' from the lumbar arteries which arise from the posterior aspect of the aneurysm sac. These need to be promptly undersewn. The native aorta may be very friable and surgical haemostasis may be difficult to achieve when suturing anastomoses. In addition blood loss can result from malpositioned clamps. Homologous blood transfusion can be minimised by acute normovolaemic haemodilution and intraoperative cell salvage (ICS) [15]. Predonation, although available via the National Blood Transfusion Service, is not a cost-effective option in the UK. Elective aortic surgery is ideally suited to ICS which should be mandatory. This technique provides red cells suspended in normal saline with normal concentrations of 2,3-diphosphoglycerate, free from anticoagulant. Since vascular patients have a high incidence of coronary artery disease the target haematocrit should be maintained at more than 27% (haemoglobin >90 g/l). Accurate bedside haemoglobin measurements can be made by a Hemocue®. Massive haemorrhage can produce a dilutional coagulopathy, requiring fresh frozen plasma, cryoprecipitate and platelet transfusions. Early liaison with the blood transfusion laboratory is essential if excessive bleeding occurs to ensure adequate supplies of blood and blood products. Appropriate administration of blood products is best guided by near-patient testing, using rotational thromboelastometry. Some centres do not have this technology and have to rely on laboratory-based coagulation tests, which often lag behind the clinical picture. Appropriate goals are an international normalised ratio (INR) of less than 1.5, a platelet count of greater than 50×10^9/litre and fibrinogen concentrations greater than 1.5 g/l.

Postoperative management

Patients require close monitoring after abdominal vascular surgery. Traditionally this has been provided in an intensive care unit to allow for a short period of postoperative ventilation. However, careful patient selection following meticulous preassessment, coupled with improvements in anaesthetic and surgical techniques, allow early extubation and immediate transfer to a high-dependency unit in many patients [3].

Early enteral nutrition is encouraged to maintain gut mucosal integrity and reduce bacterial translocation. Nasogastric tubes are not routinely required. Good glycaemic control is important.

Appropriate antacid, thromboembolic and antibiotic prophylaxis should be prescribed, and early mobilisation encouraged.

Following open aortic surgery patients must be closely monitored for cardiac events with serial ECGs and troponin measurements. Approximately 50% of perioperative MIs are caused by coronary plaque rupture, with 50% caused by an imbalance between myocardial O_2 supply and demand. The management of perioperative MI differs from management of MI in the medical setting because of the risk of bleeding associated with thrombolysis. In general management involves good analgesia, rate control and antiplatelet drugs (aspirin or clopidogrel). Some patients may be suitable for immediate coronary angiography and 'rescue' balloon angioplasty. Close liaison with a cardiology colleague is essential.

The possibility of concealed postoperative bleeding must be borne in mind in the unstable patient. Drains are not routinely used in infrarenal AAA surgery; the aneurysm sac is closed around the aortic graft. Patients must be closely observed for signs of increasing abdominal distension. Deranged coagulation indices must be rapidly corrected with appropriate quantities of blood products. Rarely patients may need to return to theatre for re-exploration if blood loss continues.

Postoperative renal performance should be closely monitored [16]. The incidence of renal dysfunction after infrarenal AAA surgery is around 5%, of which 0.6% require haemodialysis. Mortality exceeds 25% if renal failure occurs. Risk factors for the development of renal failure include:

(1) Pre-existing disease:
- Renal insufficiency
- Cardiac failure
- Hypertension
- Diabetes mellitus
- Renal artery artherosclerosis/stenosis

(2) Operative factors:
- Suprarenal cross-clamp
- Prolonged cross-clamp time
- Intraoperative hypotension
- Massive blood loss

(3) Others:
- Increasing age
- Drugs (non-steroidal anti-inflammatory drugs, ACE inhibitors, aminoglycosides).

The renal medulla receives only 20% of the total renal blood flow, making it highly susceptible to hypoxic injury due to its high oxygen extraction rate. Maintaining an adequate circulating volume reduces the requirement for active reabsorption of salt and water, reducing medullary oxygen requirements and reducing the risk of perioperative renal dysfunction. Infrarenal cross-clamping reduces renal blood flow by up to 40% through the alteration of the renin–angiotensin system. This can increase renal vascular resistance, causing maldistribution of blood flow away from the medulla and deterioration in glomerular filtration rate. Loop diuretics (e.g. furosemide), dopamine, mannitol, fenoldapam and N-acetylcysteine have been proposed to protect the kidney. There is no Level 1 evidence to support their use. The mainstay of renal preservation is maintenance of oxygen delivery and the avoidance of nephrotoxic drugs.

Ischaemic colitis is a rare complication after infrarenal AAA surgery (0.6%). Sacrifice of the inferior mesenteric artery means that the descending colon, sigmoid colon and rectum are dependent on collateral circulation. If this is inadequate the bowel may become ischaemic. Risk factors include a suprarenal cross-clamp, prolonged clamp times and pre-existing mesenteric artery atherosclerosis. Ischaemic colitis presents with bloody diarrhoea, abdominal pain and unexplained fever or leucocytosis. Persistent postoperative metabolic acidosis with rising lactate concentrations which cannot be attributed to other causes should precipitate urgent surgical re-exploration.

Spinal cord ischaemia is a rare but devastating complication of infrarenal AAA repair; it is much more common after thoracic aneurysm repairs. A flaccid paraparesis with dissociated sensory loss occurs in fewer than 0.5% of elective infrarenal AAA repairs; this incidence increases in emergency aortic surgery.

The distal circulation needs to be closely monitored. Distal atheroembolism may occur which may require exploration and possible embolectomy if the viability of the lower extremity is compromised.

Postoperative analgesia

The mainstay of postoperative analgesia in the majority of patients after infrarenal AAA surgery is with an epidural infusion of low-dose local anaesthetic combined with an opioid. Multimodal analgesia is introduced as soon as possible.

Rarely the insertion of an epidural may be contra-indicated. Should this be the case anaesthesia of the anterior abdominal wall may be provided by transversus abdominis plane (TAP) blocks or rectus sheath catheters supplemented by systemic opioids administered by a patient-controlled analgesia device.

References

1. Ashton HA, Buxton MJ, Day NE, *et al*. The Multicentre Aneurysm Screening Study (MASS) into the effect of abdominal aortic aneurysm screening on mortality in men: a randomised controlled trial. *Lancet* 2002;**360**:1531–9.

2. Sakalihasan N, Limet R, Defawe O. Abdominal aortic aneurysm. *Lancet* 2005;**365**:1577–89.

3. National Confidential Enquiry into Patient Outcome and Death. *Abdominal Aortic Aneurysm: A Service in Need of Surgery?* London: NCEPOD, 2005. Available at www.ncepod.org.uk/ 2005report2/Downloads/ AAA_report.pdf

4. Poldermans D, Bax JJ, Boersma E, *et al*. Guidelines for pre-operative cardiac risk assessment and perioperative cardiac management in non-cardiac surgery. *Eur Heart J* 2009;**30**:2769–812.

5. Fleisher LA, Beckman JA, Buller CE, *et al*. ACCF/AHA focussed update on perioperative beta blockade incorporated into the ACCF/AHA 2007 guidelines in perioperative evaluation and care for non cardiac surgery. *J Am Coll Cardiol* 2009;**54**:e13–118.

6. Wilson RJT, Davies S, Yates D, *et al*. Impaired functional capacity is associated with all-cause mortality after major intra-abdominal surgery. *Br J Anaesth* 2010;**105**:297–303.

7. Hindler K, Shaw AD, Samuels J, *et al*. Improved postoperative outcomes associated with preoperative statin therapy. *Anesthesiology* 2006;**105**:1260–72.

8. POISE Study Group. Effects of sustained release metoprolol succinate on patients undergoing non cardiac surgery: a randomised controlled trial. *Lancet* 2008;**371**:1839–47.

9. Biccard BM, Rodseth RM. A meta-analysis of the prospective randomised trials of coronary revascularisation before noncardiac vascular surgery with attention to the type of coronary revascularisation performed. *Anaesthesia* 2009;**64**:1105–13.

10. Spahn DR, Howell SJ, Delebays A, Chassot PG. Coronary stents and perioperative antiplatelet regimen: dilemma of bleeding and stent thrombosis. *Br J Anaesth* 2006;**96**:675–7.

11. Ballantyne JC. Does epidural analgesia improve surgical outcome? *Br J Anaesth* 2004;**92**:4–6.

12. NICE. *The Management of Inadvertent Perioperative Hypothermia in Adults*. London: NICE, 2008. Available at www. nice.org.uk/nicemedia/live/11962/ 40429/40429.pdf

13. Frank SM, Fleisher LA, Breslow MJ, *et al*. Perioperative maintenance of normothermia reduces the incidence of morbid cardiac events: a randomized clinical trial. *JAMA* 1997;**277**:1127–34.

14. Thomas D, Wee M, Clyburn P, *et al*. Blood transfusion and the anaesthetist: management of massive haemorrhage. *Anaesthesia* 2010;**65**:1153–61.

15. Madjdpour C, Spahn DR. Allogeneic blood transfusion: efficacy, risks, alternatives and indications. *Br J Anaesth* 2005;**95**:33–42.

16. Sear JW. Kidney dysfunction in the postoperative period. *Br J Anaesth* 2005;**95**:20–32.

Anaesthesia for thoracoabdominal aortic aneurysm surgery

Carl Moores and Alastair F. Nimmo

Introduction

A thoracoabdominal aortic aneurysm (TAAA) is an aneurysm which involves the visceral arteries: the coeliac axis, superior mesenteric artery (SMA) and the renal arteries. Most TAAAs are due to degenerative aortic disease, but a significant number, 5.9–10.4%, are the result of Marfan syndrome [1,2]. The extent of surgery required and the fact that blood flow to the abdominal organs and the spinal cord is interrupted during surgery means that their anaesthetic management is particularly challenging.

Classification of thoracoabdominal aneurysms

A modification of Crawford's classification of TAAAs is commonly used, and is shown in Figure 11.1. Extent I extends from just distal to the left subclavian artery to the renal arteries; extent II extends from the left subclavian artery to the aortic bifurcation; extent III from the level of the sixth rib to the aortic bifurcation and extent IV from the diaphragm to the aortic bifurcation. To these four original classes, a fifth, extent V, was added which extends from the sixth rib to the renal arteries. There are big differences in the rates of mortality and complications from surgery on the different extents of TAAA, particularly in relation to paraplegia.

Methods of repair

Traditionally TAAAs are repaired by open surgery which involves a thoracolaparotomy, and one-lung anaesthesia, cross-clamping the thoracic aorta, incising the aneurysm and suturing a prosthetic graft within it, then reattaching visceral and intercostal arteries.

Extent IV TAAAs may also be repaired using only a laparotomy with a clamp being passed behind the diaphragm to clamp the bottom of the thoracic aorta.

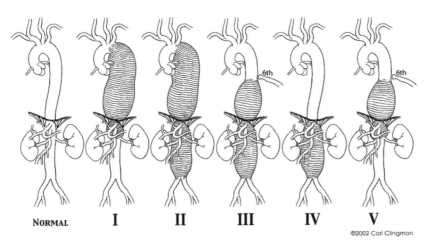

Figure 11.1 Crawford classification of thoracoabdominal aortic aneurysms. Reproduced with permission from *Annals of Surgery* 2003;**238**:372–81.

NORMAL   I   II   III   IV   V

©2002 Carl Clingman

Core Topics in Vascular Anaesthesia, ed. Carl Moores and Alastair F. Nimmo. Published by Cambridge University Press.
© Cambridge University Press 2012.

A prosthetic graft is then anastomosed obliquely to the anterior part of the upper abdominal aorta.

Stent grafts for endovascular repair of TAAAs have been developed in recent years, but excluding the aneurysm so that is does not continue to expand while simultaneously maintaining blood flow into the visceral arteries is technically challenging and blood flow cannot be restored to intercostals arteries covered by the stent. The rates of death and short- and long-term complications after endovascular repair of TAAAs are considerably higher than after endovascular repair of AAAs.

An alternative approach is a 'hybrid' repair – a combination of open surgery and endovascular repair. For example aortic visceral debranching may be undertaken – a four-branched bypass graft is performed surgically from the lower abdominal aorta or an iliac artery to the coeliac axis, SMA and both renal arteries which are then oversewn at their origins from the aorta. A stent-graft which covers the origins of these vessels can then be inserted without causing visceral ischaemia (but may cause spinal cord ischaemia). The hybrid repair involves periods of renal, hepatic and bowel ischaemia which are shorter than in conventional TAAA repair but it is nevertheless a major procedure with a high incidence of complications including paraplegia.

Endovascular and hybrid repair is covered in more detail in Chapter 12. In the remainder of this chapter we will discuss conventional open surgery.

Surgery for TAAAs was pioneered by Stanley Crawford in Houston, Texas. Crawford did not use heparin or a bypass circuit. After clamping the thoracic aorta, the abdominal viscera and spinal cord became ischaemic and it was necessary to anastomose the graft to the thoracic aorta and reattach visceral and intercostals artery origins to windows cut out of the graft very quickly if multiple organ failure and paraplegia were to be avoided.

Distal aortic perfusion

During open repair of all but extent IV aneurysms, it is now usual to use a bypass pump to maintain blood flow to the distal aorta while the surgeon performs the thoracic aortic anastomosis between two clamps. Two common techniques are employed: left heart bypass and femoro-femoral bypass.

In left heart bypass, a cannula is inserted via one of the pulmonary veins into the left atrium from

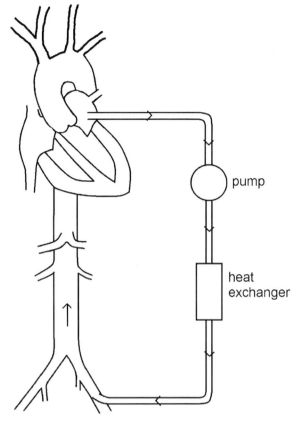

Figure 11.2 Partial left heart bypass. See text for details.

where blood is pumped by a centrifugal pump to the left femoral artery. Oxygenation of the blood is not usually required but a heat exchanger is often included in the circuit in order that the patient may be cooled as part of a strategy for visceral organ and spinal cord protection (Figure 11.2). In femoro-femoral bypass, a cannula is passed via a femoral vein into the inferior vena cava and blood is pumped through an oxygenator and heat exchanger to the left femoral artery. In both cases, blood passes up the abdominal aorta perfusing the abdominal viscera, the iliac and lumbar arteries and, depending on the position of the thoracic aortic clamps, lower intercostals arteries. The left ventricle continues to pump blood to the vessels proximal to the thoracic clamp including the coronary and carotid arteries.

Heparin is given before instituting distal aortic perfusion. However, the use of tubing and a heat exchanger/oxygenator with an antithrombotic coating and the absence of a reservoir in the circuit enables a lesser degree of anticoagulation to be used than is required for full cardio-pulmonary bypass. For example, the activated clotting time (ACT) may be maintained over 200 seconds.

Before reattachment of the visceral arteries to the aortic graft, a clamp is placed across the abdominal aorta below the renal arteries. Blood pumped from the bypass pump into the femoral artery then no longer perfuses the abdominal viscera. Some surgeons connect branches from the bypass pump to cannulae placed in the ostia of the coeliac axis, SMA and renal arteries, allowing blood to be supplied to them during part of the period during which the visceral anastomoses are being performed. However, this technique can introduce complications of its own such as dissection of the visceral arteries.

Extent I, II, III and V repair

The surgical repair of the more extensive TAAAs is via a thoracoabdominal incision with the patient in the right lateral position. The surgeon first exposes the entire aneurysm. In the chest, during one-lung anaesthesia with the left lung collapsed, the aneurysm is dissected free and is separated from the diaphragm. In the abdomen, the surgeon needs to approach the aneurysm posteriorly in order to perform the visceral anastomosis. To achieve this, the surgeon carries out a *medial visceral rotation*. The spleen and the left kidney are dissected free and retracted over to the right. As the patient is in the right lateral position this means that the left kidney comes to lie almost next to the right kidney and posterior wall of the abdominal part of the aneurysm is exposed. If distal aortic perfusion is to be used, this is instigated at this point and flow to the distal aorta established (see above).

A process of 'serial clamping' is usually employed. For example, in repair of an extent II aneurysm, the aorta is first clamped above the aneurysm and the aneurysm itself is clamped in the chest. Although the thoracic aorta is now clamped, blood flow to the viscera and spinal cord is maintained via the distal aortic perfusion. The aortic sac is opened, the aorta is transected above the aneurysm and the proximal end of the graft is sewn into place. After the proximal anastomosis has been completed the aortic graft is clamped and the upper aortic clamp is released.

The lower clamp is then moved down to the level of the diaphragm, the lower thoracic portion of the aneurysm is opened and any large intercostal arteries

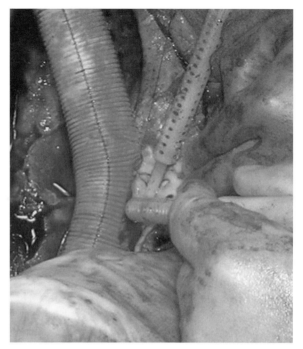

Figure 11.3 Visceral anastomosis during a thoracoabdominal aneurysm repair. The ostia of the visceral vessels, viewed from within the lumen of the aorta, are visible near the surgical suckers. An aperture has been cut in the graft, which is about to be sewn over the visceral vessels.

are reattached to the graft in order to reduce the risk of paraplegia. The graft is then flushed and clamped distal to the intercostal anastomoses before releasing the upper clamp on the graft to perfuse the reattached intercostals arteries.

The surgeon now performs the visceral anastomosis. The aneurysm is clamped below the visceral arteries. The aneurysm sac is opened to expose the ostia of the visceral arteries in its anterior wall. If the surgeon is using selective perfusion of visceral vessels from the bypass pump (see above), this is established now. The surgeon then cuts an aperture in the aortic graft which should ideally be large enough to include the ostia of all the visceral vessels. The aperture in the graft is then sewn onto the anterior wall of the sac, so that the visceral vessels are contained within it (Figure 11.3). The graft is then flushed, clamped distally and the proximal graft clamp is released. At this point, blood flows through the graft into the visceral arteries and the abdominal organs are reperfused. It is important that the period of visceral ischaemia is kept to a minimum, ideally less than an hour. If the coeliac axis and SMA are not perfused for much longer than this there is a high risk of death and complications. It is not always possible to include the left renal artery within the visceral anastomosis, in which case it is attached separately to the aortic graft via a short jump graft. With the viscera reperfused, the surgeon now performs the distal anastomosis of the graft to the aortic bifurcation.

Extent IV TAAA repair may be undertaken in many patients by a total abdominal approach, i.e. by laparotomy rather than thoracolaparotomy. Although access to clamp the distal part of the thoracic aorta is required, this is achieved from the abdomen by separating the crura of the diaphragm. The top end of the graft is often cut obliquely so that an anastomosis is formed between the graft posteriorly and the anterior part of the native aorta containing the orifices of the visceral arteries. Distal aortic perfusion is not usually used.

Preoperative assessment

Thoracoabdominal aortic aneurysm surgery involves a huge wound and extensive surgical dissection in a patient who is typically elderly and often has cardiac, respiratory or renal disease. Unlike AAA surgery where only the pelvis and lower limbs become ischaemic, TAAA repair also involves ischaemia of the bowel, liver, kidneys and often spinal cord. Massive haemorrhage from a combination of surgical bleeding and severe coagulopathy is common. It is not surprising that mortality and morbidity rates are much higher than for AAA repair and very careful assessment of a patient's fitness is required before embarking on surgery.

Mortality rates for TAAA repair have been reported as 5–14% but the mortality is higher for more extensive (extent I and II) TAAAs, and for emergency surgery [1,3–7]. This surgery should only be undertaken in specialist centres by an experienced team who undertake these procedures regularly.

The principles of preoperative risk assessment outlined in Chapter 2 apply. The risks of an individual patient dying or suffering major complications as the result of TAAA surgery will be much higher than if the same patient underwent AAA surgery. In some cases the combination of the patient's age and coexisting disease indicate a very high risk of perioperative death and complications and that if the patient survives surgery, recovery to the point where he or she feels well is likely to be very prolonged. Conservative

management may be more appropriate than surgery in this situation.

Particular concerns during assessment are the presence of coronary artery disease or cardiac failure, respiratory disease and renal impairment. Published studies on the risk of cardiac complications in vascular surgery patients and the benefits of coronary artery bypass grafting (CABG) before surgery in patients having AAA surgery or lower limb revascularisation cannot necessarily be extrapolated to TAAA surgery. In our experience the presence of significant multi-vessel coronary artery disease is associated with a high incidence of cardiac complications during surgery. Therefore, in addition to cardiopulmonary exercise testing, we routinely undertake CT coronary angiography and sometimes also dobutamine stress echocardiography, and patients with cardiac disease are reviewed by a cardiologist with a special interest in cardiac disease in vascular surgery patients. Where severe coronary artery disease is present, preoperative CABG or conservative management of the aneurysm may be considered.

Anaesthetic management

Anaesthesia for TAAA surgery cannot satisfactorily be undertaken by one anaesthetist working alone. Profound falls in blood pressure may suddenly occur as a result of haemorrhage and/or reperfusion of ischaemic tissues and can progress to cardiac arrest unless treated very rapidly. Management of this situation requires large-bore peripheral venous cannulae and central venous catheters, rapid infusion systems and the presence of at least two senior anaesthetists. Red cell salvage and retransfusion is used to reduce allogeneic blood transfusion. We use two cell salvage machines with the red cells being pumped into the reservoir of a rapid infusion system.

Surgery for TAAA may be undertaken either under general anaesthesia or combined general and epidural anaesthesia. The advantage of inserting an epidural catheter is that good analgesia with little sedation may be achieved after surgery by infusing local anaesthetic (alone or with a low concentration of opioid) and the risk of postoperative respiratory failure may be reduced. On the other hand, motor block from the local anaesthetic may be confused with leg weakness resulting from spinal cord ischaemia. It is the authors' practice to insert a mid or lower thoracic epidural catheter and at the same time to insert a

Table 11.1 Recommended additional monitoring during TAAA repair

A second invasive blood pressure

Transoesophageal echocardiography

Point-of-care monitoring of arterial gases, haemoglobin and electrolytes including calcium, glucose

Point-of-care monitoring of coagulation with thromboelastometry/thromboelastography

Depth of anaesthesia monitoring

Neuromuscular transmission monitoring

Cerebral oximetry

lumbar cerebrospinal fluid (CSF) drain (except for extent IV operations where the risk of postoperative paraplegia is lower). A double-lumen tracheal tube (usually left-sided) is inserted except where repair of an extent IV aneurysm without thoracotomy is planned.

Monitoring

Routine monitoring includes invasive arterial (radial or brachial) and central venous pressure monitoring. A pulmonary artery catheter may be inserted and can be used to measure cardiac output and mixed venous oxygen saturation in addition to pulmonary artery pressures. Additional recommended monitoring is shown in Table 11.1.

Blood loss can be sudden, large and rapid. The effect of hypovolaemia on the arterial blood pressure in the upper body is exaggerated if distal aortic perfusion is being used because the pump 'steals' the venous return to the heart resulting in an empty ventricle and little cardiac output. Rapid fluid administration and temporary reduction in pump flow is required to restore the cardiac output and upper body blood pressure A second radial (or brachial) arterial cannula enables blood pressure to be monitored continuously including during blood sampling for point-of-care testing. Some centres also monitor femoral arterial pressure if distal aortic perfusion is used.

Transoesophageal echocardiography (TOE) is a useful monitor of both ventricular filling and ventricular function and can alert the anaesthetist to new areas of ventricular wall motion abnormality which suggest myocardial ischaemia. Further, TOE

can be a particularly valuable aid to diagnosis when severe hypotension occurs during surgery and the cause is not clear.

Frequent near-patient testing during surgery (for example every 30 minutes) is an invaluable guide to appropriate treatment and should include monitoring of coagulation with thromboelastometry/thromboelastography (see Chapter 8). We routinely take samples for coagulation testing from one arterial cannula and samples into a syringe containing heparin for arterial gas analysis from the other arterial cannula to avoid the possibility of heparin contamination of the coagulation samples.

Hypothermia, periods of liver and renal ischaemia and hypoperfusion, and massive haemorrhage can profoundly alter the pharmacokinetics and pharmacodynamics of anaesthetics, opioids and muscle relaxants. Monitoring of the depth of anaesthesia assists the anaesthetist to avoid excessive doses of anaesthetic whilst ensuring that awareness is unlikely.

During repair of extent I and II TAAAs the surgeon may have to cross-clamp the aorta close to, or even proximal to, the origin of the left common carotid artery. Monitoring of cerebral oximetry with a left frontal sensor can provide a warning that blood supply to the left cerebral cortex may be inadequate. Raising the upper body blood pressure in this situation may improve collateral flow.

Intraoperative management

Moderate hypothermia e.g. to 32 °C may be used to reduce the oxygen consumption of organs that will become ischaemic during surgery. If distal aortic perfusion is used, a heat exchanger in the bypass circuit can be used to cool the patient before aortic clamping and to rewarm after the completion of the anastomoses. Cooling and warming may also be achieved by altering the temperature of the operating room, underbody water-filled blankets and an over-body blanket into which room temperature air is pumped for cooling or warm air for warming.

Visceral ischaemia, which typically lasts between 30 minutes and 1 hour, results in a severe metabolic acidosis and hyperglycaemia. Sodium bicarbonate and insulin infusions are guided by the results of point-of-care testing. Patients also develop hypocalcaemia and hypomagnesaemia, and it is the authors' practice to infuse these ions continuously during the procedure.

Large changes in blood pressure are common during TAAA surgery as a result of aortic clamping, blood loss and reperfusion of ischaemic tissues. Maintaining an acceptable blood pressure is challenging. After clamping of the thoracic aorta it is desirable to maintain a relatively high upper body arterial pressure to increase collateral flow to the anterior spinal artery. Indeed the spinal cord may remain vulnerable to ischaemia as a result of hypotension throughout the rest of surgery and postoperatively. The anaesthetist should be prepared to rapidly infuse fluid at any point during the procedure and also to manage the blood pressure pharmacologically. For example, intravenous infusions of norepinephrine, dobutamine, esmolol and glyceryl trinitrate may be primed and connected so that they can be started without delay.

Cerebrospinal fluid drainage is carried out in most centres during TAAA surgery to reduce the risk of spinal cord ischaemia (see below). We employ prophylactic CSF drainage for all except extent IV TAAAs (which have a lower risk of paraplegia). Strategies vary, but it is the authors' practice to drain CSF at 10 mm Hg above heart level during most of the procedure, decreasing this to 0 mm Hg during the period of thoracic aortic clamping. We continue to drain CSF at 10 mm Hg for 48 hours postoperatively, although in some centres, CSF is not routinely drained postoperatively unless there is evidence of spinal cord injury.

It is essential that coagulation abnormalities have been corrected by the end of surgery and that there is no significant ongoing bleeding when the chest and abdomen are closed.

Preventing spinal cord ischaemia

Paraplegia is a particularly devastating complication of TAAA surgery. It is a consequence of spinal cord ischaemia during and/or after surgery. Lower intercostal and lumbar arteries arising from the posterior wall of the aneurysm form an important component of the blood supply to the anterior spinal artery (see Chapter 12). When the thoracic aorta is clamped, blood flow into these segmental arteries distal to the clamp ceases and cord ischaemia or infarction may occur. Typically, this injury affects only the anterior part of the spinal cord. It therefore predominantly involves the anteriorly placed descending motor tracts, while sparing the ascending sensory tracts

which are found more posteriorly. Patients therefore develop weakness of one or both legs without a sensory loss (anterior spinal artery syndrome). Intercostal and lumbar arteries may be reattached to the aortic graft during surgery but cord perfusion after surgery may remain precarious so that ischaemia develops if the blood pressure falls.

The likelihood of spinal cord damage and postoperative paraplegia increases the more extensive the surgery and the greater the number of segmental vessels that are affected. It is therefore greatest with extent I, II and III repairs. Spinal cord injury is also more likely with emergency surgery and with aortic dissections. Crawford was the first to report paraplegia in a large series of TAAA repairs, with an incidence of 38% among more extensive extent I and II repairs. With advances in spinal cord protection, the incidence of paraplegia, even in the more extensive TAAA repairs, has fallen. Contemporary reports suggest an incidence of paraplegia of 4–15% [1–3,5–7].

A number of different strategies have been adopted in an effort to reduce the incidence of paraplegia. These include surgical re-anastomosis of large intercostal or lumbar arteries to the aortic graft, distal aortic perfusion during the thoracic anastomosis (see above), CSF drainage, hypothermia (of the CSF or the patient generally), and pharmacological methods.

Surgical strategies to reduce spinal cord injury

Where possible, the surgeon connects larger lower intercostal and upper lumbar arteries to aortic graft. In some centres, an attempt is made to identify radiologically before surgery which vessels are likely to be most important in supplying the spinal cord in order to guide the surgeon. Alternatively, intraoperative monitoring may be used as a guide to whether further vessels need to be reanastomosed.

Intraoperative monitoring of spinal cord function

Intraoperative monitoring of spinal cord function can alert the anaesthetist and surgeon to the presence of spinal cord ischaemia. Treatment can then be instigated; for example mean arterial pressure can be increased and, if a patient is on left heart bypass, the flow to the distal aorta can be increased.

Somatosensory evoked potentials (SEPs) and motor evoked potentials (MEPs) have both been used to monitor spinal cord function. Motor evoked potentials have the advantage that they monitor the function of the anterior part of the spinal cord, which is the part of the cord most likely to be affected by ischaemia. Monitoring of MEPs is discussed further in Chapter 12.

Jacobs published a series of 52 patients who underwent extent I and II TAAA repair with spinal cord monitoring using MEPs [11]. Where MEPs indicated spinal cord ischaemia, this was reversed by increasing distal aortic perfusion or reimplanting intercostal or lumbar arteries into the aortic graft. No patients in the series developed leg weakness.

Cerebrospinal fluid drainage

Cerebrospinal fluid drainage is one of the most widely practised techniques to reduce the incidence of paraplegia during aortic surgery.

It is known that CSF pressure increases in response to aortic clamping, and this decreases the spinal cord perfusion pressure. Decreasing the CSF pressure should therefore increase the cord perfusion pressure and reduce the risk of cord ischaemia. Studies in dogs showed that aortic clamping was associated with a reduction in blood flow in the thoraco-lumbar spinal cord to 2.4 ml/100 g per minute and that this increased to 6–10 ml/100 g per minute in response to CSF drainage. This increase in blood flow was sufficient to prevent paraplegia in response to partial spinal cord ischaemia applied for up to 1 hour [12]. This led to the adoption of CSF drainage in a number of centres, although the success of this in reducing paraplegia rates in TAAA surgery was initially mixed.

Crawford performed a prospective trial in 1991 in which 100 patients were randomised into a treatment group receiving CSF drainage and a control group who did not [13]. No difference in the incidence of neurological deficit was found between the treatment group (30%) and the control group (33%). However, CSF was only drained intraoperatively, and the total volume of CSF drained was limited to 50 ml.

Coselli published a study in 2002, in which 156 patients undergoing extent I and extent II TAAA aneurysm repairs were randomised to receive CSF drainage or not. Mild hypothermia, left heart bypass and the reimplantation of critical intercostal or lumbar vessels were employed. Cerebrospinal fluid was drained to a pressure of 10 mm Hg for 48 hours postoperatively (or longer if a neurological deficit was present). A mean of 64 ml of CSF was drained intra-operatively and 260 ml postoperatively. In the CSF drainage group the incidence of paraplegia was 2.7%, compared to 13.3% in the control group [2].

In a systematic review of published literature Cinà identified three randomised controlled trials looking at the effect of CSF drainage on spinal cord injury in patients with extent I and II TAAA [14]. These included the two studies mentioned above and a third by Svensson et al., in which the treatment group received intrathecal papaverine as well as CSF drainage. Combining these studies in a meta-analysis, Cinà found an incidence of lower limb neurological deficit of 12% in patients treated with CSF drainage, compared with 33% in control patients. He also found a similar reduction in the incidence of neurological deficit in cohort studies.

As well as providing protection against neurological deficit, there are many published examples of CSF drainage being successfully instigated to treat late-onset neurological deficit following TAAA repair. Nevertheless, the paucity of well-conducted, prospective randomised controlled trials of CSF draining in TAAA surgery led the authors of a *Cochrane Review* on the subject to conclude only that 'there is limited evidence that perioperative CSF drainage appears to reduce the rate of paraplegia after repair of type I and II TAAA'.

Drainage of CSF is achieved by the insertion of a needle into the lumbar subarachnoid space, confirmed by the free flow of CSF. A catheter is then threaded through the needle. Purpose-designed lumbar CSF drainage kits are available and these larger catheters drain CSF more effectively than epidural catheters. Cerebrospinal fluid drainage manometers allow the drainage pressure to be adjusted – when CSF pressure reaches the limit that has been set it spills over into a collecting chamber. It is the authors' practice to drain CSF at 10 mm Hg during surgery and for 48 hours postoperatively, reducing this to 0 mm Hg during aortic clamping. We set the zero point of 0 mm Hg at heart level.

Cerebrospinal fluid drainage is not without complication, however. Haematomas may occur within the spinal cord itself or within the spinal canal leading to neurological complications [15,16]. Cerebrospinal fluid drainage is also associated with intracranial bleeding. In a series of 230 patients undergoing TAAA repair, Dardik reported six cases of postoperative subdural haematoma detected prior to discharge from hospital, three of whom died. There were a further two cases where subdural haematoma occurred several months after CSF drainage. Subdural haematoma appeared to be associated with large volumes of CSF drained [17]. In a series of 648 patients undergoing TAAA repair, Wynn performed a CT scan in 24 patients who had bloodstained CSF in their drains. Of these, 14 had had an intracranial bleed, either subdural, subarachnoid or intraparenchymal. Only three of these patients had neurological symptoms. She suggested that CSF hypotension may result in a caudal displacement of the brain which may lead to tears in the intracranial venous sinuses or blood vessels [18].

Hypothermia

Hypothermia reduces the metabolic requirements of nervous tissue and may therefore protect against the effects of ischaemia. Spinal cord hypothermia can be achieved either by cooling the patient as a whole or by attempting to cool the spinal cord alone.

Marsala showed that cooling the spinal cord, by infusing cold saline into the epidural space, was effective in preventing spinal cord injury in a dog model of spinal cord ischaemia [19]. This has led to a number of centres using epidural or CSF cooling, by the infusion of cold fluids. For example, Cambria infused cold saline and local anaesthetic drugs into the epidural space, monitoring temperature and pressure via a catheter placed in the CSF. Typically, they achieved a CSF temperature of 23–25 °C with an infusion rate of 4–5 ml/minute, and aimed to maintain a gradient of 40 mm Hg between arterial pressure and CSF pressure. They have reported an incidence of paraplegia of 10.6% in patients undergoing epidural cooling during repair of extent I and II TAAA, compared to 19.8% in historical controls [3].

Drugs used for spinal cord protection
Naloxone

It is known that extracellular levels of excitatory amino acids (EAAs) such as glycine, glutamate and taurine are elevated in models of brain ischaemia and it is thought that these EAAs may contribute to neurotoxicity (excitotoxicity). Drugs such as naloxone, which reduce extracellular concentrations of EAAs, might therefore be neuroprotective. Kunihana has shown that in patients undergoing TAAA repair, CSF levels of EAAs are higher in patients who suffered spinal cord injury compared to those who

did not. He has also shown that intravenous naloxone significantly reduces CSF levels of EAAs [20].

In a series of 110 patients undergoing thoracic and thoracoabdominal aneurysm repair, some of whom received naloxone, Acher reported one case of spinal cord injury out of 61 patients in the naloxone group compared with 11 cases out of 49 patients in the control group [21].

On the other hand, it is possible that opioid drugs may contribute to spinal cord injury. In an animal model of spinal cord ischaemia, the administration of opioid drugs worsened neurological injury [22]. Kakinohana reported a case where epidural morphine was administered post TAAA repair. The patient developed a paraparesis which was reversed with naloxone [23].

Papaverine

Svensson has suggested that the intrathecal administration of the vasodilator papaverine reduces the incidence of spinal cord injury in TAAA surgery [24]. He published a series in which there were no neurological deficits in 11 patients undergoing extent I and II TAAA repair with CSF drainage and papaverine compared to 8 patients with neurological deficits in a similar group of 19 patients in whom these interventions were not used. It is difficult to know how much of this benefit was due to CSF drainage but the assumption is that the vasodilator may further increase blood flow in the spinal cord, thereby reducing ischaemia.

Reducing renal injury

Patients undergoing TAAA surgery suffer renal injury as a result of ischaemia to the kidneys. The incidence of postoperative renal failure requiring dialysis is reported as 4.8–15% [1–3,5,7]. Postoperative renal failure has been reported to be associated with preoperative renal insufficiency, a prolonged period of aortic clamping, extensive atherosclerosis, the need for separate left renal artery attachment to the aortic graft and, interestingly, some authors have found an association between the use of distal aortic perfusion and renal failure. Postoperative renal failure is associated with a worse outcome after surgery [8–10].

In order to reduce the magnitude of the perioperative renal injury, the period of renal ischaemia should be as short as possible, nephrotoxic drugs should be avoided and hypotension and low cardiac output avoided after renal reperfusion.

A number of additional strategies have been tried in an attempt to reduce renal injury during TAAA repair. Selective perfusion of the kidneys with blood from the distal aortic perfusion pump may be employed. An alternative strategy is to infuse cold crystalloid solution, typically at $4\,^{\circ}C$, into the renal arteries in order to reduce the metabolic demands and oxygen consumption of the kidneys. Köksoy randomised 30 patients undergoing extent II TAAA repair to receive renal artery perfusion with either Ringer's lactate solution at $4\,^{\circ}C$ or normothermic blood from the left heart bypass circuit. The incidence of acute renal dysfunction, defined as a serum creatinine rise of greater than 50% above baseline, was 63% in the blood group compared to 21% in the cold crystalloid group [25]. Lemaire randomised patients to undergo renal perfusion with either cold crystalloid solution or cold blood, but found that cold blood was not superior to cold crystalloid solution in preventing renal injury [26].

Postoperative management

In some centres, patients who have undergone repair of an extent IV TAAA via a total abdominal approach may be woken up and have the tracheal tube removed in the postanaesthesia care unit after an hour or two of postoperative lung ventilation. In other hospitals they are routinely transferred to the intensive care unit (ICU) after surgery with the tracheal tube in place.

Patients who have had a thoracolaparotomy have the double-lumen tracheal tube changed to a single-lumen tube after surgery and are transferred ventilated to the ICU. If the face is oedematous an airway exchange catheter can be used to facilitate the change of tracheal tube.

The anaesthetist's aim is that when the patient is transferred to the ICU, he or she is cardiovascularly stable with a satisfactory blood pressure, no coagulopathy or signs of ongoing bleeding, good gas exchange, normothermic and not acidotic.

Postoperative respiratory failure and difficulty weaning from lung ventilation is a common complication after TAAA repair involving thoracolaparotomy. Factors contributing to this include preoperative lung diseases – typically chronic obstructive pulmonary disease, the large thoracolaparotomy wound, surgical trauma to the diaphragm, prolonged one-lung anaesthesia, pulmonary remote reperfusion injury,

massive transfusion of blood components, postoperative pleural effusion and pneumonia. Respiratory function frequently deteriorates a day or two after surgery so caution is required before early weaning from ventilation and removal of the tracheal tube. Tracheostomy is appropriate if a prolonged period of lung ventilation appears likely to be required.

A vitally important aspect of postoperative management is that the patient is only lightly sedated so that movement of the lower limbs can be regularly assessed and charted. Our practice is to use low-dose infusions of propofol and remifentanil in combination with a dilute local anaesthetic infusion through a mid-thoracic epidural catheter. We have found that patients are usually sufficiently awake to move their legs to command within 1 hour of ICU admission. Spinal cord ischaemia may occur and result in weakness of one or both legs days or even weeks after surgery, often in association with hypotension. Therefore regular assessment and charting of power in the lower limbs must continue throughout the patient's hospital admission. Hypotension must be avoided and during the first 24 hours after repair of TAAAs (apart from extent IV) we maintain the mean arterial pressure (MAP) above 80 mm Hg.

If leg weakness develops, treatment involves raising the MAP and lowering the CSF drainage pressure (or reinserting a CSF drain if it has been removed). If there is uncertainty about whether epidural local anaesthetic is contributing to leg weakness, the epidural infusion should also be turned off for long enough for any local anaesthetic effect to wear off.

We routinely drain CSF at a pressure of 10 mm Hg above heart level for 48 hours after surgery if there is no leg weakness then stop draining CSF but leave the catheter in place for a further 24 hours before removing it if lower limb movements remain normal.

Fluid balance needs to be carefully managed postoperatively. There will be continuing fluid losses after surgery as a result of the extensive surgical dissection and trauma. Sufficient fluid, for example in the form of boluses of colloid, should be given to maintain an adequate circulating volume and cardiac filling. However hypotension after surgery is often the result of a combination of hypovolaemia and vasodilation and its management typically requires the combination of intravenous fluid and a vasoconstrictor infusion. Postoperative atrial fibrillation frequently occurs but appears to be less common in patients who are receiving a beta-blocker.

Coagulation should be monitored and any coagulopathy treated. If satisfactory haemostasis is present surgically and on point-of-care testing at the end of the operation then there is often little requirement for further blood components after surgery. A rise in creatinine is to be expected after surgery and in a minority of patients a period of renal replacement therapy will be required.

References

1. Coselli JS, Bozinovski J, LeMaire SA. Open surgical repair of 2286 thoracoabdominal aortic aneurysms. *Ann Thorac Surg* 2007;**83**:S862–4; discussion S890–2.

2. Coselli JS, LeMaire SA, Köksoy C, *et al.* Cerebrospinal fluid drainage reduces paraplegia after thoracoabdominal aortic aneurysm repair: results of a randomized clinical trial. *J Vasc Surg* 2002;**35**:631–9.

3. Cambria RP, Clouse WD, Davison JK, *et al.* Thoracoabdominal aneurysm repair: results with 337 operations performed over a 15-year interval. *Ann Surg* 2002;**236**:471–9; discussion 479.

4. Coselli JS, Conklin LD, LeMaire SA. Thoracoabdominal aortic aneurysm repair: review and update of current strategies. *Ann Thorac Surg* 2002;**74**:S1881–4; discussion S1892–8.

5. Coselli JS, LeMaire SA, Miller CC, *et al.* Mortality and paraplegia after thoracoabdominal aortic aneurysm repair: a risk factor analysis. *Ann Thorac Surg* 2000;**69**:409–14.

6. Grabitz K, Sandmann W, Stuhmeier K, *et al.* The risk of ischemic spinal cord injury in patients undergoing graft replacement for thoracoabdominal aortic aneurysms. *J Vasc Surg* 1996;**23**:230–40.

7. Schepens MA, Heijman RH, Ranschaert W, *et al.* Thoracoabdominal aortic aneurysm repair: results of conventional open surgery. *Eur J Vasc Endovasc Surg* 2009;**37**:640–5.

8. Jacobs MJ, Statius van Eps RG, De Jong DS, *et al.* Prevention of renal failure in patients undergoing thoracoabdominal aortic aneurysm repair. *J Vasc Surg* 2004;**40**:1067–73; discussion 1073.

9. Kashyap VS, Cambria RP, Davison JK, *et al.* Renal failure after thoracoabdominal aortic surgery. *J Vasc Surg* 1997;**26**: 949–55; discussion 955–7.

10. Safi HJ, Harlin SA, Miller CC, *et al.* Predictive factors for acute renal failure in thoracic and thoracoabdominal aortic aneurysm surgery. *J Vasc Surg* 1996;**24**:338–44; discussion 344–5.

11. Jacobs MJ, Meylaerts SA, de Haan P, *et al.* Strategies to prevent neurologic deficit based on motor-evoked potentials in type I and II thoracoabdominal aortic aneurysm repair. *J Vasc Surg* 1999;**29**:48–57; discussion 57–9.

12. Bower TC, Murray MJ, Gloviczki P, *et al.* Effects of thoracic aortic occlusion and cerebrospinal fluid drainage on regional spinal cord blood flow in dogs: correlation with neurologic outcome. *J Vasc Surg* 1989;**9**:135–44.

13. Crawford ES, Svensson LG, Hess KR, *et al.* A prospective randomized study of cerebrospinal fluid drainage to prevent paraplegia after high-risk surgery on the thoracoabdominal aorta. *J Vasc Surg* 1991;**13**:36–45; discussion 45–6.

14. Cina CS, Abouzahr L, Arena GO, *et al.* Cerebrospinal fluid drainage to prevent paraplegia during thoracic and thoracoabdominal aortic aneurysm surgery: a systematic review and meta-analysis. *J Vasc Surg* 2004;**40**:36–44.

15. Murakami H, Yoshida K, Hino Y, *et al.* Complications of cerebrospinal fluid drainage in thoracoabdominal aortic aneurysm repair. *J Vasc Surg* 2004;**39**:243–5.

16. Weaver KD, Wiseman DB, Farber M, *et al.* Complications of lumbar drainage after thoracoabdominal aortic aneurysm repair. *J Vasc Surg* 2001;**34**:623–7.

17. Dardik A, Perler BA, Roseborough GS, Williams GM. Subdural hematoma after thoracoabdominal aortic aneurysm repair: an underreported complication of spinal fluid drainage? *J Vasc Surg* 2002;**36**:47–50.

18. Wynn MM, Mell MW, Tefera G, *et al.* Complications of spinal fluid drainage in thoracoabdominal aortic aneurysm repair: a report of 486 patients treated from 1987 to 2008. *J Vasc Surg* 2009;**49**:29–34; discussion 34–5.

19. Marsala M, Vanicky I, Galik J, *et al.* Panmyelic epidural cooling protects against ischemic spinal cord damage. *J Surg Res* 1993;**55**:21–31.

20. Kunihara T, Shiiya N, Wakasa S, *et al.* Assessment of hepatosplanchnic pathophysiology during thoracoabdominal aortic aneurysm repair using visceral perfusion and shunt. *Eur J Cardiothorac Surg* 2009;**35**:677–83.

21. Acher CW, Wynn MM, Hoch JR, *et al.* Combined use of cerebral spinal fluid drainage and naloxone reduces the risk of paraplegia in thoracoabdominal aneurysm repair. *J Vasc Surg* 1994;**19**:236–46; discussion 247–8.

22. Kakinohana M, Nakamura S, Fuchigami T, *et al.* Mu and delta, but not kappa, opioid agonists induce spastic paraparesis after a short period of spinal cord ischaemia in rats. *Br J Anaesth* 2006;**96**:88–94.

23. Kakinohana M, Marsala M, Carter C, Davison JK, Yaksh TL. Neuraxial morphine may trigger transient motor dysfunction after a noninjurious interval of spinal cord ischemia: a clinical and experimental study. *Anesthesiology* 2003;**98**:862–70.

24. Svensson LG, Stewart RW, Cosgrove DM, *et al.* Intrathecal papaverine for the prevention of paraplegia after operation on the thoracic or thoracoabdominal aorta. *J Thorac Cardiovasc Surg* 1988;**96**:823–9.

25. Köksoy C, LeMaire SA, Curling PE, *et al.* Renal perfusion during thoracoabdominal aortic operations: cold crystalloid is superior to normothermic blood. *Ann Thorac Surg* 2002;**73**:730–8.

26. LeMaire SA, Jones MM, Conklin LD, *et al.* Randomized comparison of cold blood and cold crystalloid renal perfusion for renal protection during thoracoabdominal aortic aneurysm repair. *J Vasc Surg* 2009;**49**:11–9; discussion 19.

Chapter 2

Anaesthesia for endovascular aortic repair surgery

Maged Argalious

Introduction

Despite numerous advances in surgical and monitoring techniques that resulted in improved overall survival in patients with thoracoabdominal aneurysm undergoing open surgical repair [1], the open surgical approach with its associated aortic cross-clamp, large surgical incision and massive fluid shifts is still accompanied by a high incidence of postoperative 30-day mortality of 19% and a 1-year mortality as high as 31%. Postoperative morbidity involves multiple organ systems, and includes thrombotic events (myocardial infarction, deep venous thrombosis, pulmonary embolism, stroke), postoperative pulmonary complications (atelectasis, pneumonia, acute respiratory distress syndrome) and renal failure.

In 1991, the first cases of endovascular repair of the abdominal aorta, using a synthetic tube graft were described [2]. Despite the smaller surgical incision, the absence of aortic cross-clamping and a dramatic decline in fluid shifts, a large proportion of patients with thoracoabdominal aneurysms were not candidates for endovascular exclusion of their aortic aneurysms, mainly due to challenges in creating an adequate seal with these stents to avoid continuous aneurysm expansion (endoleaks), while avoiding the risk of graft migration and major vessel occlusion.

In the last 20 years several generations of endovascular stent-grafts by several manufacturers have helped extend the inclusion criteria to elective and emergent repair of thoracoabdominal aneurysms (Figure 12.1) [3], type B aortic dissections [4] and traumatic aortic injuries.

Evolution and types of endovascular aortic grafts

Endovascular stent-grafts are fabric or synthetic tube grafts reinforced by a wire frame that can be collapsed within a catheter for delivery and deployed within the aortic lumen via expansion with a ballooning catheter.

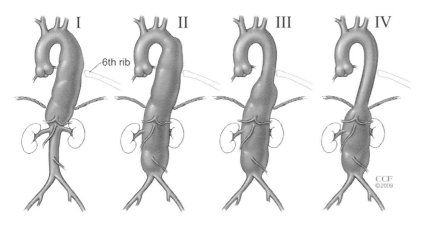

Figure 12.1 Crawford classification of thoracoabdominal aneurysms.

Core Topics in Vascular Anaesthesia, ed. Carl Moores and Alastair F. Nimmo. Published by Cambridge University Press.
© Cambridge University Press 2012.

The endovascular stent-graft is designed to be deployed within the aorta to span the length of the aneurysm and exclude blood flow into the aneurysm cavity.

Endovascular stent repair requires the existence of a 1-cm long non-tapered region of aorta on either end of the aneurysm, often called the aneurysm neck, to provide a landing zone for each end of the graft. Furthermore, aneurysms that span aortic branch vessels require either extra-anatomic bypass (also called aortic debranching) or coverage of the branch vessels to accomplish endovascular stent repair.

Endovascular aortic repair (EVAR) in the thoracic location is typically referred to as TEVAR (thoracic endovascular aortic repair) while EVAAR refers to endovascular abdominal aortic repair.

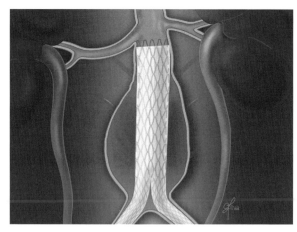

Figure 12.2 Modular bifurcated stent graft in the infrarenal aorta. See plate section for colour version.

Tube grafts

The first 'endografts' were aorto-aortic tube grafts with balloon-expandable stents stitched to either end [2]. These were effective in the short term but implantation sites in the distal aorta proved to be subject to a high failure rate due to underestimation of atheromatous disease in the aorto-iliac segment and continued expansion of the distal aorta.

Aorto-uni-iliac stent-grafts

This triggered the use of aorto-uni-iliac stent-grafts which required simultaneous occlusion of the contralateral iliac segment combined with a femoro-femoral cross-over graft to maintain blood flow to the contralateral leg.

Modular bifurcated stent-grafts

In the mid-1990s, modular bifurcated endografts were developed to preserve the normal anatomic configuration of the aorto-iliac segments and to enable devices to be applied to a wide range of vascular anatomy by allowing the pairing of different iliac sizes with each modular 'body' section (Figure 12.2). They may consist of two or three components (modules), depending on whether one or both iliac limbs are modular. Proximal fixation may consist of an infrarenal sealing stent (with or without hooks) or a suprarenal bare stent to provide 'transrenal fixation'.

Fenestrated stent-grafts

Endovascular grafts with fenestrations, which are openings within the graft fabric to accommodate visceral arteries, have been developed to improve the proximal seal by incorporating segments of the visceral arteries into the proximal sealing zone.

Fenestration refers to the creation of a hole within the stent-graft. The challenge is to line up this hole with the orifice of the branch artery, thereby maintaining end-organ perfusion while excluding the aneurysm. The addition of a nitinol ring to support the circumference of the fenestrations improves the seal between the aortic component and branched vessel grafts by mating the stent-graft and the nitinol ring reinforcing the fenestration.

Branched stent-grafts

Branched stent-grafts are used in the endovascular repair of aortic aneurysms that involve the origins of vital arteries (e.g. abdominal viscera) (Figure 12.3).

While fenestrated stent-grafts have no branches at all, just holes (i.e. fenestrations) in the wall of the primary graft, branches are added at the time of insertion when covered stents are used to bridge the gap between each fenestration and each target artery.

Branched stent-grafts can be categorised according to the type of connection between the trunk of the graft and its branches. The branches of a uni-body stent-graft are permanently attached to the trunk. They are pushed or pulled into the target arteries at the time of deployment using catheters and wires. The branches of a cuffed stent-graft are also attached to the trunk of the stent-graft, but they are not long enough to reach the target arteries without the addition of overlapping extensions in the form of covered stents.

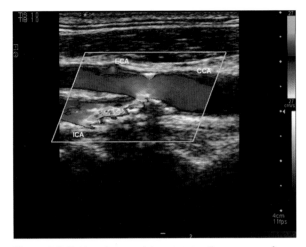

Figure 1.2 Duplex ultrasound demonstrates the presence of plaque at the carotid bifurcation.

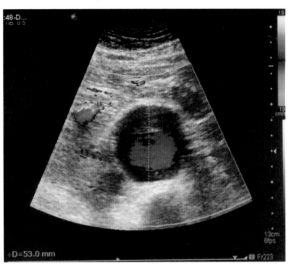

Figure 1.3 Ultrasound scan of abdominal aortic aneurysm.

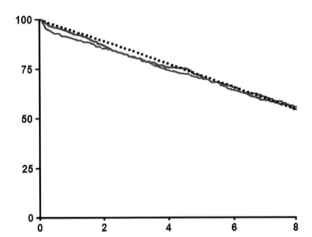

Figure 2.1 Survival 8 years after random allocation to open (blue line) or endovascular (red line) AAA repair: EVAR I study. The superimposed black dotted line is expected survival for a 77-year-old population, matched for fe/male proportions and median year of recruitment to EVAR I. Reproduced with permission from reference [3].

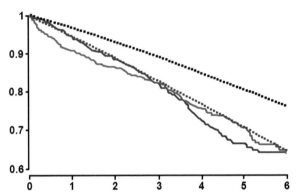

Figure 2.2 Survival 6 years after random allocation to open AAA repair (red line) or surveillance until AAA >5.4 cm diameter (blue line): UK small aneurysms study. The black dotted line is expected survival for the recruited population, matched for fe/male proportions and reported morbidities (equivalent to a 70-year-old population). The observed survival matches to a 75-year-old population (purple dotted line). Reproduced with permission from reference [5].

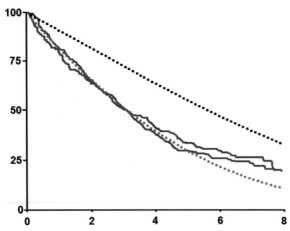

Figure 2.3 Survival 8 years after random allocation to endovascular AAA repair (red line) or no surgery (blue line): EVAR II study. The black dotted line is expected survival for the recruited population, matched for fe/male proportions and reported morbidities (equivalent to an 83-year-old population). The observed survival matches to a 91-year-old population (red dotted line). Reproduced with permission from reference [6].

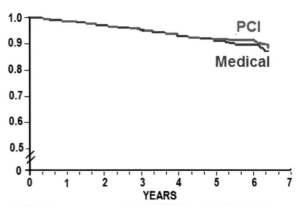

Figure 3.2 Equivalent survival in populations with stable ischaemic heart disease randomly allocated to early percutaneous coronary intervention, PCI (red line), of drugs (blue line). Reproduced with permission from reference [9].

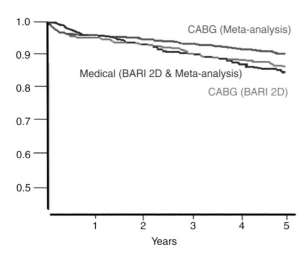

Figure 3.3 Survival in patients with stable coronary artery disease treated with drugs (blue line) or coronary artery bypass grafting (CABG). The red CABG survival curve is reproduced with permission from an early meta–analysis [10] and the orange CABG survival curve is reproduced with permission from reference [11].

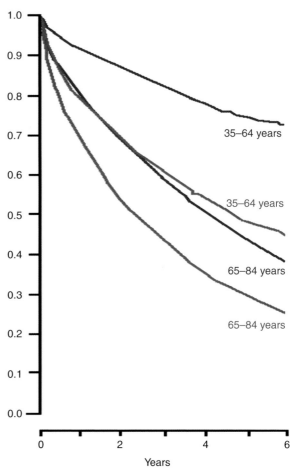

Figure 3.4 The improved survival of heart failure patients between 1988 and 2000 (lower and upper curves respectively), categorised according to age group (35–64 years in blue, 65–84 years in red). Reproduced with permission from reference [26].

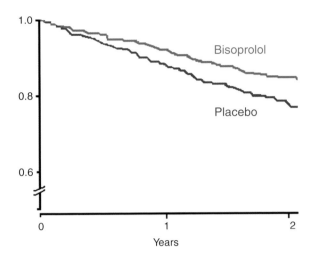

Figure 3.5 Survival improved by bisoprolol in heart failure patients with reduced ejection fractions. Reproduced with permission from reference [27].

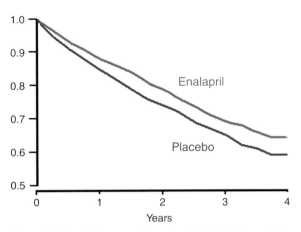

Figure 3.6 Survival improved by enalapril in heart failure patients with reduced ejection fractions. Reproduced with permission from reference [28].

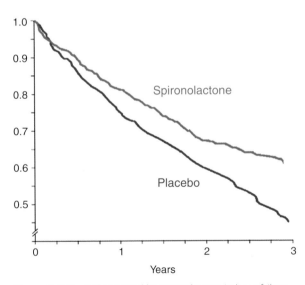

Figure 3.7 Survival improved by spironolactone in heart failure patients with reduced ejection fractions. Reproduced with permission from reference [29].

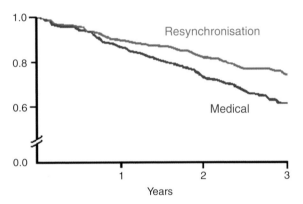

Figure 3.8 Survival improved by cardiac resynchonisation in heart failure patients with reduced ejection fractions (<25%). Reproduced with permission from reference [30].

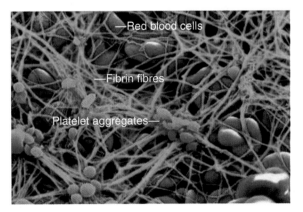

Figure 8.1 Scanning electron micrograph of a blood clot formed in vitro showing fibrin fibres, platelet aggregates and trapped red blood cells. From Veklich Y, Weisel JW. *Nature* 2001;**413**:6855 – cover illustration; with permission.

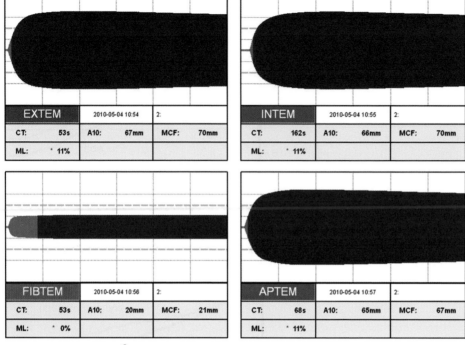

Figure 8.9 Normal ROTEM® results. Four tests have been performed simultaneously on one blood sample. The colour of the trace changes from purple to blue when its amplitude reaches 20 mm.

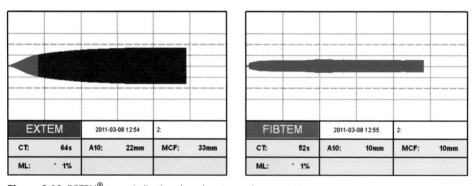

Figure 8.10 ROTEM® traces indicating thrombocytopaenia – see text.

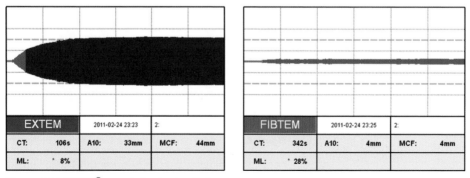

Figure 8.11 ROTEM® traces indicating low fibrinogen concentration – see text.

DIAGNOSIS

1. Clot firmness
- in the presence of heparin use the HEPTEM result
- if there is hyperfibrinolysis (ML > 15 %) use the APTEM result

CLOT FIRMNESS		A10 in EXTEM / INTEM / HEPTEM / APTEM		
		< 22 mm	22-38 mm	≥ 39 mm
A10 in FIBTEM	< 5 mm	Low fibrinogen Low platelets	Low fibrinogen (†platelets - see below)	Low fibrinogen
	5-7 mm	Low platelets Low fibrinogen	Low platelets Low fibrinogen	Clot firmness appears satisfactory. See Sections 2, 3 & blue box below. (If bleeding isn't controlled consider: -raising fibrinogen (FIBTEM A10>10mm) -in patients on aspirin* or clopidogrel* giving platelets and/or desmopressin).
	≥ 8 mm	Low platelets	Low platelets	

†Typically fibrinogen < 1.5 g/l & platelets 50-100. Also consider giving platelets if ongoing bleeding

2. Clotting time
- in the presence of heparin run a HEPTEM test

Causes of a prolonged CT	
Fibtem A10 < 5 mm	= Low fibrinogen
CT prolonged in Intem but normal in Heptem	= Heparin effect
Fibtem A10 ≥ 5 mm and no heparin effect	= Low coagulation factors

When to treat CT		
CT in Intem / Heptem > 300	or	CT in Extem / Aptem > 100s
CT in Intem / Heptem 240 - 300 s	or	CT in Extem / Aptem 80 - 100s
CT in Intem / Heptem < 240 s	or	CT in Extem / Aptem <80 s

3. Hyperfibrinolysis

Lysis of clot within 20 mins	Fulminant lysis
Lysis of clot within 20 – 40 mins	Early lysis
Lysis of clot after more than 40 mins	Late lysis - ?treat

Repeat Rotem tests including Aptem after treatment (or if no treatment is given)

TREATMENT

Treat	Treat if bleeding / high risk of bleeding	See below*

Low fibrinogen – FFP or fibrinogen concentrate or cryoprecipitate
Low platelets – platelets
Low coagulation factors – FFP or PCC   Heparin – protamine (if reversal appropriate)
Hyperfibrinolysis – tranexamic acid (1 g – 2 g bolus)

* IMPORTANT
Rotem® does not detect the effect of aspirin, clopidogrel or Reopro® on platelets
Rotem® is not a sensitive test for some anticoagulants e.g. warfarin, LMWH
Rotem® does not detect von Willebrand factor deficiency

Figure 8.12 Example of a guideline which uses the ROTEM® results to diagnose and treat impaired haemostasis during surgery.

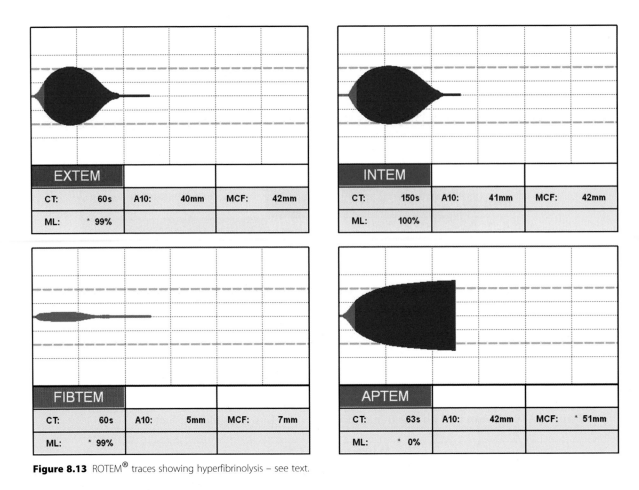

Figure 8.13 ROTEM® traces showing hyperfibrinolysis – see text.

Figure 8.14 Multiplate® impedance aggregometry results in a patient taking aspirin – see text.

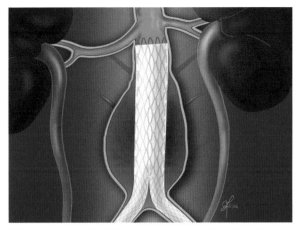

Figure 12.2 Modular bifurcated stent graft in the infrarenal aorta.

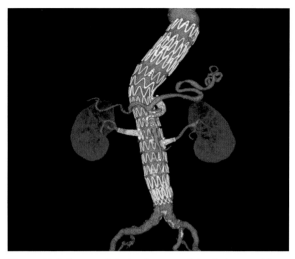

Figure 12.3 Stent-graft in the thoracocoabdominal aorta with branched visceral vessels.

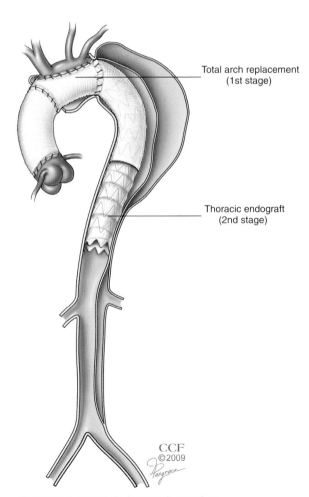

Total arch replacement (1st stage)

Thoracic endograft (2nd stage)

Figure 12.4 Staged elephant trunk procedure.

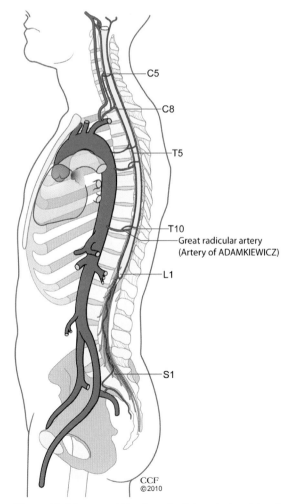

C5

C8

T5

T10
Great radicular artery (Artery of ADAMKIEWICZ)

L1

S1

Figure 12.6 Segmental blood supply of the spinal cord showing the origin of artery of Adamkiewicz.

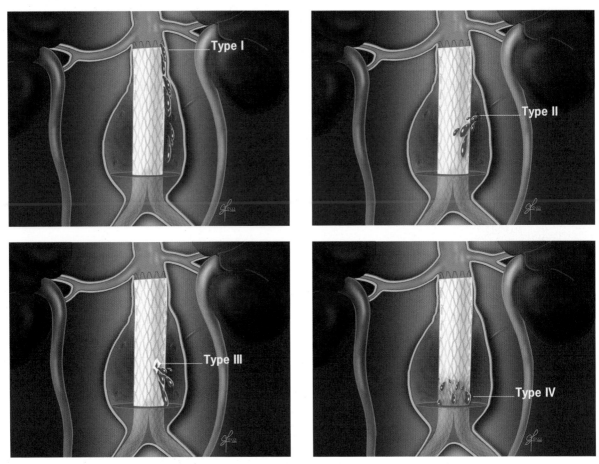

Figure 12.7 Types of endoleaks. While types II and IV are considered benign, especially if not associated with an increase in aneurysm sac diameter, types I and III require interventions such as placement of extension cuffs to prevent aneurysm rupture.

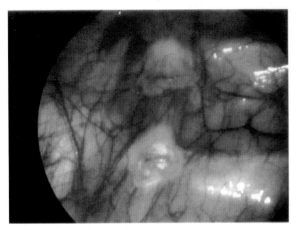

Figure 17.2 Thoracoscopic sympathectomy. The thoracoscope is looking at the posterior wall of the thorax. The second and third ribs are the whitish structures on the right. The thoracic sympathetic chain has been divided as it passes over the ribs.

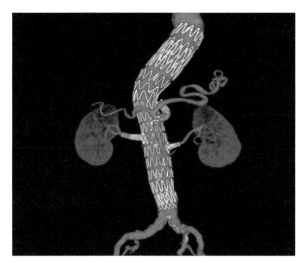

Figure 12.3 Stent-graft in the thoracocoabdominal aorta with branched visceral vessels. See plate section for colour version.

Directional branches are longer, custom-designed cuffs that are permanently attached to the main aortic trunk. They provide a longer area of seal (overlap) between the small vessel branch and the aortic component [5]. These branches are utilised in preference to a reinforced fenestrated design when there is a large aortic lumen or angulation of the aorta in the region of a critical branch, since these directional branches should allow any angulation between the aorta and branch to be gently accommodated, thereby improving flow dynamics. In addition, directional branches allow the use of the more versatile self-expanding branch vessel grafts (rather than the stiffer, balloon-expandable stent-grafts). However, these endografts require custom design and production according to each patient's three-dimensional aortic imaging (computed tomography or magnetic resonance angiography) and reconstruction [6]. They are therefore more expensive, require extensive surgical expertise and may increase fluoroscopic as well as contrast dye load exposure as a result of the longer procedure time.

Surgical procedures to expand the eligibility for endovascular stent-grafting

Retroperitoneal incision/approach

While conventional endografts are generally introduced via the femoral vessels, introduction via the iliac vessels or the infrarenal aorta may be necessary if the femoral vessels are small in diameter, are heavily calcified or highly tortuous. In these cases, a Dacron graft conduit is generally sewn onto the common iliac artery or aorta via a retroperitoneal approach to allow stent-graft introduction; the conduit is usually over-sewn at the end of the case. If needed, it can also be used as a bypass to the femoral system to treat concomitant occlusive disease

Hybrid procedures

In cases of aortic aneurysms involving major branches that originate from the aorta, adequate sealing of the aneurysm requires coverage of the major aortic branches that are involved in the aneurysm. To avoid ischaemic complications that occur as a result of coverage of these vessels, 'hybrid' approaches, i.e. a combination of open surgical and endovascular stenting procedures, have been developed to expand the 'anatomical' suitability for endovascular stenting [1,7]. Even though these procedures involve open surgical procedures, they are typically thought to be less invasive than traditional open surgical repair of aortic aneurysms and do not involve aortic cross-clamping, a major cause of surgical morbidity (stroke, renal failure, paraplegia) in the open surgical approach.

Hybrid procedure can either be staged or can be done simultaneously in the same operative setting. Common hybrid approaches are:

Left carotid subclavian bypass

Up to 40% of patients undergoing TEVAR have lesions requiring coverage of the ostium of the left subclavian artery (LSA) to obtain proximal seal (proximal landing zone). In these patients as well as in selected patients who have an anatomy that compromises perfusion to the brain, spinal cord, heart, or left arm, routine preoperative LSA revascularisation is strongly recommended prior to TEVAR. Table 12.1 lists some of the conditions that require LSA revascularisation, commonly performed using a left carotid to left subclavian artery bypass.

Staged elephant trunk procedures

For patients with aneurysms involving the transverse arch with no adequate proximal landing zone but adequate distal landing zone, a first-stage total arch replacement (stage I elephant trunk procedure) (Figure 12.4) may be performed to treat the proximal

Table 12.1 Conditions requiring preoperative LSA revascularisation prior to TEVAR [7]

Patients who need elective TEVAR where achievement of a proximal seal necessitates coverage of the LSA
Presence of a patent left internal mammary artery to coronary artery bypass graft
Termination of the left vertebral artery at the posterior inferior cerebellar artery or other discontinuity of the vertebrobasilar collaterals
Absent or occluded right vertebral artery
Functioning arteriovenous shunt in the left arm
Prior infrarenal aortic repair with ligation of lumbar and middle sacral arteries
Planned long-segment (20 cm) coverage of the descending thoracic aorta at the origin of critical intercostal arteries
Hypogastric artery occlusion
Presence of early aneurysmal changes that may require subsequent therapy involving the distal thoracic aorta

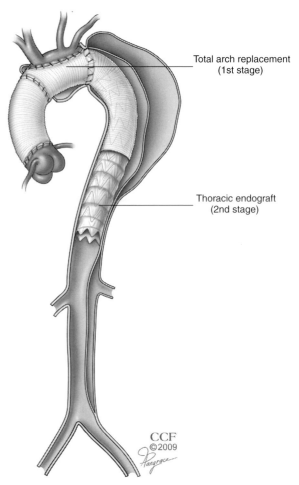

Figure 12.4 Staged elephant trunk procedure. See plate section for colour version.

aortic pathology and create a proximal landing zone using cardiopulmonary bypass and deep hypothermic circulatory arrest. This is followed at a later setting with the second stage endovascular repair utilising the elephant trunk graft as the proximal landing zone [8].

Aortic visceral debranching

To allow for endovascular stenting of aortic aneurysms that involve major visceral branches such as the coeliac, superior mesenteric, inferior mesenteric vessels and renal vessels without the need for conventional open repair that involves aortic cross-clamping, a visceral debranching procedure can be used, either at the same setting immediately prior to endovascular stenting or as a first part of a 'staged' procedure [1]. Following a midline laparotomy, and systemic heparinisation to a goal activated clotting time (ACT) >300 seconds, the visceral debranching procedure is performed using a custom designed multibranch graft with distal anastomoses to the left renal artery, superior mesenteric artery, coeliac axis, and right renal artery. Inflow for visceral debranching is typically performed via a single proximal anastomosis from the left iliac system, infrarenal aorta or existing infrarenal aortic graft.

The distal anastomoses to the abdominal vessels are performed in an end-to-end manner with the proximal vessels being divided and oversewn at their origins from the aorta to prevent retrograde type II endoleak.

Thoracic endovascular aortic repair is performed immediately following completion of the debranching portion of the procedure or can be performed in a separate operating room setting typically within the same hospitalisation.

Indications and contraindications to endovascular aortic repair

Elective surgical intervention is usually indicated for abdominal aortic aneurysms more than 5 cm in diameter (>5.5 cm for thoracoabdominal aortic aneurysm, TAA), those growing by more than 1 cm yearly

Table 12.2 Assessment of EVAR eligibility by imaging (ultrasound, computed tomography, magnetic resonance angiography)

1 Proximal aneurysm neck:
Length: >15 mm
Diameter: <30 mm
Angulation: <60° angulation in long axis
Thrombus: <2 mm layer of mural thrombus

2 Distal landing zone: adequate diameter and length

3 Iliac arteries: absence of aneurysms and occlusive disease

4 Access arteries: adequate diameter, absence of occlusive disease

Table 12.3 Common (traditional) contraindications for EVAR

Aortic aneurysm involving major aortic branches (left subclavian, celiac, superior mesenteric, inferior mesenteric, renal)

Short proximal neck

Thrombus presence in proximal landing zone

Conical proximal neck

Greater than 120° angulation of the proximal neck

Critical inferior mesenteric artery

Significant iliac occlusive disease

Tortuosity of iliac vessels

(3 mm yearly for TAA) as well as for symptomatic aortic aneurysms.

Patients with significant comorbid medical diseases (also referred to as physiological risk) are typically considered for endovascular grafting due to the high surgical morbidity and mortality associated with open surgical repair in that patient population.

Endovascular stent-grafting is specifically recommended for patients with degenerative or traumatic aneurysms of the descending thoracic aorta exceeding 5.5 cm, saccular aneurysms or postoperative pseudo-aneurysms [9].

Aortic imaging as well as angiographic 'roadmapping' is important for assessment of EVAR eligibility (also referred to as anatomic risk) (Table 12.2). Aortic imaging can identify patients with aortic anatomy that either precludes the use of endovascular stents, requires the use of custom fenestrated or branched stent-grafts, or necessitates the use of staged and/or hybrid procedures.

Table 12.3 lists the traditional criteria that precluded the use of EVAR. The introduction of fenestrated and branched stent-grafts, as well as the use of aortic debranching procedures, has reduced the contraindications for endovascular stent-grafting.

Preoperative evaluation and preparation of patients undergoing endovascular aortic repair

Patients presenting for EVAR typically have a high incidence of medical comorbidities (cardiac, pulmonary, renal, neurological).

Table 12.4 Indications of non-invasive stress testing in patients undergoing elective EVAR (high-risk surgery)

Patients with active cardiac conditions such as unstable coronary syndrome, decompensated congestive heart failure, significant arrhythmias, and severe valvular heart disease

Patients with low (< 4 metabolic equivalents) or unknown functional capacity with one or more clinical risk factors according to Lee's revised cardiac risk index (history of ischaemic heart disease, history of compensated or prior heart failure, history of cerebrovascular disease, diabetes mellitus and renal insufficiency) [11]

Despite the fact that EVAR is associated with less fluid shifts, absence of aortic cross-clamping and a smaller surgical incision, it should be considered a high-risk surgery (based on a perioperative risk of major adverse cardiac events > 5%) and patients should undergo functional testing when indicated based on the American College of Cardiology/American Heart Association (ACC/AHA) guidelines for preoperative evaluation of patients undergoing non-cardiac surgery, especially if the results of functional testing will alter management (Table 12.4) [10].

Perioperative renal protection

Acute kidney injury (AKI) following EVAR is multifactorial in nature and can occur as a result of hypoperfusion, mechanical encroachment of the stent graft on the renal vessels and emboli to the renal arteries.

Table 12.5 Strategies to reduce the incidence of acute kidney injury following EVAR

Ensure perioperative euvolaemia

Maintain cardiac output and blood pressure

Limit contrast dye exposure

Use iso-osmolar non-ionic contrast dye

Pharmacologic strategies especially in patients with baseline chronic kidney disease:

N-Acetylcysteine

Sodium bicarbonate

Statin drugs

Table 12.6 Factors affecting the use of local anaesthesia for EVAR

Patient is able to lie in the supine position for 1–2 hours (no orthopnoea)

Patient cooperation and understanding that a 'deep level of monitored anaesthesia care' will not be feasible, since patients will be periodically asked to hold their breath during angiography

Favourable iliofemoral anatomy making a retroperitoneal incision for iliac artery access unlikely

Favourable aneurysm anatomy (no need for fenestrated or branched stent-grafts), with an expected surgical duration less than 2 hours

One of the most common causes of AKI in patients undergoing EVAR is radiographic contrast-induced nephropathy and occurs in 2–10% of patients exposed to intavascular radiographic contrast agents. Reduced glomerular filtration rate is an independent predictor of mortality in patients undergoing EVAR [12].

Contrast nephropathy results from a combination of medullary ischaemia and direct tubular toxicity. Increased plasma concentrations of endothelin, a potent vasoconstrictor, following contrast exposure, supports its role in medullary ischaemia. An additional potential mechanism is generation of reactive oxygen species, whether due to contrast-mediated injury to the glomerulus or due to direct generation of free radicals by the contrast medium itself.

Various strategies have been used to reduce the incidence of contrast-induced AKI [13], including limiting the exposure to contrast dye, the use of iso-osmolar and non-ionic contrast dye, as well as pharmacologic agents reported to reduce the incidence of contrast-dye-induced AKI, including N-acetylcysteine, sodium bicarbonate and statin drugs [14]. Nevertheless, perioperative hydration and maintenance of a normal cardiac output and stable haemodynamics appears to be the most important strategy in preventing contrast-induced AKI (Table 12.5).

Choice of anaesthetic management

Endovascular aortic repair has been safely done using local infiltration anaesthesia, central neuraxial blockade (spinal, epidural) as well as general anaesthesia.

Local anaesthesia with monitored anaesthesia care

Several centres perform EVAR cases safely under local anaesthesia [15]. It is important to note that the mode of anaesthesia should not reduce the level of perioperative monitoring (see section on choice of intraoperative monitoring). Table 12.6 lists the conditions that should be present before local anaesthesia for EVAR is attempted.

Central neuraxial blockade

Both spinal and lumbar epidural anaesthesia has been safely used in EVAR cases [16]. Some centres have reported beneficial effects with the use of regional anaesthesia, e.g. less vasopressor use, shorter intensive care unit and hospital stay. Other studies have reported equal efficacy and safety when compared to general anaesthesia [16]. It is likely that there is a selection bias in the non-randomised trial documenting better outcomes with regional anaesthesia since patients with fewer comorbidities undergoing 'straightforward' EVAR are more likely to receive central neuraxial anaesthesia.

Intrathecal drainage catheters (see below) can be used for spinal drug delivery as well as for cerebrospinal fluid (CSF) drainage. This technique has the advantage of allowing intrathecal drug dose titration to the target dermatomal levels (T10) to be blocked while avoiding the sympathectomy caused by a high level of spinal anaesthesia. This technique requires the avoidance of CSF drainage for 30–40 minutes after intrathecal drug delivery (e.g. bupivacaine 5 mg) to

Table 12.7 Factors influencing the choice of central neuraxial anaesthesia for EVAR (in addition to the factors influencing the choice for local anaesthesia)

No contraindications to central neuraxial blockade, e.g. patient approval, patient not on anticoagulation or platelet inhibitors (thienopyridines)

No need for transoesophageal echocardiography

No need for motor evoked potential (MEP) or somatosensory evoked potential (SSEP) monitoring

No need for measures to achieve a motionless field (use of adenosine or transvenous pacing) during stent deployment

Table 12.8 Factors influencing the choice of general anaesthesia for EVAR

Complicated EVAR with planned fenestrated or branched endografts due to the expected long duration

Need for iliac artery access (through a retroperitoneal incision) since a high level of central neuraxial blockade is necessary which increases the respiratory side-effects

Planned use of transoesophageal echocardiography

Planned haemodynamic manipulations to create a motionless field during stent deployment

Planned SSEP and/or MEP monitoring

History of difficult airway especially if EVAR procedures are performed outside the operating room suite (i.e. interventional radiology or cardiology suite) where immediate expert help may not be available and access to the airway may be delayed by the fluoroscopy machine

avoid drainage of the intrathecally administered local anaesthetics.

Lumbar epidural anaesthesia allows the administration of titrated doses to avoid a sympathectomy and subsequent hypotension. It also allows the use of short- and intermediate-acting local anaesthetics (lidocaine, mepivacaine) so that postoperative neurological examination for absence of lower extremity neurological deficits can be performed as early as possible. Lumbar epidural catheters can be placed in the 'ready rooms' with epidural anaesthetics only administered in the operating room 10–15 minutes prior to the start of the procedure. The epidural catheter is typically removed in the recovery room after confirmation of a normal coagulation profile, since minimal postoperative analgesia is typically required after EVAR (small bilateral groin incisions) (Table 12.7).

General anaesthesia

Factors influencing the choice of general anaesthesia are listed in Table 12.8. Regardless of the mode of anaesthesia, the intraoperative anaesthetic goals during EVAR are to maintain haemodynamic stability, and preserve perfusion to vital organs including the brain, heart, spinal cord, kidney and splanchnic vessels. Avoidance of hypertension and tachycardia reduces the imbalance in myocardial oxygen supply demand relationship and avoids the resultant ischaemic acute coronary events. In addition, avoidance of hypertension and tachycardia are essential in reducing rate of rise of left ventricular pressure (dP/dt) in patients with both aortic aneurysms and dissections.

During induction of general endotracheal anaesthesia, blunting of the haemodynamic response to intubation can be accomplished with short-acting beta-blockers such as esmolol. Newer agents such as the short-acting dihydropyridine clevidipine can reduce the blood pressure without a reflex increase in heart rate. It is important to avoid long-acting antihypertensive agents since postinduction hypotension commonly occurs in this patient population.

Maintenance of intravascular volume and early identification and management of bleeding is essential, especially as most bleeding in EVAR is concealed under the drapes.

It is not uncommon for the surgical team to access one or both brachial arteries in addition to accessing the femoral vessels to aid stent deployment during EVAR. Accidental withdrawal of a vascular sheath out of a major vessel while surgeons are monitoring the fluoroscopic screens is a major cause of acute hypovolaemic shock. Vigilance of the anaesthetist in observing all the access sites and early identification (and notification of the surgeon) of the source of surgical bleeding is essential. Other causes of acute blood-loss anaemia can occur due to rupture of the femoral or external iliac artery during attempts to introduce a large vascular sheath through a small-diameter iliofemoral vessel. This complication may require an emergent laparotomy if the proximal portion of the transected vessel retracts into the abdominal cavity. An unexplained drop in haematocrit should alert to a possible retroperitoneal bleed/haematoma. This occurs more commonly in the setting of a retroperitoneal incision to create an iliac artery conduit (see above), especially in that patients are anticoagulated to maintain an ACT >300 seconds before stent introduction, which promotes the expansion of any haematoma across the retroperitoneal plane.

While rupture of an aneurysm is an ever-present possibility during EVAR, other aforementioned aetiologies occur more commonly. Nevertheless, one of the most important roles of the anaesthetist in EVAR is to be prepared with adequate intravenous access, and to embrace the possibility of aneurysm rupture. Preparation for the possible use of cell salvage in case of unexpected bleeding in EVAR could reduce exposure of patients to the risk of allogeneic red cells.

Following endovascular stenting and removal of the vascular sheaths, re-establishing blood flow to the lower extremities is associated with 'reperfusion hypotension' due to 'washout' of the metabolic acid load into the systemic circulation, causing systemic vasodilation and possible myocardial stunning.

Communication between the surgeon and the anaesthetist is particularly important during EVAR and a basic knowledge of the steps involved during EVAR helps the anaesthesiologist in the safe perioperative management of patients undergoing EVAR.

For example, endoluminal balloon inflation to seal the balloon-expandable endograft to the aortic wall mimics an aortic cross-clamp and causes an acute abrupt rise in blood pressure. Communication of this step avoids the unnecessary administration of hypotensive agents, since the balloon inflation is only temporary for 30–60 seconds and is followed by balloon deflation, which can result in intractable hypotension if hypotensive agents are administered. Table 12.9 lists common causes of hypotension during EVAR by pathophysiological mechanism.

Choice of intraoperative monitoring
Cerebrospinal fluid drainage

Cerebrospinal fluid drainage theoretically increases spinal cord blood flow by decreasing CSF pressure resulting in an increased spinal cord perfusion pressure. Spinal cord perfusion pressure is defined as distal mean aortic pressure minus CSF pressure.

The blood supply of the spinal cord is made up of two posterior spinal arteries (originating from the vertebral or posterior inferior cerebellar artery) and one anterior spinal artery (Figure 12.5). From the caudal end, the anterior spinal artery receives arterial collateral supply from the internal iliac artery and its branches, the middle sacral artery and the inferior mesenteric artery, while the thoracic portion of the anterior spinal artery is supplied by radicular branches of the intercostal arteries.

The largest of the radicular branches, the artery of Adamkiewicz (arteria radicularis magna), arises directly from the aorta at T9–T12 in the majority of cases, but can arise anywhere between T5 and L5 (Figure 12.6). Exclusion of this artery during aneurysm stenting can result in paraplegia (Table 12.10). Other postulated mechanisms are the occurrence of hypoperfusion as a result of hypotension as well as thrombosis or embolisation of the arteries supplying the anterior spinal artery. The injury seen after ischaemia of the spinal cord (anterior spinal artery syndrome) is manifested by loss of motor function and pinprick sensation and preservation of vibratory and position sense.

While several randomised controlled trials and meta-analyses documented the efficacy of CSF drainage (to a pressure of 10 mm Hg) in reducing the incidence of spinal cord ischaemia after open thoracoabdominal repair [17], evidence to support the efficacy of lumbar CSF drainage to decrease the incidence of spinal cord ischaemia after EVAR procedures is limited (Table 12.11) [18]. There are, however, multiple reports of reversal of paraplegia after institution of CSF drainage in patients undergoing TEVAR. In light of proven efficacy in the open thoracic repair literature, it is unlikely that randomised controlled trials will be conducted to prove efficacy in EVAR.

Lumbar CSF drainage catheters are typically placed preoperatively under local anaesthesia through 14 G Tuohy needles. The CSF drainage catheters are advanced 10–20 cm into the subarachnoid space under strict aseptic conditions and are taped to the patient's back. Care should be avoided to avoid kinking of the catheters during taping and a trial of 'passive' drainage of CSF after the patient is in the supine position ensures free flow of CSF when drainage is initiated.

Prophylactic drainage of CSF to a pressure of <10 mm Hg is typically done by connecting the catheter to a drainage system set to a pressure of 10 mm Hg, so that any rise in CSF pressure above 10 mm Hg results

Table 12.9 Causes of intraoperative hypotension during EVAR (TEVAR and EVAAR)

Hypovolaemia
Absolute hypovolaemia due to surgical bleeding (may be occult)
Iliac artery rupture during device introduction (more in females with small iliofemoral diameter)
Accidental withdrawal of the device during fluoroscopic manipulation resulting in bleeding from the femoral artery under the drapes (may also occur during brachial artery access)
Rupture of the aortic aneurysm
Retroperitoneal bleeding especially following retroperitoneal dissection for iliac artery conduit
Relative hypovolaemia due to lactic acidosis
Reperfusion of lower extremities following stent deployment and device withdrawal after endovascular aortic repair
Visceral ischaemia during branched stent-graft introduction (caeliac, superior mesenteric) or coverage during TEVAR
Reperfusion syndrome following endovascular repair of acute aortic type B dissection
Cardiogenic
Guidewire manipulation near the aortic arch (aortic baroreceptors) with resultant arrhythmias
Overadvancement of guidewire into the left ventricle resulting in hemopericardium and cardiac tamponade
Retrograde type A aortic dissection during TEVAR
Perioperative myocardial ischaemia
Iatrogenic
Intra-arterial injection of nitroglycerin (per surgeon) into major aortic branches (e.g. renal vessels) to prevent vasospasm
Intravenous contrast-dye-induced allergic/anaphylactic reactions
Manoeuvres to temporarily interrupt blood flow and create a motionless field during device deployment:
Intravenous injection of adenosine
Rapid ventricular pacing to create a motionless field during device deployment
Right atrial inflow occlusion
Neurogenic
Acute spinal artery syndrome causing paraplegia and neurogenic shock
Distributive: abdominal compartment syndrome following TEVAR for type B aortic dissection
Re-establishing blood flow to ischaemic gut with massive oedema exacerbated by massive fluid resuscitation to treat hypotension → can result in a vicious cycle until the abdomen is opened surgically to relieve the pressure

in drainage of CSF into a sealed collection system. Caution should be taken to ensure that the zero point of the transducer is set at the patient's midaxillary line or external auditory meatus while patient is in the supine position.

Since CSF overdrainage carries its own risks (see below), therapeutic CSF drainage to a lower CSF pressure (as low as 5 mm Hg) is only undertaken if the patient develops paraparesis perioperatively as evidenced by clinical examination or MEP monitoring.

The CSF drainage catheter is typically left in place for 48–72 hours and gradual increase in CSF pressure as well as capping of the catheters for a few hours prior to the catheter's removal is recommended. This is done to allow CSF re accumulation and to evaluate the onset of any paraparesis or paraplegia prior to actual CSF drainage catheter removal. If patients develop any lower extremity neurological deficits, reinstitution of CSF drainage is undertaken, vasopressor therapy is initiated to raise mean arterial

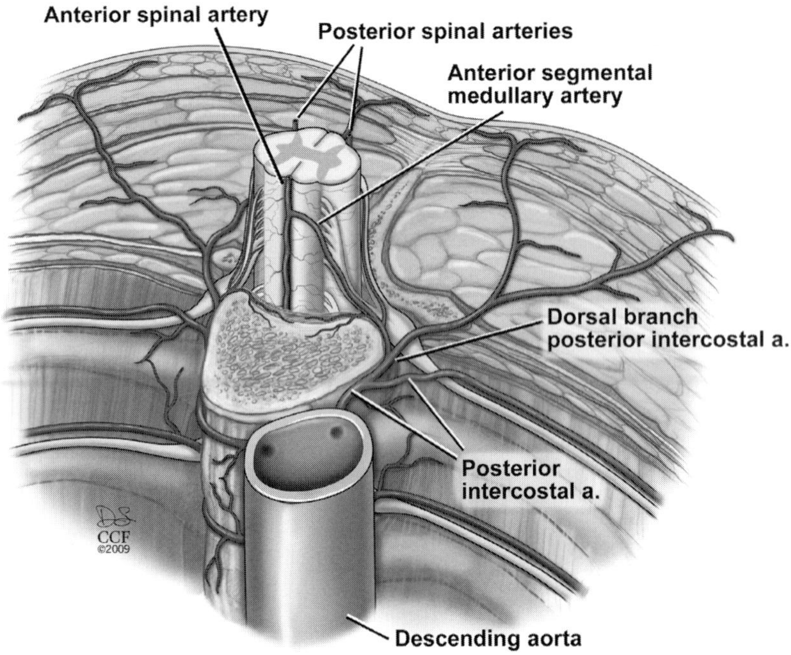

Figure 12.5 Blood supply of the spinal cord.

Anterior spinal artery

Posterior spinal arteries

Anterior segmental medullary artery

Dorsal branch posterior intercostal a.

Posterior intercostal a.

Descending aorta

pressure and serial neurological examination are performed for evidence of reversal of neurological deficits (Table 12.12).

In these cases, gradual increase in CSF pressure may avoid recurrence of neurological deficits and allows time for 'adaptation' of the remaining collateral circulation.

Complications associated with lumbar CSF catheters include meningitis, epidural abscess, persistent CSF leak and intracranial hypotension (temporal downward herniation with kinking of the posterior cerebral artery resulting in an acute brain infarction or death, breakage or retention of catheter fragments, intradural spinal, epidural haematoma, subdural or intracerebellar haematoma.

Somatosensory and motor evoked potential monitoring

Motor (MEP) and somatosensory evoked potential (SSEP) monitoring is utilised in patients undergoing EVAR with a high risk for postoperative paraplegia whether due to a planned long-segment thoracic exclusion (type I and II Crawford classification) or due to limited collateral circulation in patients with prior open or endovascular aortic repair.

The main goal of intraoperative neurophysiologic monitoring is to ensure adequate spinal cord

perfusion throughout the EVAR procedure and to immediately identify spinal cord ischaemic changes that require prompt intervention, typically by augmenting mean arterial blood pressure and instituting CSF drainage. The detection of reversible transient spinal cord ischaemic changes by intraoperative monitoring may also identify patients at risk for delayed postoperative paraplegia.

Intraoperative monitoring of SSEPs is performed by placing stimulating electrodes on the skin adjacent to peripheral nerves in the arms or legs. Electrical stimulation of the peripheral nerves in the limbs generates action potentials that can be measured from recording electrodes over the lumbar plexus, brachial plexus, spine, brainstem, thalamus and cerebral cortex.

A major limitation of SSEP monitoring is that it is more likely to detect posterior column ischaemia and may therefore miss spinal cord ischaemia which is typically confined to the anterior spinal cord and causes a selective motor deficit with intact sensation. As a result, paraplegia can occur despite normal SSEP signals.

Motor evoked potentials elicited through transcortical electrical stimulation have also been advocated for the detection of intraoperative spinal cord ischaemia. To monitor MEPs, electrical stimulation to the scalp overlying the motor cortex

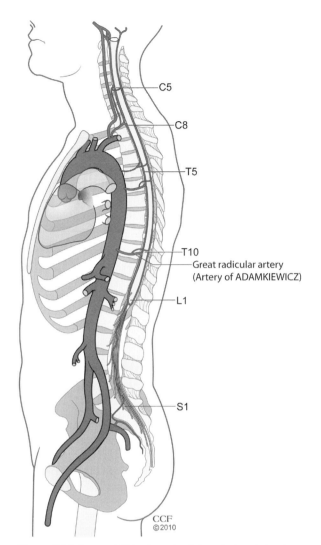

Figure 12.6 Segmental blood supply of the spinal cord showing the origin of artery of Adamkiewicz. See plate section for colour version.

Table 12.10 Factors believed to cause or contribute to the development of spinal cord ischaemia after TEVAR

The extent of the descending thoracic aorta covered by graft due to exclusion of critical intercostal arteries at the T6–T12 vertebral levels that supply the anterior spinal artery

Previous abdominal aortic aneurysm repair explained by compromised collateral vascular supply to the spinal cord from the pelvic and hypogastric circulation as a consequence of prior sacrifice of the inferior mesenteric artery or sacrifice of the median sacral artery

Injury to the external iliac artery from intravascular delivery of the stent or severe pre-existing occlusive disease of the femoral or iliac arteries, because spinal cord collaterals originating from the iliac arteries may be compromised

Hypotension associated with an occult retroperitoneal bleed due to reduction in CSF perfusion pressure

Severe atherosclerosis of the thoracic aorta due to the increased risk of emboli to the anterior spinal artery

Table 12.11 Indications of CSF drainage in TEVAR

Long-segment thoracic aortic exclusion especially close to T6–T12 (types I–III Crawford classification)

Prior open or endovascular abdominal or thoracic repair due to limited remaining collateral circulation

Table 12.12 Management of paraplegia following TEVAR

Elevation of mean arterial blood pressure (>80 mm Hg) using alpha agonist, e.g. norepinephrine or phenylephrine)

   Improves spinal cord perfusion pressure

   Counteracts neurogenic shock caused by autonomic dysfunction as a consequence of spinal cord ischaemia

Therapeutic CSF drainage (5–10 mm Hg)

Repeated neurological examination for evidence of reversal of paraplegia

Avoid abrupt cessation of CSF drainage by allowing gradual increase in CSF pressure followed by capping of CSF catheter prior to its removal

results in evoked potentials that travel from the motor cortex, through cortical spinal tracts, anterior horn cell and peripheral nerve, and finally to muscle. An interruption in this pathway will result in the loss or reduction of amplitude in the MEPs. Stimulation of the motor cortex with sensing over the popliteal nerve is the most commonly employed technique [19].

Central neuraxial anaesthesia is contraindicated if SSEP or MEP monitoring are planned. During general anaesthesia, inhaled anaesthetic concentrations should be maintained at 1/2 minimum anaesthetic concentration (MAC) when performing SSEP monitoring since high inhaled anaesthetic concentrations attenuate cortical signals and neuromuscular blocking drugs should be avoided when performing MEP neuromonitoring. Hypothermia attenuates signals with MEPs and SSEPs and should be avoided.

129

Loss of SSEP and MEP signals is not specific to spinal cord ischaemia and can also occur as a result of peripheral nerve ischaemia and lower extremity vascular malperfusion whether due to arterial cannulation or atheroemboli to lower extremities.

Since most endovascular stents are non-retrievable (cannot be retrieved once deployed), some centres do not use intraoperative SSEP or MEP monitoring and rely on early postoperative identification and management of neurological deficits.

However, the inflation of a balloon in the intended area of aortic segment exclusion can mimic stent deployment and can identify the occurrence of SEP and or MEP changes before permanent endovascular stenting, triggering early augmentation of spinal cord perfusion pressure (by increasing mean arterial blood pressure and reducing CSF pressure).

Site of invasive arterial monitoring

Invasive arterial blood pressure monitoring is essential in EVAR cases. In addition to the ever-present risk of aneurysm rupture and the potential for massive blood loss, medical comorbidities of patients presenting for EVAR dictate a continuous monitoring technique. More importantly, the possibility for the use of hypotensive agents during stent deployment makes an intra-arterial catheter indispensable. For TEVAR procedures in particular, the site of arterial cannulation has to be discussed with the surgeon, since right or left brachial artery access may be required to aid in stent deployment. In addition, the surgeons may elect to advance a 'pigtail' catheter through the left brachial artery for accurate identification of the take-off of the left subclavian vessel from the aorta to avoid encroachment of the stent graft on the origin of the vessel during deployment.

Indications and applications of transoesophageal echocardiography in endovascular aortic repair

Although the primary diagnosis of aortic aneurysm or aortic dissection will have already been established in patients undergoing EVAR in the abdominal or thoracic location, transoesophageal echocardiography (TOE) has multiple roles in the perioperative management of these patients [20]. The TOE probe may have to be withdrawn into the pharynx during deployment of thoracic endografts since the TOE probe is radio-opaque and may interfere with the surgeon's visualisation of aortic landmarks during TEVAR. Care should be taken during repeated withdrawal and reinsertion of the probe into the oesophagus and stomach to avoid causing trauma (lip, dental, oesophageal) especially in the setting of systemic anticoagulation.

Avoidance of high-contrast dye load exposure

One of the major roles of TOE is to avoid or reduce the use of contrast dye in patients with reduced preoperative glomerular filtration rate, since pre-existing renal disease is one of the most important predictor of perioperative contrast-induced AKI and carries a higher mortality.

Diagnosis of aortic pathology

In addition to confirming the diagnosis, TOE is used to screen the aorta for evidence of further pathology including the presence and severity of atheroma, the presence of other concomitant aneurysms as well as the relationship of aortic aneurysms to major vessels.

Identification of guidewire, sheath and endograft location within the aorta

The guidewire typically appears as a bright echodense structure within the aortic lumen. The sheath, while also echodense, is typically thicker in diameter. A deployed endograft can be seen as a circumferential echodense structure lining the inner diameter of the aortic lumen in short axis.

In cases of aortic dissection, identification of the location of the guidewire, its presence in the true lumen (versus false lumen) as well as detection of the entry site of dissection (intimal flap) can be invaluable in aiding the deployment of the endograft into the true lumen to re-establish blood flow to ischaemic vessels. Intravascular ultrasound (IVUS) has also been increasingly utilised for the identification of true versus false lumen in cases of aortic dissection.

Detection of endoleaks

It has been shown that TOE is more sensitive than angiography in the detection of endoleaks.

A 'swirling' appearance in the excluded aneurysm sac after endograft deployment or the appearance of spontaneous echo contrast (smoke) denoting persistence of 'low flow' should trigger the use of color-flow Doppler to look for evidence of persistence of blood flow in the aneurysm sac. The early detection of endoleaks allows for their prompt management and avoids the undetected continuous expansion of the aneurysm sac which can eventually lead to aneurysm rupture (see section on endoleaks).

Cardiac assessment

In addition to the overall evaluation of fluid status and assessment of biventricular function, TOE can aid in the early identification and management of myocardia ischaemia.

Balloon occlusion of the aorta for 30 seconds to seal the aortic endograft to the aortic wall (endoluminal balloon inflation) is associated with a marked increase in left ventricular afterload and can result in the acute onset of left ventricular failure due to ischaemic cardiomyopathy or worsening of diastolic dysfunction. New regional wall motion abnormalities (NRWMA) can be detected by TOE, as well as acute reduction in biventricular systolic and or diastolic function that persist after aortic balloon deflation and aid in the early institution of pharmacologic therapy.

Further, TOE can aid in the diagnosis of new-onset (iatrogenic) retrograde aortic dissections, as well as identify aortic valve and coronary artery involvement in patients with known aortic dissections.

Unexpected complications, such as acute cardiac tamponade due to overadvancement of the guidewire resulting in endocardial wall perforation have also been diagnosed with TOE.

Haemodynamic manipulation during aortic endograft deployment

Newer generations of self-expanding aortic endografts only require a temporary reduction in mean arterial pressure and heart rate during stent deployment. It is important to note that the goal is not to reduce blood pressure per se but to temporarily reduce blood flow (cardiac output) in the aorta during deployment until maximum expansion, apposition and sealing of the endograft against the aortic wall occurs. The titrated use of short-acting agents to reduce heart rate (e.g. esmolol with a target heart rate of 50–60 beats per minute) and systemic blood pressure (e.g. sodium nitroprusside, nitroglycerin, clevidipine with a target mean arterial pressure of 60–70 mm Hg) can safely achieve this goal while avoiding

residual postdeployment hypotension with its deleterious effects on end-organ perfusion (including spinal cord perfusion).

For endograft deployment in the proximal descending thoracic aorta, as well as for newer endograft technique involving the aortic arch and the ascending aorta, endograft deployment requires an entirely 'motionless' field. The rationale for this approach is threefold:

- once deployed, almost all thoracic endografts cannot be repositioned
- proximal and distal landing zones of thoracic and aortic arch endografts are typically dangerously close to major vessels originating from the aorta (aortic branch vessels) with catastrophic effects if stent migration or encroachment occurs
- Even with the stent-graft perfectly positioned, deployment of the graft can be complicated secondary to the high volume of blood flow in the thoracic aorta and the potential for the 'windsock effect', which is the tendency for the graft to be pulled distally before deployment is complete.

Techniques used to achieve a motionless field include the use of adenosine, transvenous pacing as well as right atrial inflow occlusion [21].

Use of intravenous adenosine

To achieve a motionless field, some centres utilise adenosine in a dose of 6–12 mg intravenously (preferably through central intravenous access due to its short half-life of <10 seconds), causing a transient atrioventricular heart block [22]. General anaesthesia is typically preferred for patients receiving adenosine since its side-effects, facial flushing, dyspnoea, chest tightness, bronchospasm and a sense of 'impending death', can cause patient discomfort, confusion and may result in abrupt patient movement if the drug is administered while patients are awake (cases done under MAC or regional anaesthesia). The adenosine dose may be increased in patients on theophylline since methylxanthines prevent binding of adenosine at receptor sites. The dose is often decreased in patients on dipyridamole and diazepam because adenosine potentiates the effects of these drugs. The main disadvantage of adenosine is that bradyasystole is not reliably achieved with the aforementioned doses and may require higher doses.

Rapid ventricular pacing

Ventricular pacing at a rate of 150–180 beats per minute results in loss of atrioventricular synchrony, resulting in a reduction of ventricular filling time, decreased left ventricular preload, stroke volume and cardiac output [23]. The systolic pressure will drop down immediately and markedly once pacing is initiated, and will immediately return to normal after inactivation of the pacemaker.

In order to achieve rapid ventricular pacing, a bipolar cardiac pacing catheter is positioned in the right ventricular apex via the femoral or jugular vein and the pacing threshold checked once installed. An acceptable threshold was 1 mV with the pacemaker output set to 4–5 mV. Rapid ventricular pacing is tested after insertion to ensure effectiveness. The main advantages of rapid ventricular pacing are that it is reproducible, predictable and can be terminated instantaneously.

Right atrial inflow occlusion

This method relies on reduction of cardiac preload and by using a compliant occlusion balloon introduced through the femoral or jugular vein into the right atrium to inflate in the inferior or superior vena cava [24]. Potential complications of this technique include balloon rupture or migration and intracranial venous hypertension in the case of occlusion of the superior vena cava.

Complications of endovascular aortic repair

Early complications

Early complications include iliofemoral lacerations, AKI, pelvic and lower extremity ischaemia, myocardial ischaemia, paraplegia, stroke and postimplantation syndrome.

Postimplantation syndrome occurs during the early postoperative period and is characterised by leucocytosis, fever and elevation of inflammatory mediators such as C-reactive protein, interleukin-6 and tumour necrosis factor. It is thought to be due to endothelial activation by the endoprosthesis. The lack of knowledge of this physiological entity might lead to unnecessary interventions.

For TEVAR, development of either unilateral or bilateral reactive pleural effusions is not uncommon, with a reported incidence of 37% to 73%.

While cases of thrombocytopenia as a result of 'consumption' of platelets in the fabric graft have been reported, clinically significant thrombocytopenia, coagulopathy and fibrinolysis after EVAR are rare.

Late complications

Late complications include device migration, endoleaks with resultant aneurysm rupture, endograft infection, as well as long-term effects of radiation exposure (carcinogenesis, skin burns).

Endoleak is defined as the persistence of blood flow outside the lumen of the endograft but within an aneurysm sac or adjacent vascular segment being treated by the graft.

Classification of endoleaks

Endoleaks can be classified as shown in Figure 12.7.

Type I endoleak Involves the proximal or distal seal zones. Further ballooning or placement of another graft may be necessary to achieve seal. Vigorous proximal ballooning may be hazardous; retrograde proximal aortic dissection has been reported.

Type II endoleak Unusual in the thoracic aorta, but due to retrograde flow from intercostal arteries into the sac. Typically resolves with conservative management.

Type III endoleak Occurs with inadequate overlap and seal between modular components. Usually responds with further ballooning or additional graft or stent placement.

Type IV endoleak Occurs due to porosity of the graft, which is a rare occurrence with current generation devices.

Type V endoleak Otherwise known as 'endotension', occurs in the setting of continued sac expansion despite absence of an identifiable endoleak on subsequent imaging studies and may be due to the limitations in imaging technology.

Endoleaks are also classified on the basis of timing of occurrence. Endoleaks detected within the first 30 days of deployment are considered 'primary', whereas those detected later in the postoperative period are termed 'secondary'. Secondary endoleaks are typically types I or III and require intervention to prevent aneurysm rupture.

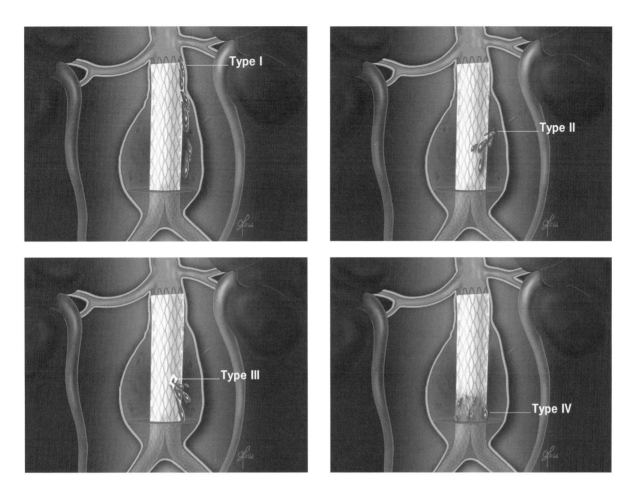

Figure 12.7 Types of endoleaks. While types II and IV are considered benign, especially if not associated with an increase in aneurysm sac diameter, types I and III require interventions such as placement of extension cuffs to prevent aneurysm rupture. See plate section for colour version.

Following EVAR, protocol-driven routine surveillance imaging – at regular intervals – is mandatory for the early detection and management of endoleaks and patients should be informed that continued surveillance will be a feature of their lives after EVAR.

Outcomes

Most trials comparing EVAAR with open surgery have shown a reduction in short term (perioperative and or 30-day) mortality [25–29]. Most studies show that the beneficial mortality trend is lost over time, as early as at 1 year [30] in some trials and as late as at 4 years in others [28]. In a recent study, however, the early perioperative mortality advantage was not offset by increased morbidity and mortality in the first 2 years after repair [29]. Longer-term data are needed to fully assess the relative merits of the two procedures.

The Dutch Randomized Endovascular Aneurysm Management (DREAM) trial randomly assigned 351 patients with asymptomatic abdominal aortic aneurysms (AAAs) greater than 5 cm in diameter with anatomy suitable for EVAR to open or endovascular repair. A strong trend toward a 30-day benefit in mortality favoured EVAR in this study (1.2% for EVAR vs. 4.6% for open surgery; $p = 0.10$) [25]. Two-year follow-up data demonstrated that by 1 year, this trend toward improved survival was lost, with no mortality benefit using EVAR [30].

The EVAR Trial 1 (EVAR I), compared EVAR to open surgical repair in 1082 patients with suitable EVAR anatomy and aneurysms ≥5.5 cm [26]. Blood product use and length of hospital stay favoured EVAR, as did perioperative mortality (1.7% for EVAR vs. 4.7% for open surgery; $p = 0.009$) [27]. However, the primary end-point of all-cause mortality did not show a lasting benefit for EVAR at the 4-year study conclusion.

Long-term complication and reintervention rates also were higher in the EVAR group, but a reduction in aneurysm-related death was noted (3.5% for EVAR vs. 6.3% for open surgery; $p = 0.02$) [26].

Using Medicare administrative data, Schermerhorn *et al.* compared patients undergoing open repair with those undergoing endovascular repair in the United States between 2001 and 2004 [28]. There were 22 830 matched patients available for study in each cohort. Perioperative mortality was 1.2% after EVAR and 4.8% after open repair (95% confidence interval (CI), 3.51–4.56; $p < 0.001$). Long-term survival rates reflected an early mortality benefit for EVAR that lasted more than 3 years, at which time mortality rates converged. By the fourth year, the rate of AAA rupture was significantly higher in the EVAR group (1.8% for EVAR vs. 0.5% for open repair; $p < 0.001$), as were reintervention rates related to AAA (9.0% for EVAR vs. 1.7% for open repair; $p < 0.001$).

Finally, Lederle *et al.*, in a multicentre clinical trial, randomized 881 veterans from 42 Veterans Affairs Medical Centers with eligible AAA to EVAR versus open repair [29]. Perioperative mortality (30-day or inpatient) was lower for endovascular repair (0.5% vs. 3.0%; $p=0.004$), but there was no significant difference in mortality at 2 years (7.0% vs. 9.8%, $p=0.13$). Patients in the endovascular repair group had reduced median procedure time (2.9 vs. 3.7 hours), blood loss (200 vs. 1000 ml), transfusion requirement (0 vs. 1.0 units), duration of mechanical ventilation (3.6 vs. 5.0 hours), hospital stay (3 vs. 7 days) and intensive care unit stay (1 vs. 4 days), but required substantial exposure to fluoroscopy and contrast. There were no differences between the two groups in major morbidity, procedure failure, secondary therapeutic procedures, aneurysm-related hospitalisations, health-related quality of life or erectile function.

Most randomised trials reporting on intermediate and long-term mortality only included EVAR in the abdominal position (EVAAR) versus open surgery and did not randomize patients with thoracoabdominal aneurysms, mainly because endografts in the thoracic position have only received US Food and Drug Administration (FDA) approval in March 2005. Despite promising results of TEVAR versus open repair in the reduction of perioperative morbidity, mid-term results are less promising and large randomised trials addressing long-term outcomes are still needed.

In a retrospective database review, Stone *et al.* compared the perioperative and 48-month mortality of patients undergoing TEVAR with those undergoing open surgery during the same time period [31]. Operative mortality was significantly lower in the TEVAR group (7.6%) versus open surgery group (15.1%) ($p = 0.09$). Survival at 48 months was similar for both cohorts (~60%). Reinterventions were required at a nearly identical rate for open repair and TEVAR (10%) and both groups experienced similar rates of spinal cord ischaemic complications (~7%)

Fenestrated and branched endografts are considered investigational devices and have not been approved for general use. In a recently published retrospective review, Bakoyiannis *et al.* reported on outcomes of 155 patients who underwent fenestrated and branched endograft insertion for thoracoabdominal aneurysms [32]. The 30-day mortality was 7.1%, while the 1-year mortality was 16.1% with 18.4% patients developing type I endoleak, 5.8% developing renal failure and 3.2% of patients developing permanent lower extremity neurological deficits, highlighting the high morbidity and mortality associated with these procedures.

With the advancement in technology that increases patients' anatomical suitability for EVAR through various modifications in endograft designs, as well as improvement in imaging modalities and surgical expertise, the hope is that resultant endovascular exclusion of thoracoabdominal aneurysms will translate into a lesser incidence of endoleaks, a lower reintervention rate and ultimately a reduction in long-term aneurysm-related morbidity and mortality and improved survival.

References

1. Derrow AE, Seeger JM, Dame DA, *et al.* The outcome in the United States after thoracoabdominal aortic aneurysm repair, renal artery bypass, and mesenteric revascularization. *J Vasc Surg* 2001;**34**:54–61.

2. Parodi JC, Palmaz JC, Barone HD. Transfemoral intraluminal graft implantation for abdominal aortic aneurysms. *Ann Vasc Surg* 1991;**5**:491–9.

3. ACCF/AHA/AATS/ACR/ASA/ SCA/SCAI/SIR/STS/SVM. Guidelines for the Diagnosis and Management of Patients with Thoracic Aortic Disease: Executive Summary. A Report of the American College of Cardiology Foundation/American Heart Association Task Force on Practice Guidelines, American Association for Thoracic Surgery, American College of Radiology, American Stroke Association,

Society of Cardiovascular Anesthesiologists, Society for Cardiovascular Angiography and Interventions, Society of Interventional Radiology, Society of Thoracic Surgeons, and Society for Vascular Medicine. *Anesth and Analg* 2010;**111** • Number 2

4. Nienaber CA, Rousseau H, Eggebrecht H, *et al.* The INvestigation of STEnt Grafts in Aortic Dissection (INSTEAD) Trial *Circulation* 2009;**120**:2519–28.

5. Greenberg RK, West K, Pfaff K, *et al.* Beyond the aortic bifurcation: branched endovascular grafts for thoracoabdominal and aortoiliac aneurysms. *J Vasc Surg* 2006;**43**:879–86.

6. Greenberg RK, Sternbergh WC, 3rd, Makaroun M, *et al.* Intermediate results of a United States multicenter trial of fenestrated endograft repair for juxtarenal abdominal aortic aneurysms. *J Vasc Surg* 2009;**50**:730–7.

7. Matsumura JS, Lee WA, Mitchell RS, *et al.* The Society for Vascular Surgery Practice Guidelines: Management of the left subclavian artery with thoracic endovascular aortic repair. *J Vasc Surg* 2009;**50**:1155–8.

8. Greenberg RK, Haddad F, Svensson L, *et al.* Hybrid approaches to thoracic aortic aneurysms: the role of endovascular elephant trunk completion. *Circulation* 2005;**112**:2619–26.

9. Svensson LG, Kouchoukos NT, Miller DC, *et al.* Expert consensus document on the treatment of descending thoracic aortic disease using endovascular stent-grafts. *Ann Thorac Surg* 2008;**85**:S1–41.

10. ACC/AHA. Guidelines on Perioperative Cardiovascular Evaluation and Care for Noncardiac Surgery: A Report of the American College of Cardiology/American Heart Association Task Force on Practice Guidelines (Writing Committee to Revise the 2002 Guidelines on Perioperative Cardiovascular Evaluation for Noncardiac Surgery). *Circulation* 2007;**116**:e418–e500.

11. Lee TH, Marcantonio ER, Mangione CM, *et al.* Derivation and prospective validation of a simple index for prediction of cardiac risk of major non cardiac surgery. *Circulation* 1999;**100**:1043–9.

12. Azizzadeh A, Sanchez LA, Miller CC, *et al.* Glomerular filtration rate is a predictor of mortality after endovascular abdominal aortic aneurysm repair. *J Vasc Surg* 2006;**43**:14–18.

13. Barrett BJ, Parfrey PS. Preventing contrast nephropathy induced by contrast medium. *N Engl J Med* 2006;**354**:379–86.

14. Diaz-Sandoval LJ, Kosowsky BD, Losordo DW. Acetylcysteine to prevent angiography-related renal tissue injury (the APART trial). *Am J Cardiol* 2002;**89**:356–8.

15. Verhoeven EG, Cina CS, Tielliu IF, *et al.* Local anaesthesia for endovascular abdominal aortic aneurysm repair. *J Vasc Surg* 2005;**42**:402–9.

16. Ruppert V, Leurs LJ, Steckmeier B, Buth J, Umscheid T. Influence of anaesthesia type on outcome after endovascular aortic aneurysm repair: an analysis based on EUROSTAR data. *J Vasc Surg* 2006;**44**:16–21.

17. Coselli JS, LeMaire SA, Köksoy C, Schmittling ZC, Curling PE. Cerebrospinal fluid drainage reduces paraplegia after thoracoabdominal aortic aneurysm repair: results of a randomized clinical trial. *J Vasc Surg* 2002;**35**:631–9.

18. Hnath JC, Mehta M, Taggert JB, *et al.* Strategies to improve spinal cord ischemia in endovascular thoracic aortic repair: outcomes of a prospective cerebrospinal fluid drainage protocol. *J Vasc Surg* 2008;**48**:836–40.

19. Cheung AT, Pochettino A, McGarvey M, *et al.* Strategies to manage paraplegia risk after endovascular stent repair of descending thoracic aortic aneurysms. *Ann Thorac Surg* 2005;**80**:1280–9.

20. Swaminathan M, Lineberger CK, McCann RL, Mathew JP. The importance of intraoperative transesophageal echocardiography in endovascular repair of thoracic aortic aneurysms. *Anesth Analg* 2003;**97**:1566–72.

21. Qu L, Raithel D. Techniques for precise thoracic endograft placement. *J Vasc Surg* 2009;**49**:1069–72.

22. Plaschke K, Böckler D, Schumacher H, Martin E, Bardenheuer HJ. Adenosine-induced cardiac arrest and EEG changes in patients with thoracic aorta endovascular repair. *Br J Anaesth* 2006;**96**:310–16.

23. Pornratanarangsi S, Webster MW, Alison P, Nand P. Rapid ventricular pacing to lower blood pressure during endograft deployment in the thoracic aorta. *Ann Thorac Surg* 2006;**81**:e21–3.

24. Lee WA, Martin TD, Gravenstein N. Partial right atrial inflow occlusion for controlled systemic hypotension during thoracic endovascular aortic repair. *J Vasc Surg* 2008;**48**:494–8.

25. Prinssen M, Verhoeven EL, Buth J, *et al.* A randomized trial comparing conventional and endovascular repair of abdominal aortic aneurysms (DREAM–1). *N Engl J Med* 2004;**351**:1607–18.

26. EVAR Trial Participants. Endovascular aneurysm repair versus open repair in patients with abdominal aortic aneurysm (EVAR trial 1): randomised controlled trial. *Lancet* 2005;**365**:2179–86.

27. Greenhalgh RM, Brown LC, Kwong GP, *et al.* Comparison of endovascular aneurysm repair with open repair in patients with abdominal aortic aneurysm (EVAR trial 1), 30-day operative mortality results: randomised controlled trial. *Lancet* 2004;**364**:843–8.

28. Schermerhorn ML, O'Malley AJ, Jhaveri A, et al. Endovascular vs. open repair of abdominal aortic aneurysms in the Medicare population. *N Engl J Med* 2008;**358**:464–74.

29. FA Lederle, JA Freischlag, TC Kyriakides, *et al.* Outcome following endovascular vs. open repair of abdominal aortic aneurysm: a randomized trial. *JAMA* 2009;**302**:1535–42.

30. Blankensteijn JD, de Jong SE, Prinssen M, *et al.* Two year outcomes after conventional or endovascular repair of abdominal aortic aneurysms (DREAM-2). *N Engl J Med* 2005;**352**:2398–405.

31. Stone DH, Brewster DC, Kwolek CJ, *et al.* Stent-graft versus open-surgical repair of the thoracic aorta: mid-term results. *J Vasc Surg* 2006;**44**:1188–97.

32. CN Bakoyiannis, KP Economopoulos, S Georgopoulos, *et al.* Fenestrated and branched endografts for the treatment of thoracoabdominal aortic aneurysms: a systematic review. *Endovasc Ther* 2010;**17**:201–9.

Anaesthesia for emergency abdominal aortic surgery

Alastair F. Nimmo

Introduction

Emergency abdominal aortic surgery may be required for a ruptured aortic aneurysm, a symptomatic aneurysm or for acute occlusion of the aorta with distal ischaemia.

The term *ruptured or leaking aneurysm* applies to the situation in which blood has escaped through a defect in the wall of the aortic aneurysm. There may initially be only a small leak of blood from the aorta, or a larger retroperitoneal haematoma (Figure 13.1) or massive intraperitoneal bleeding. Most patients who suffer a ruptured aneurysm die before reaching hospital. Of those who survive, some are shocked on arrival in hospital and others have a normal blood pressure. However, a haemodynamically stable patient with a ruptured aneurysm may lose further blood from the aorta, deteriorate and die at any moment so that repair of the aneurysm is extremely urgent.

Abdominal aortic aneurysms can cause symptoms by a variety of mechanisms including embolisation of contents of the aneurysm sac to the arteries of the lower limbs. However, the term *symptomatic aneurysm* usually refers to the situation in which a patient with an aortic aneurysm has abdominal or back pain and aneurysm tenderness and it is thought that, although the aneurysm has not yet ruptured, there is a high risk of rupture.

Ruptured aortic aneurysm

Anaesthesia for repair of ruptured abdominal aortic aneurysm (AAA) is one of the most challenging situations faced by an anaesthetist. Anaesthesia and surgery are very urgent. The patient is usually elderly and often has cardiac, respiratory or renal disease but

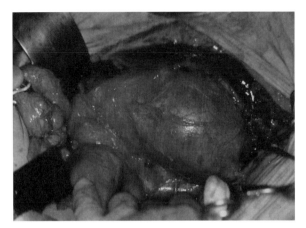

Figure 13.1 A ruptured aortic aneurysm at operation.

the information available is frequently incomplete and the time for assessment and investigations very limited.

Presentation and diagnosis

A ruptured AAA usually occurs in patients older than 60 years and in men more commonly than women (because men are more likely to have an aneurysm). The classic presentation of a ruptured AAA is the sudden onset of abdominal or back pain in association with an episode of syncope or hypotension and a pulsatile abdominal mass. However, this combination of symptoms and signs is not always present and misdiagnosis or delayed diagnosis is common. Pain may have been present for days or weeks before presentation or may not be apparent, particularly in patients presenting with confusion or an impaired conscious level. Blood pressure may be normal on admission and palpation of the aneurysm may be difficult if the patient is obese. Other symptoms such as vomiting and dizziness may be present.

Core Topics in Vascular Anaesthesia, ed. Carl Moores and Alastair F. Nimmo. Published by Cambridge University Press. © Cambridge University Press 2012.

On the other hand, a patient with a AAA which has not ruptured who has another cause of abdominal or back pain or shock such as cholecystitis or a myocardial infarction may mistakenly be thought to have a ruptured aneurysm.

A portable ultrasound examination in the Emergency Department can confirm the presence of an aneurysm but is not a reliable guide as to whether an aneurysm has ruptured. In the past it was considered inappropriate to undertake a CT scan of the abdomen if there was a high suspicion of a ruptured AAA because the delay caused by the investigation may result in the patient's condition deteriorating and death occurring before surgery. However, now that many Emergency Departments have CT scanners in or immediately beside the department, a CT scan can often be undertaken very quickly and if endovascular repair of a ruptured AAA is contemplated, a preoperative CT scan is usually required to decide if that approach is possible and to plan the procedure.

Occasionally AAAs rupture into the inferior vena cava to produce an aortocaval fistula or into the bowel, resulting in an aortoenteric fistula. An aortocaval fistula may be diagnosed before surgery – from clinical signs of venous engorgement, high-output cardiac failure and a continuous 'machinery' abdominal murmur or thrill, or on CT scan – or it may be a surprise finding during surgery. A primary aortoenteric fistula occurs when the aneurysm erodes into bowel, usually into adherent duodenum. A secondary aortoenteric fistula is a complication of previous aortic surgery and usually there is erosion of the proximal aortic suture line into the duodenum. In both types, minor episodes of gastrointestinal haemorrhage may occur initially followed by massive exsanguinating haemorrhage hours to weeks later.

Management options

There are three options for management of a ruptured AAA:

(1) open surgical repair
(2) endovascular repair
(3) conservative management, i.e. palliative care.

The patient may have been previously assessed for elective repair of an asymptomatic AAA and the decision made at that time that the risks of surgery exceeded the benefits. It does not necessarily follow that an attempt to repair the aneurysm is inappropriate

Table 13.1 Edinburgh Ruptured Aneurysm (ERA) score [1]. One point is allocated for each preoperative variable that fulfils the criterion resulting in a score of between 0 and 3 points

Preoperative variable	Score
Haemoglobin <90 g/l	1
Best recorded in-hospital Glasgow Coma Scale of <15	1
Recorded in-hospital Blood pressure of <90 mm Hg	1

now that it has ruptured. Rupture of an AAA is almost always fatal if repair is not undertaken so the balance of risk and benefit may now be very different.

However, repair of ruptured AAA is associated with a high rate of death and complications and may be considered inappropriate in some patients – for example:

- patients with underlying medical conditions that preclude any significant long-term survival (e.g. terminal cancer)
- patients with underlying conditions that already result in poor quality of life (e.g. demented elderly nursing home patient)
- patients in whom a combination of age, comorbidity, clinical presentation and, when known, aneurysm extent (i.e. suprarenal or thoracoabdominal aneurysm) makes survival with a reasonable quality of life appear unlikely.

Various scoring systems have been used as an aid to predicting the outcome of ruptured AAA repair [1]. Those that rely on the results of laboratory investigations such as serum creatinine have the disadvantage that the required information may not be available at the time the decision as to whether or not to attempt to repair the aneurysm is made. Incorporating preoperative haemoglobin into a score is less of a problem because point of care measurement of haemoglobin is commonly available in the Emergency Department. An example of such a scoring system, the Edinburgh Ruptured Aneurysm (ERA) score, is shown in Table 13.1. In a prospective study of several scoring systems, 27 of 111 patients with a diagnosis of ruptured AAA did not undergo attempted operative repair [1]. In 13 of these cases the reason for not attempting repair was refractory cardiac arrest/loss of consciousness. The remaining

84 patients underwent open surgery. The 30-day or in-hospital mortality was 26% in patients with an ERA score of ≤ 1, 59% in patients with a score of 2 and 82% in patients with a score of 3.

The commonest operation for a ruptured AAA is open surgery with a transperitoneal approach through a midline or transverse abdominal incision to an aneurysm that has ruptured retroperitoneally. The posterior peritoneum, often distended with haematoma, is exposed before dissecting and clamping the neck of the aneurysm – usually below the renal arteries. There is a risk of tearing the left renal vein or its tributaries during the dissection and the resulting venous bleeding can be difficult or impossible to control. Sometimes the aorta is clamped above the renal arteries or above the coeliac axis. After clamping the neck of the aneurysm, both common iliac arteries are clamped, the aneurysm is opened and its contents evacuated. Bleeding occurs from the orifices of lumbar arteries in the posterior wall of the aneurysm and these are oversewn. The inferior mesenteric artery, if patent, is usually tied off.

A prosthetic tube or Y-shaped graft is sutured end-to-end to the neck of the aneurysm to form the top anastomosis, then a clamp is applied to the graft and the upper aortic clamp is removed to test the anastomosis. The lower end of the graft is then sutured to the aortic bifurcation in the case of a tube graft, or in the case of a Y-graft to the bifurcation of each common iliac artery. The graft is thoroughly flushed to remove any clot before the lower anastomosis is completed and the clamps on the iliac arteries are released one side at a time.

Endovascular repair of ruptured AAAs has become a common technique in some centres in recent years. A contrast-enhanced CT scan is usually undertaken to determine if endovascular repair is possible and the size of the stent-graft(s) required. At the start of the procedure a balloon may be inserted via the femoral artery into the supracoeliac aorta and inflated to produce temporary control of bleeding until the stent-graft is deployed. Two types of stent-graft are available for this procedure. Modular bifurcated stent-grafts may be used, as are commonly used for elective endovascular repair. A main aortic body with ipsilateral iliac leg is inserted through one femoral artery. The other iliac leg is inserted through the contralateral femoral artery and attached to the main body to form a Y-shaped graft. It is necessary to have a large variety of sizes of the modular stent-graft components in stock to ensure that suitable sizes are immediately available.

Alternatively, an aorto-uni-iliac stent-graft can be inserted through one femoral artery to exclude the aneurysm from the circulation. This may be inserted more quickly than a bifurcated stent-graft and a smaller selection of graft sizes needs to be stocked. However, after insertion of an aorto-uni-iliac stent it is necessary to occlude the contralateral iliac artery to prevent retrograde flow into the aneurysm sac and then an open surgical femoro-femoral bypass graft is required to restore the circulation to the contralateral leg.

Conventional open surgery is typically associated with an operative (30-day or in-hospital) mortality rate of around 40–50%. This figure is affected by a hospital's policy on the selection of patients for surgery and tends to be higher in units that operate on almost all patients with ruptured aneurysms than in those that elect not to operate on moribund patients. A number of case series of endovascular repair of ruptured AAA report lower mortality rates than this. However, patients selected for endovascular repair were typically haemodynamically stable and had 'favourable anatomy' for endovascular repair, i.e. with an infrarenal neck of the aneurysm long enough for the top of the stent-graft to obtain a seal and without severe iliac artery disease. These factors would also tend to result in a lower mortality rate for open surgical repair. Some centres have reported reduced overall mortality rates after adopting a policy of endovascular repair for suitable patients with ruptured AAA [2,3]. However, there may be publication bias with hospitals whose results improve being more likely to publish than those whose results remain unchanged or get worse. A multicentre randomised trial of open surgery versus endovascular repair for ruptured AAA, the IMPROVE trial, is currently under way.

Assessment

When it has been decided that surgery should be undertaken to repair a suspected ruptured AAA, the patient should be transferred to the operating room as quickly as possible because their condition may rapidly deteriorate at any moment leading to cardiorespiratory arrest. Investigations should not delay transfer to theatre except when it has been decided that an emergency CT scan is appropriate. Nor should transfer be delayed by attempts to insert an arterial cannula or central venous catheter. Oxygen should be given by face-mask and at least one large peripheral intravenous cannula inserted if possible in the Emergency Department. Blood samples should be taken when the cannula is inserted for a full blood count, coagulation screen, urea and electrolytes and glucose and for blood transfusion but there is no need to wait for the results of blood tests before surgery. If point-of-care testing is available, rapid results of for example the haemoglobin concentration may be obtained. Blood components, e.g. 10 units of red cells, 4 units of fresh frozen plasma (FFP) and 2 standard adult doses of platelets, should be requested for issue as soon as possible. An ECG and portable chest X-ray and insertion of a urethral catheter can be performed very quickly in most Emergency Departments and may well already have been done by the time the decision is made that the patient should have surgery. If not, they should not be allowed to delay transfer to theatre.

A brief assessment of the patient should be undertaken before or during transfer to theatre. A history of the previous state of health and any drugs being taken (e.g. oral anticoagulants or dual antiplatelet therapy) may be obtained from the patient, relatives or any case notes that are available. A brief clinical examination should include assessment of the heart rate and rhythm, blood pressure, peripheral perfusion, conscious level, whether dentures are present and whether there is likely to be any difficulty with tracheal intubation. Vascular surgery patients may have a significant difference in blood pressure between the two arms, usually because of a subclavian artery stenosis, and if this is the case the higher reading should be regarded as being correct [4]. The results of any investigations that are available should be reviewed. A chest X-ray may reveal that the aneurysm extends to involve the thoracic aorta.

Analgesia may be required if the patient is in severe pain and small doses of intravenous fentanyl are appropriate in this situation. However, shocked elderly patients may be very sensitive to the effects of opioids which may decrease blood pressure, depress conscious level and result in airway obstruction. Therefore, the aim should be to relieve severe pain while getting the patient to theatre as quickly as possible, rather than making the patient completely comfortable, unless it has been decided that surgery is inappropriate.

Preoperative fluid resuscitation

It is common practice to avoid or restrict giving intravenous fluids to a patient with a ruptured AAA until anaesthesia is induced and surgery is about to start even if the patient is hypotensive. The rationale for this 'permissive hypotension' or 'hypotensive resuscitation' is that after initial bleeding from the aortic aneurysm, clot formation, retroperitoneal tamponade and hypotension may be important in limiting further haemorrhage. Fluid resuscitation to restore blood pressure before the aorta is clamped may dislodge clot and overcome tamponade. It may result in further haemorrhage and in dilutional anaemia and coagulopathy. There have been no randomised trials of preoperative fluid resuscitation (nor of anaesthetic techniques) in ruptured AAA patients. However, a randomised trial in hypotensive patients with penetrating torso injuries found that mortality and complication rates were reduced by not giving intravenous fluid until the patients reached the operating room [5]. Animal models of aortic haemorrhage have also provided support for a policy of hypotensive resuscitation [6].

In practice, hypotensive resuscitation may involve either maintaining an arbitrary minimum value of blood pressure, e.g. a systolic of 70 mm Hg, or not giving any intravenous fluids unless hypotension is producing cerebral or myocardial ischaemia. It is essential that any delay before surgery is minimised to avoid a prolonged period of preoperative hypotension. If intravenous fluids are given before surgery red cells may need to be given as well as clear fluids to avoid a severe dilutional anaemia.

Management in the operating theatre: open repair

General anaesthesia is required for open repair of a ruptured aneurysm and the insertion of an epidural catheter before surgery is not appropriate. The patient should be transferred directly into the operating room as rapidly as possible and not into an anaesthetic induction room. Anaesthesia is usually induced after the surgeons have disinfected and draped the abdomen so that the operation can start as soon as the patient is asleep. (Occasionally tracheal intubation is required before this for airway protection or to assist ventilation in the unconscious moribund patient and if surgery is considered appropriate in this situation little anaesthesia may be required before aortic clamping.)

Table 13.2 Minimum requirements for satisfactory management of the start of anaesthesia for a ruptured AAA

Two anaesthetists

At least one, preferably two, large intravenous cannulae

Rapid fluid infuser and warmer

Red cell concentrate in theatre

Anaesthetic drugs for rapid sequence induction

Vasoconstrictor/inotrope drugs, e.g. syringes of ephedrine, phenylephrine, and epinephrine 1 in 100 000

Monitoring: five-lead ECG and ST segments, blood pressure, O_2 saturation

Preparation

Two experienced anaesthetists are required for satisfactory management of the patient. The drugs and equipment that are required at induction of anaesthesia are shown in Table 13.2. Red cells should be in the operating theatre, ready to transfuse before anaesthesia is induced, but surgery should not be delayed by waiting for blood grouping, antibody screens or cross-matching. Emergency group O blood should be used if group-specific blood is not yet available.

Invasive blood pressure monitoring at the time of induction is useful because severe hypotension may occur at this stage and progress to cardiac arrest. If an arterial cannula is in place before induction a sample may be taken for point-of-care testing of haemoglobin. The arterial cannula should be inserted in an upper limb artery, usually radial or brachial. However, if the blood pressure is low, it may be difficult to insert an arterial cannula and prolonged attempts should not be allowed to significantly delay surgery. It is desirable to position one or both of the upper limbs on arm boards at 90° to the body so that there is access during surgery to existing intravenous and arterial cannulae or for the insertion of new ones. If a urethral catheter is not already in place it may be inserted before induction. A central venous catheter is not required before surgery unless it has proved impossible to insert a large peripheral venous cannula, in which case a large central venous catheter is useful. Depth of anaesthesia monitoring of both induction and maintenance of anaesthesia is a useful aid to avoiding awareness while not giving unnecessarily large doses of anaesthetic agents. A shocked elderly patient may require much lower doses of anaesthetic than are typically used.

Induction

A rapid sequence induction should be performed. Etomidate or ketamine are appropriate for induction if the patient is hypotensive; thiopentone may be considered if the blood pressure is normal. The use of propofol for induction is not appropriate. Unless the patient has already received opioid analgesia or is profoundly hypotensive, intravenous opioid should be given before induction to reduce the risk of a hypertensive response to laryngoscopy causing further bleeding. Fentanyl is appropriate but morphine should be avoided because renal failure may occur, impairing the excretion of the active metabolite morphine-6-glucuronide.

A large fall in blood pressure may occur on induction because of vasodilation, reduction in sympathetic tone and circulating catecholamine levels, reduced venous return secondary to positive pressure ventilation and abdominal muscle relaxation reducing tamponade and allowing further bleeding. The anaesthetist should aim to maintain the blood pressure around the preinduction level (unless the preinduction blood pressure was considered to be unacceptably low), avoiding or correcting large falls in pressure but not raising the blood pressure of a patient who was hypotensive before induction to normal until the aorta is clamped. Rapid infusion of fluids and sometimes also the administration of vasoconstrictor or inotrope drugs may be required to maintain the blood pressure at an acceptable level. If the hypotension is severe the operating table should be tilted head down and only gentle positive pressure ventilation given. If continuous invasive blood pressure monitoring is not possible at induction, palpation of the carotid pulse and observation of the capnography trace may give an early indication of a profound fall in blood pressure and cardiac output. Rapid infusion of clear fluids can very quickly result in a severe dilutional anaemia. Therefore, unless the haemoglobin concentration is known to be high, red cells should also be given.

Maintenance

Surgery may commence as soon as the patient is unconscious. If suxamethonium was given for muscle relaxation during induction, a non-depolarising relaxant should be given as soon as the tracheal tube is in place. The surgeon faces a difficult enough task without having to contend with a patient coughing or

Table 13.3 Recommended further monitoring during repair of ruptured AAA

Temperature

Urine output

Depth of anaesthesia monitoring

Monitoring of cardiac output/cardiac filling

Point-of-care monitoring of haemoglobin, blood gases, electrolytes, coagulation

straining as the effect of the suxamethonium wears off. Maintenance of anaesthesia may be either with a volatile anaesthetic or a propofol infusion. A low concentration of volatile anaesthetic/low target concentration or infusion rate of propofol will be appropriate initially if the blood pressure is low and depth of anaesthesia monitoring is very useful for guiding appropriate adjustment.

Once the surgeon has clamped the aorta, blood pressure usually rises and the aim should now be to maintain a blood pressure around normal. Severe hypertension and/or signs of myocardial ischaemia may require treatment during aortic clamping. Further opioid analgesia and an increase in the depth of anaesthesia may be given as may specific treatment with an intravenous beta-blocker or an infusion of glyceryl trinitrate (GTN). Intravenous beta-blocker, e.g. atenolol 2.5 mg, may be given if tachycardia is associated with ECG signs of ischaemia.

Monitoring

Additional monitoring that is recommended during emergency abdominal aortic surgery is shown in Table 13.3. If not already in place an arterial cannula, central venous catheter, nasogastric tube and nasopharyngeal temperature probe should now be inserted. Central venous pressure (CVP) monitoring is of limited value in determining how much intravenous fluid is required [7]. While a low CVP during surgery suggests hypovolaemia, CVP may also be normal or high in this situation. Other monitors of cardiac output or filling or aortic flow are more useful as a guide to intravenous fluid administration. Examples include pulse contour analysis of the arterial pressure waveform, transoesophageal echocardiography and oesophageal Doppler. Pulse contour analysis has the advantage of being quick to set up and not requiring any additional probe to be inserted.

The displayed absolute values of stroke volume and cardiac output are unlikely to be accurate in the presence of the marked haemodynamic changes that occur during aneurysm repair. However, the percentage increase in stroke volume in response to an intravenous fluid challenge may give a useful indication of whether hypovolaemia is present, as may the pulse pressure variation or stroke volume variation over the respiratory cycle (see also Chapter 6).

Temperature should be monitored and attempts made to maintain or restore normothermia by raising the temperature in the operating room, warming intravenous fluids, forced-air warming of the upper body and under-body warming of the upper body, and ensuring the head is wrapped or covered. Warming of the lower limbs, which will be ischaemic during the period of aortic clamping, should be avoided.

Point-of-care monitoring of haemoglobin, coagulation, arterial gases and acid–base status, electrolytes and glucose is extremely useful in guiding the appropriate administration of blood components and the correction of acid–base and electrolyte abnormalities during surgery.

Transfusion and correction of coagulopathy

Sufficient red cells should be transfused to avoid the development of severe anaemia, e.g. the haemoglobin should be maintained above 80 g/l. The use of intraoperative red cell salvage reduces the need for allogeneic blood transfusion.

Patients having surgery for a suspected ruptured AAA may have massive haemorrhage and severe coagulopathy, or a small contained rupture with little blood outside the aorta or indeed be found to have an aneurysm which hasn't in fact ruptured. There is, therefore, great variation in the presence and severity of abnormalities of haemostasis between patients and there may also be rapid changes during surgery. For example a patient with a ruptured AAA may have relatively normal coagulation at the start of surgery but develop a severe coagulopathy during the operation. In general, the greater the blood loss and the greater the degree of shock, the more severely coagulation is impaired.

It is not uncommon for patients presenting with a ruptured AAA, particularly patients with atrial fibrillation, to be taking warfarin and this should be reversed with prothrombin complex concentrate.

Dual antiplatelet therapy, for example with aspirin and clopidogrel, is another cause of excessive bleeding.

Once the aorta is clamped, the surgeon may be able to assess whether or not there is diffuse microvascular bleeding. Point-of-care testing of coagulation with thromboelastometry/thromboelastography is extremely useful and permits the rapid identification and treatment of abnormalities such as a low fibrinogen concentration, thrombocytopaenia or excessive fibrinolysis. (See Chapter 8 for a description of point-of-care monitoring of coagulation.)

If there are clinical signs of severe coagulopathy with diffuse bleeding and point-of-care testing is not available, it is preferable to treat the problem empirically, e.g. with transfusions of FFP and platelets, rather than waiting for laboratory results.

Heparin is not usually given to patients with a ruptured AAA if the clinical picture is of significant bleeding and impaired coagulation or if point-of-care testing indicates a coagulopathy. However, if there has been little blood loss and there is no evidence of impaired coagulation clinically or on point-of-care testing, intravenous heparin may be given before aortic clamping.

Renal function

Renal dysfunction is common after ruptured AAA repair. In addition to the causes of renal dysfunction after elective aneurysm repair discussed in Chapter 10, there may also have been a period of preoperative renal ischaemia as a result of haemorrhagic shock. Measures that reduce the incidence or severity of renal dysfunction are avoiding or minimising the duration of suprarenal aortic clamping, maintaining an adequate blood pressure and cardiac output (after any initial period of permissive hypotension) by giving sufficient intravenous fluid, and the avoidance of nephrotoxic drugs. No specific pharmacological measures have been shown to be of benefit.

Clamp release

A large fall in blood pressure may occur when the iliac clamps are released, reperfusing the ischaemic pelvis and lower limbs. Cardiac arrest may occur at this stage. The hypotension results from a combination of hypovolaemia as the vasodilated vessels of the lower body are refilled with blood (and bleeding from anastomoses may also occur), and the effects of ischaemic metabolites returning from the lower body causing pulmonary hypertension and reduced myocardial contractility.

Intravenous fluid loading before clamp release reduces the fall in blood pressure. It is important that the surgeon gives the anaesthetist advance warning of clamp release to permit fluid loading and so that the anaesthetist is ready to treat marked hypotension with further rapid intravenous fluid infusion and/or the intravenous injection of a vasoconstrictor/inotrope such as ephedrine. The clamps should be released slowly, reperfusing one leg at a time, and if the fall in blood pressure is excessive clamps may be reapplied or the iliac arteries temporarily compressed by the surgeon.

Other changes that occur on clamp release include a temporary fall in oxygen saturation, an increase in arterial and end-tidal carbon dioxide concentration and a worsening of the metabolic acidaemia that is usually already present. Minute ventilation should be increased provided that there is not severe hypotension.

If there is little or no fall in blood pressure or rise in carbon dioxide when the circulation to a leg is restored, the possibility that blood flow to the limb is obstructed by thrombus or emboli should be considered. If the leg appears ischaemic the surgeon may pass an embolectomy catheter into the femoral artery.

Postoperative care

It is important that satisfactory haemostasis has been obtained before the abdomen is closed. If there is significant ongoing bleeding after surgery it is unlikely that the patient will survive. Securing haemostasis requires both that the surgeon has stopped sources of surgical bleeding and that the anaesthetist has corrected coagulopathy that is causing diffuse microvascular bleeding. Point-of-care testing with thromboelastometry/thromboelastography enables the rapid diagnosis and appropriate treatment of the causes of a coagulopathy.

After repair of a ruptured AAA, the patient should be transferred to the intensive care unit for further care. Postoperative complications are common and include abdominal compartment syndrome, myocardial ischaemia and infarction, cardiac failure, respiratory failure, renal failure, colonic ischaemia, lower limb ischaemia, stroke and paraplegia. However, in most published series, the majority of patients who are alive after repair of a ruptured AAA survive to leave hospital.

Anaesthesia for endovascular repair of ruptured abdominal aortic aneurysm

Endovascular repair of a ruptured AAA may be undertaken under local (infiltration) anaesthesia or general anaesthesia. A combined technique may be used – the initial part of the procedure is performed under local anaesthesia and then, after the stent-graft has been deployed and the patient is haemodynamically stable, general anaesthesia is induced. If an aorto-uni-iliac stent-graft is deployed followed by a surgical femoro-femoral cross-over graft, the latter procedure is likely to be poorly tolerated by a patient under local anaesthetic because of ischaemic leg pain. The use of spinal or epidural anaesthesia has been described but has the disadvantages that coagulopathy may increase the risk of an epidural haematoma and that the sympathetic block may worsen hypotension before surgery, resulting in intravenous fluid administration and in uncertainty about whether the fall in blood pressure is the result of the anaesthetic or further bleeding from the aneurysm.

Much of the discussion above about management of open AAA repair applies to management of endovascular repair. Permissive hypotension is commonly employed before deployment of the stent and any delay before repair of the aneurysm must be minimised. The assessment of blood loss and clinical assessment of coagulopathy is made more difficult when the abdomen has not been opened. Intravenous heparin is given in some centres and avoided in others.

Whether the overall mortality and complication rate is reduced by endovascular repair of ruptured AAA is uncertain. Common complications after endovascular repair include abdominal compartment syndrome and renal failure. Decompression laparotomy may be required to treat abdominal compartment syndrome [8].

Symptomatic abdominal aortic aneurysm

A symptomatic AAA is one which is causing abdominal or back pain, is tender and is thought to be at a high risk of rupturing soon. Mortality rates from repair of symptomatic aneurysms are substantially higher than from elective aneurysm repair. The term, however, covers a spectrum of different presentations from the patient with a slightly tender aneurysm when seen at the outpatient clinic who the surgeon decides it is wise to admit with a view to repair on the next available elective operating list to a patient whose symptoms and signs may in fact be the result of a contained rupture. The appropriate anaesthetic management will also vary, therefore, from management similar to that of an elective AAA repair to management similar to that of a ruptured aneurysm. The urgency with which surgery is planned may be a guide as to the likelihood that a contained rupture has already occurred or is imminent but may be influenced by factors other than the patient's condition – for example by the surgeon's schedule and when the next available space on an elective list is available. A CT scan will usually have been undertaken before repair of a symptomatic aneurysm but a contained rupture can sometimes be difficult to identify.

An important decision that the anaesthetist managing a patient who is to have repair of a symptomatic aneurysm may have to make is whether or not to insert an epidural catheter before surgery. If immediate surgery is planned, insertion of an epidural catheter may cause some delay and if local anaesthetic (even a 'test dose') is injected through the catheter there is potential for confusion and misdiagnosis if hypotension then occurs because it may be the result of vasodilation from the epidural or of rupture of the aneurysm. Insertion of an epidural catheter is best avoided if the patient has had an episode of severe pain, syncope or hypotension and there is concern that this might have been the result of aneurysm rupture. On the other hand, if there is no history of these events, the CT scan suggests that it is unlikely the aneurysm has ruptured and coagulation is normal, then insertion of an epidural catheter is reasonable.

Acute aortic occlusion

Acute aortic occlusion may result from a saddle embolus – an embolus (usually of cardiac origin) which impacts at the aortic bifurcation – or from thrombosis in an atherosclerotic aorta, an aortic aneurysm or an aortic graft. It presents with sudden ischaemia of both lower limbs leading to symptoms and signs which may include pain, paralysis, numbness, paraesthesia, mottling, pallor or cyanosis. Paralysis and sensory loss may lead to misdiagnosis as a primary neurological problem. Femoral pulses are absent. Patients often have cardiac disease and/or peripheral arterial disease.

Treatment for the aortic occlusion may involve transfemoral embolectomy using Fogarty balloon catheters, aortobifemoral bypass or axillobifemoral bypass. Lower limb fasciotomy or amputation may be required. Intravenous heparin infusions are commonly given before and after surgery.

Patients with an acute aortic occlusion are severely ill and there is a high incidence of perioperative death, cardiac complications and renal failure. While transfemoral embolectomy can be performed under local (infiltration) anaesthesia, an experienced anaesthetist should be present to monitor the patient, provide analgesia and sedation if appropriate, give appropriate intravenous fluids and treat other conditions such as fast atrial fibrillation. Admission to the intensive care or high-dependency unit after surgery is appropriate.

References

1. Tambyraja AL, Lee AJ, Murie JA, Chalmers RT. Prognostic scoring in ruptured abdominal aortic aneurysm: a prospective evaluation. *J Vasc Surg* 2008;**47**:282–6.

2. Moore R, Nutley M, Cina CS, *et al*. Improved survival after introduction of an emergency endovascular therapy protocol for ruptured abdominal aortic aneurysms. *J Vasc Surg* 2007;**45**:443–50.

3. Wibmer A, Schoder M, Wolff KS, *et al*. Improved survival after abdominal aortic aneurysm rupture by offering both open and endovascular repair. *Arch Surg* 2008;**143**:544–9.

4. Frank SM, Norris EJ, Christopherson R, Beattie C. Right- and left-arm blood pressure discrepancies in vascular surgery patients. *Anesthesiology* 1991;**75**:457–63.

5. Bickell WH, Wall MJ, Jr, Pepe PE, *et al*. Immediate versus delayed fluid resuscitation for hypotensive patients with penetrating torso injuries. *N Engl J Med* 1994;**331**:1105–9.

6. Roberts K, Revell M, Youssef H, Bradbury AW, Adam DJ. Hypotensive resuscitation in patients with ruptured abdominal aortic aneurysm. *Eur J Vasc Endovasc Surg* 2006;**31**:339–44.

7. Gelman S. Venous function and central venous pressure: a physiologic story. *Anesthesiology* 2008;**108**:735–48.

8. Djavani Gidlund K, Wanhainen A, Björck M. Intra-abdominal hypertension and abdominal compartment syndrome after endovascular repair of ruptured abdominal aortic aneurysm. *Eur J Vasc Endovasc Surg* 2011;**41**:742–7.

Anaesthesia for aorto-iliac occlusive disease and lower limb revascularisation procedures

Alastair J. Thomson

Patients with peripheral arterial disease (PAD) are often elderly, and frequently have several co-existing medical problems and a limited functional reserve. As a result, they are at high risk of significant complications and death following lower limb revascularisation surgery. The anaesthetist caring for patients with PAD plays a key role in minimising these risks around the time of surgery.

Pathophysiology of peripheral arterial disease

Peripheral arterial disease is a common manifestation of generalised atherosclerosis and the pathogenic processes underlying the disease are the same as those which affect the coronary and cerebral circulations. Multiple causes including dyslipidaemia, endothelial dysfunction, inflammation, immunological factors, oxidative stress, hypercoagulabilty and chronic infection have all been implicated in its development [1].

Atherosclerotic plaques form in medium- and large-sized arteries – the aorta and lower limb vessels can be affected. These plaques can cause a number of clinical syndromes including a chronic, slowly progressive reduction in size of the vessel lumen that leads to exercise-induced symptoms of tissue ischaemia; or sudden, acute occlusion of vessels, due to plaque rupture and thrombosis, that may lead to tissue infarction and limb loss.

Epidemiology of peripheral arterial disease

The prevalence of PAD increases with age from 3–10% in middle-aged populations to 15–20% in people over 70 years [2]. However, many of these individuals are asymptomatic, with only one in every three or four patients with PAD experiencing intermittent claudication (IC), the classic symptom of lower limb PAD. In addition, many patients with IC never consult a doctor regarding their symptoms. This is important as PAD confers a similar risk of death from cardiovascular causes as does a history of coronary or cerebrovascular disease. It is therefore important that patients with PAD are recognised, and that risk factors are managed aggressively at as early a stage as possible. It is also important to appreciate that there is a strong association between the presence of PAD and coronary artery disease (CAD).

Risk factors for peripheral arterial disease

Smoking

The association between tobacco smoking and PAD is even stronger than that between smoking and CAD. Heavy smokers are four times more likely to develop PAD than non-smokers.

Diabetes mellitus

Patients with diabetes mellitus are twice as likely to have PAD compared with non-diabetic subjects, with poor glycaemic control being particularly associated with PAD. In addition, the disease process behaves more aggressively in diabetic patients with amputation being required five to ten times more frequently compared with those patients without diabetes.

Dyslipidaemia

High levels of total cholesterol, low-density lipoprotein (LDL) cholesterol and triglycerides and low levels of high-density lipoprotein (HDL) cholesterol are associated with an increased likelihood of developing

Core Topics in Vascular Anaesthesia, ed. Carl Moores and Alastair F. Nimmo. Published by Cambridge University Press.
© Cambridge University Press 2012.

PAD. It is also now appreciated that treatment of hypercholesterolaemia may reduce the progression of the disease in patients with PAD.

Hypertension

Elevated blood pressure is a risk factor for many types of cardiovascular disease including PAD. However, diabetes mellitus and smoking are relatively stronger risk factors for developing PAD.

Hyperhomocysteinaemia

Hyperhomocysteinaemia is common in patients with PAD and is now considered to be an independent risk factor for cardiovascular disease.

Chronic kidney disease

A strong association exists between chronic renal insufficiency and PAD.

Ethnicity

Black ethnicity doubles the likelihood of developing PAD.

Natural history of peripheral arterial disease

Unfortunately, the progression of the PAD process is similar no matter whether patients experience leg symptoms or not. The main determinant of whether symptoms are experienced is the level of activity adopted. Thus, active patients may experience troublesome claudication symptoms that significantly affect their quality of life, whilst the first presentation of PAD in sedentary individuals may be with critical limb ischaemia.

For the majority of patients with PAD, claudication symptoms stabilise over time due to development of collateral blood vessels, or to metabolic adaptations within the affected muscles. However, in the remaining 20% of patients, claudication symptoms worsen. In these patients, particularly when the ankle–brachial index (ABI) is <0.50 and deteriorating, invasive therapies may be required. Nevertheless, most patients with IC (except those with diabetes) can be reassured that amputation is required relatively rarely (2–3% risk over 5 years) [2]. Unfortunately, the same is not true for the small number of patients (1–2% risk over 5 years) who progress to critical limb

ischaemia (CLI). This is usually signified by the development of non-healing ulceration, severe rest pain or gangrene. These patients require urgent revascularisation therapy, but despite this still have a 25% risk of amputation and 25% risk of death over a 1-year period [3].

Symptoms and signs of peripheral arterial disease

Intermittent claudication

The classic symptom of PAD is intermittent claudication (IC). Patients experience painful, aching, cramping, or numb sensations in one or more muscle groups of the leg that are induced by exercise and relieved by rest. Intermittent claudication is caused by an inadequate supply of oxygenated blood to meet the metabolic demands of the affected muscles. The location of pain often correlates with the site of the arterial stenosis. Thus, buttock claudication is commonly due to aorto-iliac occlusive disease whilst calf claudication occurs secondary to obstruction of the superficial femoral or popliteal arteries. However, thigh claudication can be caused by either aorto-iliac or common femoral artery disease. The severity of IC experienced depends not only on the degree of the arterial stenosis, but also on the extent of any collateral circulation, and the quantity of exercise carried out. It should also be appreciated that not all patients with PAD experience classical claudication symptoms and that many atypical variations exist. For example, pains may not always be relieved by rest. Alternatively, some patients experience claudication symptoms that do not require cessation of exercise.

A number of conditions can cause symptoms that are similar to IC (Table 14.1); however, by far the most common cause is atherosclerosis. The clinical history can often act as a guide to identify some of the less common causes of IC from atherosclerosis. For example, in a young patient with no risk factors for atherosclerosis a diagnosis of popliteal entrapment syndrome may be more likely.

Critical limb ischaemia

Critical limb ischaemia (CLI) is the most severe expression of PAD. It is caused by a marked reduction in the perfusion and oxygenation of the tissues of the leg. Patients present with pain at rest, non-healing ulcers, or gangrene. A *minority* of patients with IC progress to develop CLI (incidence 0.25–0.45 per 1000 patients/year). However, CLI carries a significantly increased risk of amputation and mortality compared with PAD which produces less severe symptoms.

Acute limb ischaemia

A third possible mode of presentation is with a sudden decrease in limb perfusion that causes an imminent threat to limb viability (Table 14.2). Patients tend to present soon after the occlusive event due to the lack of collateral vessels that would allow some perfusion to be maintained. An immediate assessment of the viability of the limb needs to be made. The limb is often pale and painful; pulses are absent (this needs to be assessed accurately with Doppler); and there may be evidence of altered sensation. Muscle tenderness and weakness are later signs of ischaemia that are likely to result in tissue loss.

Classification of peripheral arterial disease

Two similar systems can be used to classify PAD: the *Fontaine* and the *Rutherford* methods (Table 14.3) are both based on the severity of symptoms and the presence of tissue loss [2].

Assessment of the patient with possible peripheral arterial disease

A detailed *history* should be taken that establishes the initial distance at which claudication symptoms occur and also the maximum distance that can be walked. In addition, an assessment of the impact of claudication on functional capacity and quality of life should also be made. Risk factors for PAD should be sought.

A careful general *examination* should then be carried out with particular attention being paid to

Table 14.1 Causes of claudication symptoms

Most common cause	Other causes
Atherosclerosis	Acute arterial disease (dissection, embolism, thrombosis, trauma) Occluded aneurysms (commonly popliteal) Popliteal artery entrapment Iliac endofibrosis (in athletes) Adventitial cystic disease Aortic coarctation Arterial fibrodysplasia Radiation fibrosis Retroperitoneal fibrosis Takayasu arteritis Thromboangiitis obliterans (Buerger disease) Vasospasm

Table 14.2 Causes of acute limb ischaemia

Native thrombosis
Embolism (e.g. from the heart in a patient with atrial fibrillation)
Reconstruction occlusions/ graft thrombosis
Peripheral aneurysm with thrombosis or embolus
Trauma/iatrogenic (e.g. following arterial catheterisation)

Table 14.3 Classification of peripheral arterial disease

Fontaine		Rutherford		
Stage	Clinical	Grade	Category	Clinical
I	Asymptomatic	0	0	Asymptomatic
IIa	Mild claudication	I	1	Mild claudication
IIb	Moderate to severe claudication	I	2	Moderate claudication
		I	3	Severe claudication
III	Ischaemic rest pain	II	4	Ischaemic rest pain
IV	Ulceration or gangrene	III	5	Minor tissue loss
		III	6	Ulceration or gangrene

Table 14.4 Use of ankle–brachial index (ABI) to assess severity of peripheral arterial disease

ABI	Interpretation
>1.30	Non-compressible, calcified arteries
1.00–1.29	Normal
0.91–0.99	Borderline
0.81–0.90	Mild PAD
0.50–0.80	Moderate PAD
<0.50	Severe PAD

Table 14.5 Major objectives in treating peripheral arterial disease

Reducing overall mortality from cardiovascular disease
Maintaining functional ability
Avoiding amputation

the lower limbs. Pulses should be felt – these are often absent below the level of arterial stenoses. Any skin changes including hair loss, temperature differences and areas of ulceration should be noted. Abdominal examination may detect the presence of a large abdominal aortic aneurysm. The heart and carotid arteries should also be auscultated to establish the presence of murmurs or bruits. *Buerger's test* is often carried out – this involves passively elevating, and then placing the leg in a dependent position. Skin pallor during elevation, followed by flushing of the foot when placed in a dependent position suggests underlying arterial disease.

Ankle–brachial index

The ankle–brachial index (ABI) is a simple, non-invasive, inexpensive test for PAD. It compares the systolic blood pressure at the ankle (in either the posterior tibial, or dorsalis pedis artery) to the blood pressure in the arm (brachial artery). The blood pressure in each limb is measured by inflating an appropriately sized blood pressure cuff to a supra-systolic pressure, and then deflating it slowly whilst using a continuous wave Doppler device to detect the point at which the pulse becomes audible (systolic pressure). The ankle systolic pressure is then divided by the arm pressure to give the ABI. An ABI of <0.90 is abnormal and has a sensitivity of 95% and a specificity of 100% for detecting PAD. The severity of PAD can also be assessed from the ABI (Table 14.4). Patients with claudication typically have ABIs in the range 0.50–0.90 whilst CLI is associated with ABIs <0.50. However, heavily calcified, non-compressible vessels, especially in diabetic patients, can lead to falsely elevated recordings. In addition to aiding the diagnosis and assessing the severity of PAD, abnormal ABI is an independent predictor of cardiovascular events and mortality: the lower the ABI, the higher the risk of cardiovascular morbidity or death.

For patients with symptoms that are strongly suggestive of IC, yet have normal ABIs at rest, measurement of ABI after exercise may help clarify the diagnosis. A fall in ABI of greater than 20% post-exercise is diagnostic of PAD.

Treatments for peripheral arterial disease

Intermittent claudication

The symptoms of IC experienced by many patients with PAD can result in significant limitations of exercise capacity and functional ability. However, the main focus of treatment for these patients is not only to improve their symptoms and functional capacity, but also to modify risk factors and reduce their likelihood of suffering adverse cardiovascular events and death in the future.

Once a diagnosis of PAD has been made, initial treatment strategies are focussed on exercise programmes and medical treatments that should improve symptoms and reduce future risk. Interventional treatments (percutaneous transluminal angioplasty, stent insertion and surgical bypass) should only be considered if these conservative measures fail (Table 14.5).

Medical treatments

Smoking cessation

This is of prime importance both in terms of disease prevention, and delaying the progression of established disease. Smoking cessation reduces the risk of future amputation and increases life expectancy. Stopping smoking is also crucial to the long-term success of vascular interventions (angioplasty or surgery) as continued smoking increases the likelihood of graft failure by a factor of three. Counselling and

149

pharmacotherapeutic techniques should be used to maximise the likelihood of successful cessation.

Hypertension

A strong association exists between PAD and hypertension, with high blood pressure contributing to the pathogenesis of atherosclerosis and increasing the risk of developing PAD. In addition, high blood pressure is a strong risk factor for cardiac and cerebrovascular events. Hypertension should therefore be treated aggressively. Unfortunately, treatment is often inadequate in those with PAD. The relevant national guidelines should be followed to direct choice of medications; however, the Heart Outcomes Prevention Evaluation (HOPE) study suggested that angiotensin-converting enzyme (ACE) inhibitor treatment may be particularly effective in reducing the likelihood of future cardiovascular morbidity and mortality in patients with PAD [4].

Hyperlipidaemia

Aggressive treatment of hyperlipidaemia is also required. Statin therapy should be prescribed for all patients. This not only reduces the risk of future cardiovascular events and mortality, but may also improve claudication distance and ABI. Patients with significant hypertriglyceridaemia may require additional fibrate therapy.

Diabetic control

The duration of diabetes mellitus and the level of glycaemic control are strongly associated with the risk of developing PAD. Indeed, 20–30% of patients with PAD are diabetic. Diabetic patients with PAD are at increased risk of experiencing adverse cardiovascular and cerebrovascular events. In addition they are far more likely to require lower limb amputation than non-diabetic patients. Glycaemic control should be optimised to reduce the likelihood of future adverse cardiovascular outcomes.

Exercise

Exercise reduces claudication symptoms and increases the walking speed and distance covered. The exact mechanisms through which these functional improvements occur are poorly understood, but involve more than development of collateral blood flow. Improvement of endothelial function and alterations in muscle metabolism may be important. Evidence exists to support the use of supervised exercise programmes, including both treadmill and resistance training, for the treatment of claudication symptoms. Traditionally, patients with claudication have been encouraged to continue exercising as much as possible. However, this requires considerable motivation and produces inferior results when compared with structured programmes. The benefits of exercise build up gradually over a period of weeks so that, ideally, programmes should last a minimum of 12 weeks with at least three 45-minute sessions being completed each week. However, exercise training is not suitable for more advanced forms of PAD including CLI.

Antiplatelet agents

Patients with PAD have high levels of platelet activation that increase the risk of thrombosis. Antiplatelet therapy reduces the risk of non-fatal myocardial infarction, stroke and overall mortality and should therefore be considered for all patients with PAD.

Aspirin is the drug of first choice, and reduces the likelihood of serious cardiovascular events by 23%. A dose of 75–150 mg per day has been shown to be as effective as higher doses. Subgroup analysis of the CAPRIE trial suggested that the ADP receptor antagonist clopidogrel may be more effective than aspirin at preventing cardiovascular events in patients with PAD [5]. However, this remains to be confirmed in a trial specifically designed to address this question. At present, clopidogrel is recommended as an alternative drug when aspirin is contraindicated. Likewise, combinations of aspirin and clopidogrel (dual antiplatelet therapy) have not been shown to offer significant advantages over aspirin monotherapy except for patients who undergo lower limb revascularisation with a prosthetic graft.

Other medications used in patients with peripheral arterial disease

Cilostazol is a phosphodiesterase III antagonist that has a number of different actions including vasodilatation, antiplatelet effects and inhibition of proliferation of smooth muscle cells. It may be useful for some patients with claudication symptoms as it has been shown to increase pain-free walking distances by 40–70%. Because of pro-arrhythmic actions it is contraindicated in patients with heart failure.

Naftidrofuryl (a 5-HT$_2$ antagonist that alters platelet function and muscle metabolism) may also be used to improve walking distances in patients with IC.

Table 14.6 Factors to consider prior to interventional treatment (surgical or endovascular) for intermittent claudication

Evidence of severe disability (inability to work, or to perform activities important to the patient)

Lack of response to conservative treatments

Does the interventional treatment have an acceptable degree of risk and high likelihood of short- and long-term success?

Does the patient have other comorbidities that affect their prognosis or may limit exercise if IC is improved (e.g. severe angina)?

Source: Adapted from ACC/AHA 2005 Practice Guidelines for the Management of Patients With Peripheral Arterial Disease [3].

Pentoxifylline (a methylxanthine derivative with antiplatelet and anti-inflammatory effects) is another drug that is marketed for the symptomatic relief of IC. However, there is insufficient evidence to support its use.

Interventional treatment

For some patients with IC, conservative management, involving structured exercise and pharmacotherapy, fails to provide sufficient improvement of their symptoms or level of function. In these severely disabled patients, lower limb revascularisation procedures may be considered (Table 14.6).

Investigation of the location and extent of peripheral arterial disease

When revascularisation treatment (either endovascular or surgical) is being considered, further assessment of the anatomical location and extent of the PAD is required. This involves assessment of not only the area of stenosis, but also the arterial inflow and outflow from the affected area.

Digital subtraction angiography

Digital subtraction angiography (DSA) has historically been viewed as the 'gold standard' for the diagnosis of PAD. However, this is now rarely required for diagnostic purposes given the availability of modern, non-invasive alternatives (Duplex ultrasound and MRA). It remains part of many endovascular revascularisation procedures, however.

Duplex ultrasound

Duplex ultrasound is a technique that incorporates conventional (B-mode) ultrasonography along with colour Doppler waveform analysis. This allows visualisation of the vessel and stenotic areas and also gives information on blood flow and the systolic and diastolic arterial velocities. It is commonly used to further investigate patients with claudication and reduced ABIs. It can also be used to provide quantitative follow-up for patients who have undergone revascularisation procedures. It is an accurate, non-invasive test, but is dependent on operator skill. The accuracy of the technique can also be reduced by heavily calicified vessels, bowel gas and body habitus.

Magnetic resonance angiography and computed tomographic angiography

Magnetic resonance angiography (MRA) and computerised tomographic angiography (CTA) both allow the anatomical location and degree of stenosis of PAD to be determined non-invasively with high levels of sensitivity and specificity. There are advantages and disadvantages to each technique. Magnetic resonance angiography avoids exposure to ionising radiation. Furthermore, areas of heavy calcification within the arteries do not cause degradation of image quality. However, patients who are claustrophobic may not tolerate the examination and the test is not possible in patients with metallic implants or cardiac pacemakers. Patients with renal impairment are also at risk of developing nephrogenic systemic fibrosis following the use of gadolinium contrast in MRA. On the other hand, CTA can be performed significantly faster than MRA and produces higher-resolution images. However, it does require the use of iodinated contrast, which may cause allergic reactions and nephrotoxicity.

Revascularisation treatment options

Once the location and extent of the PAD have been established, alternative treatment options can then be considered. Unfortunately, there are few randomised clinical trials available to guide decisions on the most appropriate choice of revascularisation therapy (endovascular or surgical). Many factors including patient preference, clinician experience, likely lifespan of the selected treatment, the severity of comorbidities, and the risks of morbidity and mortality associated with the procedure may influence decisions. Two extensive guidelines that are based on the available evidence and expert opinion exist to help inform clinical decisions [2,3].

The TASC guidelines suggest that appropriate endovascular and surgical treatments can be selected based on the location and morphology of atherosclerotic lesions [2]. Thus, for disease within the iliac arteries, four types of lesions of increasing severity are described (A, B, C and D). Type A lesions are single, short areas of stenosis, whilst type D lesions are diffuse, long stenoses or occlusions, or bilateral disease of the external iliac arteries. In general, endovascular techniques are suggested for type A lesions, whilst surgical revascularisation is favoured for the more extensive type D lesions. A similar four-point scoring system (A to D) exists for atherosclerotic disease within femoropopliteal arteries. Again, endovascular treatments are recommended for simple, short segments of disease (type A lesions), whilst surgery is the preferred choice for type D lesions (complete occlusion of the common femoral artery, superficial femoral artery, or trifurcation).

Endovascular techniques

Endovascular techniques are generally based around balloon angioplasty (percutaneous transluminal angioplasty, PTA) where a catheter is fed into an appropriate location within the stenosed vessel under fluoroscopic guidance and a balloon is inflated to dilate the area of stenosis. This can be combined with insertion of stents that aim to reduce or delay the incidence of restenosis and occlusion. The duration of patency after endovascular procedures is, in general, prolonged by stent insertion compared with PTA. It is also influenced by the anatomical location, tending to be greater for proximal interventions in the iliac arteries (e.g. 1-year iliac artery stent patency rate 86%) and reducing for procedures carried out more distally (e.g. 1-year femoropopliteal stent patency rate 62%). Other anatomical factors associated with early occlusion include treatment of long segments of disease, and diffusely diseased distal vessels in addition to the presence of general risk factors including smoking, diabetes mellitus and renal impairment.

Ideally, pressure measurements should be made both pre- and post-stenosis prior to deciding to undertake endovascular treatment. This allows identification of patients with apparently major (50–75%) stenoses that are not haemodynamically significant who would be better treated by conservative means.

A number of other endovascular techniques are available including catheter-based atherectomy and thermal angioplasty. However, these treatments produce results that are inferior to PTA and stenting.

Surgical revascularisation techniques

A number of different surgical procedures are used to treat lower limb ischaemia. The most appropriate procedure for an individual patient is dependent on a number of factors – the location of the stenotic areas; the availability of suitable veins to act as bypass conduits; and the overall level of fitness of the patient and severity of comorbidities.

Surgery for aorto-iliac occlusive disease

The standard, most durable operation for aorto-iliac disease is the *aorto-bifemoral bypass graft* (or *aorto-unifemoral bypass graft* if only one iliac artery is diseased). This is a major surgical procedure that entails significant risks of perioperative morbidity (16%) and mortality (4.1%) [6]. As a result, this operation is generally reserved for younger patients who are judged to be at lower risk on preoperative assessment. Like open aortic aneurysm surgery, this operation involves a long midline or transverse abdominal incision, a full laparotomy, retroperitoneal dissection and vascular clamps being applied to the aorta and femoral arteries. An end-to-end or end-to-side anastomosis is completed between the upper end of the prosthetic (commonly Dacron) graft and the infrarenal aorta. The lower ends of the graft are then tunnelled retroperitoneally and anastomosed to either the common femoral or profunda femoris arteries in the groins.

The risks of aortofemoral grafting include those associated with any major vascular operation – infection, haemorrhage, coagulopathy, major organ dysfunction (myocardial ischaemia, acute respiratory distress syndrome, respiratory tract infection, renal impairment, cerebrovascular accident) plus surgery specific risks of limb loss, impotence and ischaemia of the pelvic contents, colon and spinal cord.

Extra-anatomical bypass grafts

Two alternatives exist to aortofemoral bypass grafting. These both involve bypassing arterial stenoses using prosthetic grafts that lie in subcutaneous, extra-anatomical locations. In general, they are performed in patients who are deemed to be unfit for the more major aortofemoral bypass procedure. Alternatively, they can sometimes be used as rescue treatments for failed grafts.

Axillo-bifemoral (or *uni-femoral*) *grafts* can be used in unfit patients with aorto-iliac occlusive disease who present with CLI. They are generally not used as a treatment for claudication as there is a significant risk of graft failure. A prosthetic reinforced polytetrafluoroethylene (PTFE) is anastomosed to one axillary artery in the infraclavicular fossa; the graft is then tunnelled subcutaneously down the side of the chest and abdomen to reach the groin where anastomosis to the femoral artery is completed. Extension of the graft to the contralateral groin can be carried out to treat bilateral iliac occlusions.

Femoro-femoral bypass grafts are used to revascularise an ischaemic leg that is caused by disease in one iliac artery when the contralateral iliac artery is relatively disease-free. A proportion of blood flow from the femoral artery on the unaffected side is diverted to the other femoral artery via a reinforced PTFE graft that is placed in a subcutaneous suprapubic position. Long-term patency rates are better for femoro-femoral bypass grafts than axillo-bifemoral grafts such that this operation can also be considered as a treatment for claudication in addition to CLI.

Surgery for infrainguinal arterial occlusive disease
Femoro-popliteal bypass and femoro-distal bypass grafting

Femoro-popliteal bypass is the most common surgical procedure performed to treat lower limb PAD. Occlusive disease often affects the middle to distal section of the superficial femoral artery (SFA). This operation bypasses the occluded segment of SFA by creating a parallel conduit for arterial blood flow. If possible, the ipsilateral long saphenous vein is used as the graft. This produces better long-term patency rates than prosthetic grafts (such as PTFE) which may have to be used when no suitable vein exists. The harvested, reversed (to remove the effect of the valves) long saphenous vein is placed in a tunnel that is created beneath the sartorius muscle in the medial part of the thigh. The upper part of the graft is then anastomosed to a division of the femoral artery (either common, superficial or profunda femoris). The lower end of the graft is anastomosed to the popliteal artery either above or below the knee. If more distal occlusive disease exists, it may be necessary to perform the lower anastomosis to one of the

crural vessels (anterior or posterior tibial, or peroneal arteries) or even to an artery at the level of the foot or ankle (these are referred to as *femoro-distal bypass grafts*). Despite the smaller surgical insult compared with aorto-bifemoral grafting, femoro-popliteal bypass grafting is associated with significant risks – when performed for CLI, the perioperative mortality rate is 6.3% [7].

Endarterectomy procedures can be performed on either the common femoral or profunda femoris arteries to improve blood flow if localised areas of stenosis exist. This operation involves removing the atheromatous material from the artery via a longitudinal arteriotomy. The endarterectomy is often combined with a *patch angioplasty* which involves patching a small piece of vein into the wall of the artery at the site of the arteriotomy. This process reduces the likelihood of narrowing the lumen of the artery during surgical closure.

Treatment of acute limb ischaemia

The most appropriate form of treatment for patients presenting with an acutely ischaemic limb depends on the underlying cause of the ischaemia. However, one of the main aims of treatment is to prevent worsening ischaemia from thrombus propagation. All patients should therefore be anticoagulated with intravenous heparin.

Catheter-directed thrombolysis can sometimes be used to treat intra-arterial thrombus that is not yet causing an immediate threat to limb viability. For more advanced cases, *surgical balloon embolectomy* will be required. *Fasciotomies* may be required to prevent the development of compartment syndromes.

Once the immediate cause of limb ischaemia has been addressed, patients with thromboembolism require long-term anticoagulation with warfarin.

Preoperative assessment and risk management

Patients undergoing operations to revascularise the lower limbs have a high incidence of perioperative complications and post-operative mortality – the American College of Cardiology (ACC) and American Heart Association (AHA) classify aortic and peripheral vascular surgery as high risk, with a combined incidence of perioperative cardiac death and non-fatal

Table 14.7 The goals of anaesthesia for lower limb revascularisation

Achieve haemodynamic stability (by minimising episodes of tachycardia and hypo- or hypertension)

Maintain cardiac output and oxygen delivery to the tissues

Avoid significant anaemia and optimise oxygen carrying capacity

Administer appropriate intravenous fluid therapy and transfuse blood/ blood products (if required)

Attenuate the stress responses to surgery

Maintain renal function

Maintain body temperature

Provide good postoperative analgesia

MI in excess of 5% [3]. This perioperative risk is mainly related to the presence and severity of underlying cardiac disease, but advanced age, and other co-existing chronic diseases also contribute. Careful preoperative assessment is therefore required. This is covered in detail elsewhere in this book.

Anaesthesia for lower limb revascularisation

After the decision has been made to proceed with surgical revascularisation a number of decisions require to be made regarding the choice of anaesthetic technique and monitoring for the surgery. A range of anaesthetic options exist, however, it should be appreciated that careful attention to detail in the preoperative assessment; ensuring that the patient is prescribed (and receives) appropriate medications; and adherence to a number of perioperative objectives (Table 14.7) are likely to make more difference to the outcome for the patient rather than choosing one anaesthetic technique over another.

Perioperative considerations

In general, efforts should be made to ensure that most chronic medications are administered throughout the perioperative period, including the day of surgery. This is particularly important for beta adrenergic blockers. It is also important that a statin and a single antiplatelet agent are given. There are notable exceptions to this rule – ACE inhibitors and angiotensin II receptor antagonists should be omitted throughout the perioperative period as they may contribute to acute kidney injury. Likewise, non-steroidal anti-inflammatory drugs should be avoided. The decision to give, or withhold, other antihypertensive medicines is in part based on the preoperative blood pressure (omit if blood pressure is very low) and the co-existence of severe coronary artery disease (give if the drugs affect coronary vascular resistance, e.g. calcium channel antagonists).

For patients with diabetes mellitus, oral hypoglycaemic drugs should be omitted for the entire perioperative period and blood sugar controlled by means of an insulin infusion. Similarly, patients on long-term insulin therapy should be converted to an insulin infusion for the time around the operation.

Anaesthetic techniques

General anaesthesia versus regional anaesthesia

Operations to revascularise the lower limb are often carried out under either general or regional anaesthesia (epidural, spinal and combined spinal/epidural), or combinations of these techniques. The relative benefits of general versus regional anaesthetic techniques for these procedures have been debated over many years with a number of studies presenting conflicting results. Some have suggested that regional anaesthesia has significant advantages over general anaesthesia by reducing both perioperative morbidity and mortality. It has also been suggested that regional anaesthetic techniques may improve recovery via superior pain control (including reduced requirements for opioids) and a decreased neuroendocrine response to surgery. They may also reduce episodes of myocardial ischaemia, pulmonary and thromboembolic complications, and lower the incidence of graft occlusion. However, a recently published *Cochrane Review* of anaesthetic techniques for infrainguinal revascularisation surgery concluded that there was no difference in mortality, or the incidence of perioperative myocardial infarction, or amputation rate in patients receiving general anaesthesia or neuraxial anaesthesia [8]. This report did, however, document a lower incidence of postoperative pneumonia in patients who received neuraxial anaesthesia. A major

Table 14.8 Summary of typical anaesthetic regimens for lower limb revascularisation procedures

Operation	Anaesthetic	Monitoring	Postoperative analgesia
Aortobifemoral bypass graft	GA (IPPV via ETT) *plus* thoracic epidural	Routine plus A-line and CV-line Consider CO monitor	Epidural for 2–3 days, then PCA opioid, then oral analgesia
Axillofemoral bypass graft	GA (IPPV via ETT)	Routine	PCA or oral opioid
Femoro-femoral / Femoro-popliteal/ Femoro-distal bypass grafts/ Femoral endarterectomy	Regional (lumbar epidural; CSE; spinal) plus sedation *or* GA (IPPV via ETT, or spontaneous ventilation via LMA)	Routine (A-line and/or CV-line *not* usually required unless specific patient features present)	Oral opioid (consider epidural infusion of LA for selected patients)
Balloon embolectomy	LA infiltration by surgeon *plus* intravenous sedation/ analgesia from anaesthetist	Routine	Simple oral analgesia ± oral opioid

A-line, arterial line; CSE, combined spinal/epidural; CV-line, central venous line; ETT, endotracheal tube; GA, general anaesthesia; IPPV, intermittent positive pressure ventilation: LA, local anaesthetic; LMA, laryngeal mask airway; PCA, patient-controlled analgesia.

limitation of this review is that only four studies were deemed worthy of inclusion. Nevertheless, infrainguinal revascularisation surgery lends itself to regional anaesthesia and despite the lack of strong evidence to support its use over general anaesthesia, many anaesthetists believe that it is the technique of choice provided that no contraindications exist.

A similar *Cochrane Review* of the use of epidural anaesthesia and analgesia in abdominal aortic surgery showed that epidurals provide superior analgesia, and also reduce cardiovascular, respiratory, gastrointestinal and renal morbidity compared with systemic opioid-based analgesia [9]. Again, no difference in mortality was noted between the techniques.

Typical anaesthetic regimens

Typical anaesthetic regimens for lower limb revascularisation procedures are summarised in Table 14.8.

Anaesthesia for aortic reconstruction surgery

Aortobifemoral bypass grafting is a major surgical procedure that is associated with risks of significant haemorrhage and haemodynamic instability. Large-bore venous access is required (commonly two 14 gauge cannulae in the upper limb veins) to allow rapid infusion of fluids. Ideally, a low thoracic epidural should be sited and an arterial line inserted prior to general anaesthesia. Induction of general anaesthesia should be carried out using drugs or techniques that minimise changes in blood pressure.

A non-depolarising neuromuscular blocking drug is given to facilitate tracheal intubation and potent opioids (such as fentanyl, alfentanil or remifentanil) are often given to obtund the pressor response to laryngoscopy. General anaesthesia is maintained by a volatile agent, or target controlled infusion of propofol. A multi-lumen central venous line is inserted prior to the start of surgery, and central venous pressure (CVP) transduced throughout the procedure. A urinary catheter allows urine output to be monitored.

Intraoperatively, a dense epidural block is established using concentrated local anaesthetic solutions (e.g. 0.5% levobupivacaine) along with adjuvants such as lipid soluble opioids (e.g. fentanyl or diamorphine) or preservative-free ketamine.

During surgery, intravenous fluids should be given via a device capable of providing rapid infusions of warmed fluids. Further efforts should be made to maintain normothermia using forced-air blankets and under-patient warming mattresses. Blood loss should be measured throughout the case and appropriate volumes of intravenous fluids given to replace this and other losses (evaporative and third space). A combination of crystalloid and colloid solutions is given by most anaesthetists, with balanced solutions preferred to 0.9% sodium chloride to minimise the likelihood of hyperchloraemic metabolic acidosis.

It is useful to make regular assessments of haemogloblin concentration throughout the surgery – this is often possible by performing arterial blood gas analysis on many modern analysers. This allows blood to be transfused at appropriate times. 'Transfusion triggers' are the subject of ongoing debate, with lower levels accepted now than previously. However, for most patients requiring revascularisation surgery, there is a relatively high likelihood that they have co-existing coronary artery disease. A lower limit of 80 g/l is therefore chosen, with a higher threshold of 90 g/l adopted for patients with a definite history of ischaemic heart disease. Ideally, intraoperative red cell salvage should be used routinely for surgery on the aorta to reduce the likelihood of allogeneic transfusion and conserve blood supplies.

At the same time as blood gas analysis is taking place, near-patient thromboelastography should be performed. This provides a functional assessment of the coagulation process and allows prompt recognition of coagulation abnormalities and appropriate treatment in the form of platelet concentrate, or fresh frozen plasma (FFP).

At the end of surgery, the patient should be haemodynamically stable, normothermic, non-coagulopathic and well analgesed. If these criteria are met, the patient can be extubated in theatre at the end of the operation.

Anaesthesia for infrainguinal arterial bypass surgery

These operations can be performed under regional anaesthesia plus sedation, or general anaesthesia. If regional anaesthesia is chosen, a low dose of intravenous sedation (ideally a target controlled infusion of propofol) is given prior to administering the regional anaesthetic. Catheter techniques (either epidural, or combined spinal and epidural) are usually preferred given the fact that many infrainguinal revascularisation operations can last for some hours and exceed the duration of single-shot subarachnoid anaesthesia. However, after discussion with the surgeon, if the length of surgery is anticipated to be relatively short (e.g. femoral endarterectomy), then subarachnoid anaesthesia may be appropriate.

Epidurals should be sited in the lumbar region and the block instituted with a concentrated solution of a long-acting local anaesthetic (e.g. 0.5% or 0.75% levobupivacaine). Epidural opioids are generally not required for this type of surgery. During the time that the block is being established, urinary catheterisation can take place. Once the block has been confirmed to be of sufficient height and density, the level of sedation can be titrated and surgery can proceed.

Infrainguinal bypass surgery is less likely to be associated with marked changes in blood pressure or significant blood loss than during aortic reconstruction. Routine invasive arterial blood pressure measurement is therefore not required, although specific patient factors (e.g. severe valvular heart disease, atrial fibrillation, cardiac failure) may make invasive blood pressure monitoring desirable. Nevertheless, the anaesthetist must be prepared for sudden, brisk arterial bleeding. At least one large-bore (14 gauge) cannula should be inserted prior to surgery. The patient should be well hydrated throughout the surgery using intravenous crystalloids and colloids. Blood transfusion is necessary occasionally with similar transfusion thresholds being used. As in aortic reconstruction surgery, efforts should be made to maintain normothermia throughout the procedure.

If general anaesthesia is selected, then the aim should be to provide as haemodynamically stable an anaesthetic as possible. Many anaesthetists choose to paralyse and intubate patients undergoing lower limb revascularisation procedures. However, for selected patients, airway management with a laryngeal mask airway (LMA) may be feasible. General anaesthesia can be maintained with either a volatile agent or propofol infusion. Over recent years, a body of evidence suggesting that volatile anaesthetic agents can provide a degree of cardioprotection against ischaemia-reperfusion injury has emerged. In the setting of cardiac surgery, this has been shown to reduce the risk of perioperative MI and mortality. However, this has not been demonstrated in the setting of non-cardiac surgery.

During the operation, some anaesthetists now choose to infuse remifentanil, the potent, short-acting opioid. This allows a high-dose opioid technique to be used that provides superior attenuation of intraoperative stress responses. If this technique is used, adequate doses of a longer-acting opioid, such as morphine, must be given prior to the end of surgery.

Intraoperative considerations
Implications of clamping and unclamping the aorta and major lower limb arteries

All of the operations performed to revascularise the lower limbs involve placing clamps across either the aorta and/or the iliac or femoral arteries to allow the graft to be anastomosed to the native vessel. This arterial clamping produces a number of effects that are most marked in patients having aortic surgery. Firstly, there is an acute increase in afterload for the left ventricle and this is a common time for myocardial ischaemia to occur. The magnitude of increase in afterload is more likely to be clinically significant for operations on the aorta than those on infrainguinal arteries. It may occasionally be necessary to use vasodilators to treat hypertension associated with application of an aortic cross-clamp, particularly in patients that do not have thoracic epidural anaesthesia. For all types of lower limb revascularisation surgery, tissues distal to the clamp inevitably become ischaemic during the time that the clamps are in place. Anaerobic metabolism continues in these non- (or poorly) perfused tissues with depletion of glycogen and high-energy phosphate stores and the accumulation of ischaemic metabolites and lactic acid. There is also increased production of cytokines, endothelial adhesion molecules and reactive oxygen species, and activation of the complement, kinin and coagulation pathways. On release of the clamps, the circulation is restored to the ischaemic areas. This commonly produces hypotension resulting from a number of mechanisms. The volume of the circulation is reduced relative to its normal state during the time that the clamps are in place. Intravenous fluid resuscitation is therefore required and should be started prior to the removal of the aortic clamp. In addition, the lactic acid and ischaemic metabolites that are washed in to the circulation cause systemic vasodilatation, pulmonary vasoconstriction and myocardial suppression. Vasocontrictors and inotropes are commonly required at this time to maintain haemodynamic stability. This whole process of ischaemia and reperfusion is a contributory factor to the systemic inflammatory response syndrome and postoperative organ dysfunction.

Myocardial ischaemia

Given the high prevalence of coronary artery disease in patients with PAD coupled with the nature of the surgery, it is not surprising that episodes of intraoperative myocardial ischaemia are relatively common. Perioperative myocardial ischaemia is associated with a significant risk of death in the short term, and also longer-term increases in morbidity and mortality. It is therefore important to attempt to prevent, or recognise and treat intraoperative ischaemia as promptly and effectively as possible. All patients should be on a statin and antiplatelet medication preoperatively to stabilise atherosclerotic plaques and reduce thrombotic risk. If signs of myocardial ischaemia (e.g. ST segment depression or elevation on ECG, or new regional wall motion abnormalities on transoesophageal echocardiography) develop intraoperatively the following options are available to help improve the situation. Firstly, oxygen delivery should be optimised by ensuring that blood is well oxygenated (normal SaO_2), an adequate concentration of haemoglobin is present (>90 g/l) and that the cardiac output is sufficient. Next, the heart rate should be considered. Higher heart rates lead to increased myocardial work and oxygen demands and are also associated with an increased risk of myocardial ischaemia, troponin release and perioperative myocardial ischaemia [10]. Heart rate should be controlled, ideally to less than 70 beats per minute, using intravenous beta-blockers. Initially a short-acting drug such as esmolol is recommended to achieve immediate control, however, a longer-acting agent (e.g. atenolol, or metoprolol) will also subsequently be required. Another possible therapeutic alternative is intravenous glyceryl trinitrate.

Postoperatively, serial ECGs and measurements of troponin should be performed to document whether any myocardial injury has occurred. If there is still evidence of ongoing myocardial ischaemia in the postoperative period, a cardiology review should be organised as coronary angiography and percutaneous intervention may be required.

Heparin

Another feature that is common to many forms of vascular surgery is the administration of intravenous unfractionated heparin prior to the application of vascular clamps. This prevents intravascular clotting during the time that vessels are clamped. Doses used typically range from 3000 to 5000 iu (approximately 70 iu/kg). It is uncommon to reverse the effects of heparin at the end of surgery. However, if an excessive heparin effect is suspected, this can be confirmed using a near-patient test of activated clotting time (ACT) or activated partial thromboplastin time (APTT) and a small dose of protamine given.

Postoperative care and complications

Patients undergoing operations for peripheral arterial disease are at significant risk of postoperative morbidity and mortality. This is due to a combination of surgical factors including the effects of clamping major blood vessels, ischaemia and reperfusion injury, and the potential for major haemorrhage and coagulopathy, alongside the presence of multiple, severe comorbidities. It is therefore important that patients receive postoperative care from medical, nursing and allied medical staff who are aware of the likely complications, in a location that has all of the appropriate monitoring and supportive equipment necessary. In addition, it is vitally important that all of the basic components of postoperative care – oxygen and fluid therapy, analgesia, physiotherapy, nutrition, pharmacotherapy and appropriate monitoring – are provided with thought and attention to detail.

Location of postoperative care

The optimal location of postoperative care depends on a number of factors, primarily the type of surgery that has been performed, but also the degree of urgency associated with the operation, the preoperative functional status of the patient and the presence and severity of comorbidities.

Patients who have had elective abdominal surgery for aorto-iliac reconstruction generally require postoperative care in a high dependency unit (level 2 care as defined by the Intensive Care Society), whilst some patients who have had urgent surgery or experienced intraoperative complications, may require intensive (level 3) care. In contrast, for most patients having elective infrainguinal revascularisation, postoperative care on a general ward will be suitable. However, additional monitoring and care (level 1 or 2) may be appropriate for some patients having emergency surgery, or for those with significant comorbidity and very poor functional capacity.

Post-operative complications following lower limb revascularisation

Myocardial infarction

Myocardial ischaemia is one of the greatest concerns after vascular surgery; indeed the incidence of postoperative myocardial infarction (MI) is at least four times greater than that in a general surgical population. Postoperative MI has a high mortality rate (15–25%) and is the leading cause of death after vascular surgery [11]. It is also associated with an increased risk of future MI and mortality. Most MIs occur within the first 3 postoperative days. A number of factors can contribute to myocardial infarction – as in the non-operative setting, plaque rupture can occur in patients with underlying coronary artery disease. However, within the early postoperative phase, an imbalance between oxygen demand and supply is likely to be the most important mechanism leading to MI. Prolonged episodes of tachycardia should therefore be avoided by ensuring that effective analgesia is provided and that beta-blockers are continued throughout the postoperative period, using intravenous preparations if necessary. Other important factors include low flow states that may be exacerbated by hypotension, hypercoagulabilty and inflammation. Continuing an antiplatelet drug and a statin may help mitigate these effects [12, 13]. Oxygen carriage should also be optimised by maintaining an acceptable haemoglobin concentration and oxyhaemoglobin saturation, whilst hyperoxia should be avoided. Patients should be monitored using 5-electrode ECG systems during the time spent in level 1, 2 or 3 care with any ST segment changes prompting the recording of a formal 12-lead ECG and measurement of troponin. A low threshold for cardiology referral should be adopted in the context of persistent ECG abnormalities or symptoms in keeping with MI.

Respiratory complications

Many patients with PAD have co-existing chronic pulmonary disease due to the high prevalence of cigarette smoking. This places them at increased risk of postoperative respiratory complications such as atelectasis and pneumonia. The incidence of respiratory complications is higher after aortic surgery (15%) than infrainguinal revascularisation (3%) [14]; nevertheless, efforts should be made to reduce the likelihood of respiratory complications in both groups by ensuring that chronic respiratory disease states are optimised prior to elective procedures and that bronchodilator drugs are continued perioperatively. In addition, good analgesia that allows effective coughing and clearing of secretions should be provided. Use of neuraxial anaesthesia reduces the likelihood of postoperative respiratory complications

[8,9]. Thoracic epidural analgesia is therefore recommended for 48–72 hours after surgery. For patients having infrainguinal revascularisation procedures, postoperative infusion of local anaesthetic via lumbar epidural can be considered for those with particularly severe respiratory disease, though this is not required routinely. All patients should receive oxygen therapy that is targeted to measured oxygen saturation [15].

Renal complications

Patients with significant PAD are at risk of renal dysfunction around the time of lower limb revascularisation. This risk is particularly high for those patients with pre-existing renal impairment. It is also greater for patients having aortic surgery than infrainguinal revascularisation procedures.

The aetiology of postoperative renal dysfunction is often multifactorial, with hypovolaemia, hypotension, atheroembolism, the systemic inflammatory response syndrome, rhabdomyolysis and nephrotoxins (including radiographic contrast media) all possible contributory factors. Unfortunately, no specific pharmacological therapies have been found that are useful in the prevention of perioperative renal impairment. However, a number of simple measures should be undertaken to reduce the likelihood of renal impairment. These include avoiding hypovolaemia by

ensuring that appropriate intravenous fluid therapy is administered. Likewise, blood pressure should be monitored carefully and episodes of hypotension treated promptly. Care should be taken when administering potentially nephrotoxic drugs in the perioperative period. Angiotensin receptor antagonists and ACE inhibitors should be omitted around the time of surgery whilst non-steroidal anti-inflammatory drugs are best avoided completely in patients with PAD.

Haemorrhage

Significant bleeding is an inevitable part of many vascular operations. However, by the end of surgery, haemostasis should have been achieved and any coagulopathy corrected. Episodes of hypotension after surgery should prompt an immediate search for any ongoing blood loss as leaking anastomoses can lead to sudden, life-threatening haemorrhage. Basic clinical observations (including pulse rate, capillary refill time and examination of the operation site) in addition to CVP measurement, and repeated haematocrit or haemoglobin estimation may aid the diagnosis of haemorrhage. If postoperative haemorrhage is suspected, urgent surgical review is required. A low threshold should be adopted for returning to theatre for surgical re-exploration.

References

1. Faxon DP, Fuster V, Libby P, *et al.* Atherosclerotic vascular disease conference. Writing group III: Pathophysiology. *Circulation* 2004;**109**:2617–25

2. Norgren L, Hiatt WR, Dormandy JA, *et al.* Inter-Society Consensus for the Management of PAD (TASC II). *Eur J Vasc Endovasc Surg* 2007;**33**(suppl 1): S1–75.

3. Hirsch AT, Haskal ZJ, Hertzer NR, *et al.* ACC/AHA 2005 Practice Guidelines for the Management of Patients with Peripheral Arterial Disease (lower extremity, renal, mesenteric, and abdominal aortic). *Circulation* 2006;**113**: e463–654.

4. Östergren J, Sleight P, Dagenais G, *et al.* Impact of ramipril in patients with evidence of clinical or

subclinical peripheral arterial disease. *Eur Heart J* 2004;**25**:17–24.

5. CAPRIE Steering Committee. A randomised, blinded, trial of clopidogrel versus aspirin in patients at risk of ischaemic events (CAPRIE). *Lancet* 1996; **348**:1329–39.

6. Chiu KWH, Davies RSM, Nightingale PG, *et al.* Review of direct anatomical open surgical management of atherosclerotic aorto-iliac occlusive disease. *Eur J Vasc Endovasc Surg* 2010;**39**:460–71.

7. Nicoloff, AD, Taylor LM, McLafferty RB, *et al.* Patient recovery after infrainguinal bypass grafting for limb salvage. *J Vasc Surg* 1998;**27**:256–66.

8. Barbosa FT, Cavalcante JC, Jucá MJ, Castro AA Neuraxial anaesthesia for lower-limb

revascularization. *Cochrane Database Syst Rev* 2010; **CD007083**.

9. Nishimori M, Ballantyne JC, Low JHS Epidural pain relief versus systemic opioid-based pain relief for abdominal aortic surgery. *Cochrane Database Syst Rev* 2008; **CD005059**.

10. Feringa HHH, Bax JJ, Boersma E, *et al.* High-dose β-blockers and tight heart rate control reduce myocardial ischaemia and troponin T release in vascular surgery patients. *Circulation* 2006;**114**:I-344–I-349.

11. Biccard BM, Rodseth RN The pathophysiology of peri-operative myocardial infarction. *Anaesthesia* 2010;**65**:733–41.

12. Burger W, Chemnitius J-M, Kneissl GD, Rücker, G. Low-dose aspirin for secondary cardiovascular

prevention: cardiovascular risks after its perioperative withdrawal versus bleeding risks with its continuation – review and meta-analysis. *J Int Med* 2005; 257:399–414.

13. Poldermans D, Bax JJ, Kertai MD, *et al.* Statins are associated with a reduced incidence of perioperative mortality in patients undergoing major noncardiac vascular surgery. *Circulation* 2003;**107**:1848–51.

14. Nowygrod R, Egorova N, Greco G, *et al.* Trends, complications, and mortality in peripheral vascular surgery. *J Vasc Surg* 2006;**43**:205–16.

15. O'Driscoll BR, Howard LS, Davison AG. British Thoracic Society Guideline for emergency oxygen use in adult patients. *Thorax* 2008;**63**(suppl VI): vi1–vi68.

Anaesthesia for lower limb amputation and the management of post-amputation pain

Charles Morton and John A. Wilson

Approximately 80% of all lower limb amputations in adult civilian practice are for peripheral arterial disease, including diabetes. Trauma and malignancy account for the majority of the remainder. This chapter will concentrate on amputation for vascular disease, but some of the practice considered, for example the management of phantom limb pain, will be relevant to amputations for other indications.

The scale of the problem

The reported incidence of amputation varies, depending on whether whole communities or specific subgroups (e.g. patients with diabetes) are studied, and there are differences between cultures, races and healthcare systems. For example, The Global Lower Extremity Amputation Study Group studied ten centres around the world (combined population >2 million) and reported that rate of lower limb amputation varied between 3 and 44 per 100 000 of population [1]. Some studies report all, and others only major, amputations. There is no universally agreed distinction between major and minor amputation but a practical approach is to consider amputations that sacrifice the ankle joint as major, and those that preserve the joint as minor (digit, ray, trans-metatarsal).

The most commonly quoted figures for the UK are that 500–1000 per million of population suffer from critical limb ischaemia and that 25% (125–250 per million) of these patients will require amputation (7500–15000 per annum for the UK as a whole). Between 1997 and 2006 a fairly consistent 4500–5000 patients were referred each year to the UK Prosthetics Services for consideration of lower limb prostheses but this figure reflects only major amputees who survived to discharge and wished to use a prosthesis.

In the most recent study in England only (2003–2008, based on the Hospital Episode Statistics database) the overall rate of *major* amputations was 5.1 per 100 000 with variations between centres [2]. Both incidence and mortality decreased over time. Overall, it seems that there are currently between 5000 and 10 000 amputations each year in the UK and approximately half of these are major.

Vascular disease

The epidemiology of vascular disease, with the background of smoking, hypertension, hyperlipidaemia, abnormal fibrinolysis and altered platelet function together with the role of diabetes is described in detail in chapter 1. Some studies have shown that the establishment of a specialist vascular surgical service increases the rate of surgical revascularisation of ischaemic limbs and reduces the rate of amputation.

Diabetes

Up to 50% of lower limb amputations are in patients with diabetes. A patient with diabetes is up to 15 times more likely to require an amputation than one without and the co-existence of diabetes and chronic kidney disease increases the likelihood even further. Diabetes is associated with a several-fold decrease in long-term survival after amputation.

Patients with diabetes may develop claudication but vascular disease in this group tends to be in arteries below the knee and a commoner presentation is foot ulceration, the incidence of which increases with advancing age, affecting up to 7% of diabetic patients over the age of 60. Neuropathy and atherosclerosis, individually or in combination both contribute to the development of foot ulceration. Sensory neuropathy may render the patient unaware

Core Topics in Vascular Anaesthesia, ed. Carl Moores and Alastair F. Nimmo. Published by Cambridge University Press.
© Cambridge University Press 2012.

of ill-fitting shoes or trauma to the foot. Autonomic neuropathy leads to loss of sweating and dry cracked skin. Motor neuropathy may cause muscle wasting and subsequent biomechanical changes can result in increased pressure on vulnerable parts of the foot (e.g. under the metatarsal heads). Once damage has occurred, the impaired neutrophil function, increased susceptibility to infection and impaired wound healing of patients with diabetes conspire to prevent satisfactory resolution. A number of studies have demonstrated that the existence of a specialist diabetes services is associated with a decrease in the rate of amputation in diabetic patients [3].

Level of amputation

Amputations may be minor (digit, ray, mid-tarsal), when the aim is to preserve limb function, or major (trans-tibial/below knee, through knee, trans-femoral/above knee) when the intention is to save the (remainder of) the limb. Amputations through the ankle joint are performed very rarely, if ever, in contemporary surgical practice. The higher the level of amputation, the harder it will be for the patient to use a prosthesis. Apart from the challenge of balance, the *additional* energy expenditure required to use a prosthesis is considerable: approximately 60% for a unilateral below-knee prosthesis, rising to 120% for unilateral above-knee and nearly 300% for bilateral above-knee prostheses. Given the age of most amputees, the incidence of co-existing disease and the inactive lifestyle associated with the development of peripheral arterial disease it is not surprising that a large number of patients who undergo amputation for vascular disease never manage a prosthesis.

Preoperative assessment

Amputation may be an appropriate first treatment for some patients but in the majority the need for amputation marks the advance of underlying disease beyond the point of tissue salvage. It follows that patients requiring amputation are likely to have widespread, advanced vascular disease. An example of the incidence of co-existing disease in patients undergoing lower limb amputation is shown in Table 15.1. This is from an American Veterans Health Administration study [4], and the detail will vary between populations, but the message is clear: evidence of diabetes, ischaemic heart disease, cardiac failure, cerebrovascular disease, renal dysfunction and, because

Table 15.1 Example of the incidence of co-existing disease in a study of patients discharged from US Veterans Health Administration hospitals after lower limb amputation

Diabetes	61%
Peripheral vascular disease	57%
Cardiac disease (other than cardiac failure)	22%
Cardiac failure	12%
Cerebrovascular disease	11%
Renal disease	10%

smoking is heavily implicated in the development of arterial disease, respiratory disease, should be sought and quantified. Poor control of diabetes may be a major contributor to the need for amputation, or may be precipitated by infection with resolution unlikely until after surgery. Glucose and insulin infusions may be required before, during and after surgery.

A significant number of patients will have been hospitalised with acute limb ischaemia, non-resolving foot infections or generalised sepsis and may be acutely unwell. Preoperative assessment may be complicated by the cognitive impairment associated with cerebrovascular disease or sepsis but, on the other hand, many patients will have had multiple previous contacts with medical services and the progression of the disease and comorbidity may already be documented.

Once the decision to proceed to amputation has been made it is rare for there to be time either for major changes in the management of co-existing disease to be instigated or for referral for specialist investigation, but the advice of specialist colleagues should be sought when necessary, particularly if their involvement will be needed after surgery.

Intraoperative care

Patients scheduled for amputation will often be on emergency lists and may be cared for by trainee anaesthetists, or those who do not regularly anaesthetise patients for vascular surgical procedures. Alternatively, they may on a planned operating list but scheduled last, because of the presence of infection. In either case, it is important to realise that despite the apparent simplicity of the operation, amputation carries a significantly higher mortality rate than most other vascular surgical procedures. The care of patients undergoing amputation requires experience, care

Table 15.2 Some advantages and disadvantages of anaesthetic techniques for lower limb amputation

Anaesthetic technique	Advantages	Disadvantages
Extradural anaesthesia	May be used for pain relief before surgery	Suitable environment for pre- and postoperative care (e.g. high dependency unit) required
	Option to establish block gradually in cardiovascularly unstable patients	Cessation of anticoagulation required in advance of surgery
		Systemic sepsis may be a contraindication
	May be used for postoperative analgesia	Extradural catheter is indwelling 'foreign body'
	Earlier return (cf. general anaesthesia) to oral intake an advantage for patients with diabetes	May be difficult to position patient for insertion
Subarachnoid anaesthesia	Rapid onset of reliable sensory and motor block	Rapid onset of autonomic block requires careful monitoring
	Reliable pain relief in early postoperative period	Cessation of anticoagulation required in advance of surgery
	Earlier return (cf. general anaesthesia) to oral intake an advantage for patients with diabetes	Systemic sepsis may be a contraindication
		May be difficult to position patient for insertion
General anaesthesia	Avoids concerns about neuraxial block and anticoagulation or sepsis	Systemic analgesia, or peripheral nerve block, required
	Complete loss of consciousness may be preferred by patients	Intubation may be required (delayed gastric emptying in patients with diabetes)
	Avoids problems with positioning for subarachnoid or extradural block	Cardiovascular changes associated with laryngoscopy and intubation
		Diabetes is a risk factor for difficult layngoscopy
		May not be preferred technique for patients with respiratory disease
		Likely slower return to oral intake

and attention to detail and should not be delegated to the most junior member of the team.

Anaesthetic technique

Most published studies have focussed on whether or not the anaesthetic technique influences the incidence of phantom limb pain (see below) but, in terms of other outcome, there is no evidence to support the use of any one technique over another. Advantages and disadvantages of extradural, subarachnoid and general anaesthesia for major lower limb amputation are summarised in Table 15.2. Major amputation under peripheral nerve blockade (sciatic, plus 'three-in-one' or psoas compartment blocks) has also been described, but block of smaller peripheral nerves (e.g. digital, metatarsal, 'ankle block') situated close to small blood vessels is probably unwise because of the risk that the increased tissue pressure will compromise the already threatened blood flow.

Anticoagulation

Anaesthetists and surgeons should agree standard policies for anticoagulation, and more importantly its cessation, in patients scheduled for amputation so as to retain the option of central neural block. Usual practice is to stop intravenous heparin 4 hours before surgery. European and North American guidelines suggest a gap of 12 (prophylactic dose) and 24 (therapeutic dose) hours between low-molecular-weight heparin (LMWH) and subarachnoid or extradural anaesthesia.

Infection

A very large proportion of patients presenting for amputation will have evidence of local infection, but this alone should not preclude subarachnoid or extradural anaesthesia. Systemic infection poses more of a problem. The presence of untreated or uncontrolled sepsis would generally be regarded as a contraindication to central neural block, unless the hazards of alternative techniques were very great, but if appropriate antibiotic therapy has been started and there are signs of improvement (e.g. reduced fever, reduced white blood cell count) there is no reason to withhold central neural block [5]. In patients not already receiving antibiotics, prophylactic antibiotics will be required around the time of induction of anaesthesia and these should be according to local policy.

If there is concern about either residual anticoagulation or infection in patients who would benefit from central neural block it would seem sensible to prefer the single injection, small needle of subarachnoid rather than the larger needle and indwelling catheter of extradural anaesthesia, although there is no published evidence to support this presumption.

Previous amputation and regional anaesthesia

In patients who have undergone amputation previously, both phantom sensation and phantom limb pain may occur during regional anaesthesia; one small prospective study reported incidences of 10% and 5% respectively. The phantom pain commonly presents soon after onset of the block, occasionally as the block recedes. There are no known preoperative predictors of the phenomenon and although phantom pain occurring in these circumstances seems to wane after approximately 20 minutes it can be extremely distressing to the patient and difficult to treat, other than by resorting to general anaesthesia. This has prompted some authors to suggest previous amputation as a contraindication to a regional block affecting the amputated limb.

Blood loss

Blood loss is variable but increases as the level of amputation rises. Between 0.5 and 1.0 litres may be lost during trans-femoral/above-knee amputation. Blood transfusion, even when corrected for existence of co-existing disease, has been reported to be associated with a higher incidence of adverse events so should not be used without a clear indication.

Monitoring

The level of monitoring will be governed by patient factors, rather than the nature of the surgery, and invasive monitoring may sometimes be required. Several intravenous drugs may be required after surgery (e.g. antibiotics, glucose and insulin) and a central venous access may be useful if peripheral venous access is likely to be unreliable.

Postoperative care

As has already been stated, lower limb amputation is associated with a high mortality (see below). This probably represents the severity of underlying disease, with amputation marking the inability of medical and surgical intervention to halt the inexorable advance of vascular disease, the effects of diabetes, or both. A high standard of postoperative care is required. Particular attention should be paid to the possibility of cardiac complications, and a period in a high dependency unit may be required.

Mortality

As with other adverse events, mortality increases with rising level of amputation, severity of co-existing disease and advancing age. An American study of nearly 1000 major amputations reported a 30-day mortality rate of 17.5% for above-knee and 4.2% for below-knee amputations, with median survivals of 20 and 52 months respectively [6]. Renal insufficiency is associated with a higher 30-day mortality, and diabetes with a worse long-term survival (32% vs. 43% 5-year survival) [7].

Immediate postoperative pain

Inevitably, immediately after surgery, or when regional block has receded, the patient is likely to experience pain at and near the site of surgery. Response to conventional analgesics can be expected and extradural infusion or peripheral nerve blocks may have a role.

Other post-amputation phenomena

Other problems are common for patients after the loss of a limb and may manifest as one or more of the following:

- Stump pain – felt in the residual region, adjacent to the amputated area.
- Phantom sensation – the sensation that the amputated part is still present in some form, but is not painful.
- Phantom pain – pain perceived to be coming from the amputated part.

Epidemiology of post-amputation phenomena

Stump pain

After the immediate postoperative period, patients may develop stump pain, with reported incidence of between 7% and 76% [8,9]. There can be a variety of causes including ill-fitting prostheses, poorly fashioned stumps, formation of neuromata, muscle spasms or the development of a chronic regional pain syndrome. Expert surgery, limb fitting and rehabilitation may have a role in prevention, otherwise treatment is aimed at the cause.

Phantom sensation

Phantom sensation is the illusion that the removed body part is present despite amputation. Intensity varies from a vague awareness of the missing part, through specific localised sensations such as itching toes, to the perception of an exact replica of the limb. After amputation these sensations are almost universal with an incidence of over 90% and they can be considered normal, but to the unprepared patient they may be alarming. Preoperative explanation and continuing postoperative reassurance are important. Over time, both duration and frequency of non-painful phantom phenomena tend to decrease; the incidence at 8 days, 6 months and 2 years in one study was 84%, 90% and 71% respectively [10]. Around 75% of patients had kinaesthetic sensations (feelings of length, volume or other spatial sensations) in the first 6 months after amputation decreasing to less than 50% later in the study.

Between one-third and two-thirds of amputees have been reported to experience shortening of the virtual limb with time, a concept known as 'telescoping' [11].

Phantom pain

Phantom pain can occur almost immediately after amputation with 75% of amputees developing pain within a few days. The incidence of phantom pain seems to be anything between 30% and 80% and is highest immediately after amputation, the frequency and duration of attacks decreasing over time, at least in the first 6 months. It is estimated that 5–10% of patients will suffer from chronic severe pain, scoring greater than 5/10 on a numerical rating scale [8]. In general terms phantom pain tends to be located to the distal part of the amputated limb, the majority of patients describing intermittent pain. The pain described is variable but typically patients feel burning, cramping, shooting or crushing pains. Intensity is extremely variable, ranging from occasional mild pain to continuous severe pain.

Factors influencing pain

The occurrence of phantom pain is independent of age, level or side of amputation, reason for amputation or prosthesis use. Phantom sensations, stump pain and pre-amputation pain, however, do have an association with phantom pain, with many studies showing a consistent association. Traditionally, it was thought that psychological factors played a major part in patients who experienced phantom limb pain. This theory postulated that, rather than being a physiological phenomenon, phantom pain may in some way be a somatisation of a grief process, say for the loss of the limb or even being a manifestation of grief for loss of a spouse. However, there does not seem to be an excess of psychiatric or psychological pathology in patients who have undergone amputation, but in common with other patients with chronic pain, they do clearly suffer from stress, anxiety and depression [12,13].

Pathophysiology of post-amputation pain

The mechanism of post-amputation pain is complex and understanding in this area is a rapidly changing and advancing field. Nerve injury may cause neuroma formation in the nerve with resultant increased excitability and ectopic discharges. There are changes in ion channel expression particularly sodium channels. The nerve phenotype changes, with resulting alteration in neuropeptide expression, neurotrophins playing a major part in these changes, and there is evidence of involvement of the sympathetic system. In addition, there are changes at the level of the spinal cord leading to long-term potentiation and central sensitisation. Dorsal horn inhibitory control is diminished and changes occur in both descending modulatory systems and the cerebral cortex.

Peripheral changes

After peripheral nerve transection, damage to primary afferent fibres results in areas of demyelination at the injury site. The nerve attempts to regenerate by axonal sprouting, resulting in a neuroma, a tangled axonal mass. Amputation of a limb will involve transaction of major nerves and this may result in a neuroma which gives rise to spontaneous neuronal activity [14]. These frequent abnormal spontaneous discharges, termed 'ectopic activity', arise not only from the neuroma, but from other parts of the nerve, including the dorsal root ganglion (DRG) [15]. Accumulation of sodium channels at the sites of ectopic discharges may result in an altered membrane threshold leading to spontaneous discharge [16]. In humans ectopic activity has been shown to correlate with pain in amputees and dysaesthesia associated with back pain and radicular pain.

Central sensitisation

Central sensitisation is an important factor in the development of chronic pain states. Sustained nociceptive input, either from nerve damage or tissue injury, results in sustained alteration in spinal cord neurones, causing prolonged and increased output from the dorsal horn. A wide range of changes can be detected including an increase in receptive field (spatial changes), increased response to afferent activity (threshold changes), increased spontaneous neuronal activity and prolonged 'after discharges' in response to transient stimuli [17].

The release of the excitatory amino acid glutamate and the subsequent activation of the N-methyl D-aspartate (NMDA) receptor are key to the development of central sensitisation [18].

Clinical relevance of central sensitisation

The post-injury hypersensitive state leads to alterations in the sensory modality of low-threshold mechanoreceptors. Pain may occur after what would normally be an innocuous stimulus (such as brushing), a condition known as allodynia. In addition the facilitated spinal processing may give rise to an exaggerated response to what would normally be a painful stimulus, a condition known as hyperalgesia.

Cortical changes

Much research on post-amputation pain has focussed on plasticity of the somatosensory cortex, the primary area of which is located in the post central gyrus [19]. This area is organised into a specific somatotopic map, known as the Penfield homunculus. It has been shown that after denervation, the cortical representation of one body part may expand into an adjacent part of the cortex representing the denervated area (in this case the cortex representing the amputated part), a concept known as cortical reorganisation. Is cortical reorganisation related in some way to phantom pain? Using brain imaging techniques, cortical remapping has been demonstrated in patients with upper limb deafferentation. The magnitude of cortical remapping was correlated with the severity of phantom pain but not phantom sensations. The mechanism behind cortical reorganisation may be multifactorial, perhaps involving potentiation of synapses, unmasking latent connections, or by growth of new neural connections. There is evidence to suggest that plasticity in the somatosensory cortex changes can occur very rapidly. For instance, referred sensations from the face have been demonstrated within 24 hours of amputation of the upper limb and cortical remapping confirmed using functional magnetic resonance imaging (fMRI) at 1 month.

Prevention of phantom limb pain

As discussed above, there are few predictive features to suggest who will suffer post-amputation pain. Consistently, though, post-amputation pain is associated with pre-amputation pain and, in general, severe acute pain is known to be a risk factor for the development of chronic pain.

Severe pre- and post-operative pain may lead to a lasting somatosensory change or 'memory' resulting in post-amputation pain. The observation that patients with little or no pain immediately before surgery were at a lower risk of post-amputation pain led to the hypothesis that rendering patients pain-free before surgery could reduce post-amputation pain. In addition, it has been suggested that prevention of central sensitisation, particularly by using NMDA receptor blockade, could have a role in preventing chronic neuropathic pain. Researchers have therefore focussed on techniques that involve continuous peripheral nerve blockade, continuous epidural analgesia and techniques utilising NMDA receptor blockade with ketamine.

Continuous peripheral nerve blockade and epidural analgesia

Several studies have investigated the role of perineural and epidural analgesia in reducing the incidence of phantom limb pain. Drugs studied in this context have included local anaesthetics, opioids, α2-agonists and NMDA antagonists, alone or in combination [20]. Good perioperative pain control has been demonstrated but, despite early promise, there is no conclusive evidence that the use of these techniques prevents or reduces the occurrence of phantom pain.

Ketamine

Activation of the NMDA receptor is a key factor in the development of central sensitisation, and animal studies suggest that NMDA antagonists given in advance of nerve damage may have a role in reducing the incidence of chronic pain. The NMDA receptor antagonist ketamine has been shown to be effective in the short-term relief of post-amputation pain in humans, but perioperative infusions of ketamine, either intravenously or epidurally, have not reduced the incidence of post-amputation pain [21,22].

Gabapentin

One trial has investigated the role of oral gabapentin, given for 30 days immediately after amputation, in the prevention of phantom pain, but did not demonstrate a reduction in its incidence [23].

Treatment of phantom pain

A survey of US war veteran amputees described more than 50 different treatments for phantom limb pain, indicating that there is no one accepted treatment and success is often poor [24]. The evidence base for the treatment of phantom limb pain treatment is limited. Up until relatively recently, many of the treatments in use were largely based on anecdote and case reports. Since phantom pain is a type of neuropathic pain, as discussed above, pharmacological approaches focus largely on accepted treatments for neuropathic pain for which several evidence-based practice guidelines have been produced.

Neuropathic pain in general

First line treatments tend to be tricyclic antidepressants (TCAs, e.g. amitriptyline), serotonergic noradrenergic reuptake inhibitors (SNRIs, e.g. venlafaxine, duloxetine) or anticonvulsants such as the gabapentinoids [25–27]. Second-line therapy is an alternate drug to the chosen first line, i.e. if a TCA was chosen then an anticonvulsant may be tried next (or vice versa). Topical lidocaine can be used for discrete areas of allodynia. Opioids, including tramadol, are used as third-line agents. NMDA antagonists are used on specialist advice. League tables of efficacy have been produced using the concept of numbers needed-to-treat (NNT) for neuropathic pain [28], rather than phantom pain specifically. Tricyclic antidepressants have NNTs of around 2.3–3.0, anticonvulsants 2.1–3.6, and intravenous lidocaine 3.0. Although these drugs have satisfactory NNT values in neuropathic pain, they are largely based on studies of patients with diabetic neuropathy or post-herpetic neuralgia. Whether these NNTs can be extrapolated to phantom limb pain is debatable, but there is no doubt that these drugs are popular first-line therapies in phantom pain.

Phantom limb pain specifically

The anecdotes and case reports alluded to above have been superseded by several small-scale randomised controlled trials (RCTs) in the treatment of phantom pain. Despite a proven track record in other types of neuropathic pain, amitriptyline in doses up to 125 mg did not show any benefit over placebo [29]. Gabapentin, on the other hand, has been shown to be superior (doses up to 2400 mg) to placebo in one small RCT [30].

Summary

In patients requiring lower limb amputation for vascular disease:

- Extensive co-existing disease is likely, with a high incidence of diabetes.

- Co-existing disease is likely to be advanced.
- No single anaesthetic technique has been shown to be superior to others.
- Both short- and longer-term mortality is high.
- Post-operative phantom sensations are almost universal.
- Post-operative phantom pain is common and up to 10% of patients will suffer persistent, severe phantom limb pain.

- The pathophysiology of phantom pain is complex.
- Efforts to reduce the incidence and severity of phantom pain have had little success.
- The evidence base for treating established phantom pain is sparse but gabapentin seems to be appropriate first-line therapy.

References

1. Comparing the incidence of lower extremity amputations across the world: the Global Lower Extremity Amputation Study. *Diabet Med* 1995;**12**:14–18.

2. Moxey PW, Hofman D, Hinchliffe RJ, *et al.* Epidemiological study of lower limb amputation in England between 2003 and 2008. *Br J Surg* 2010;**97**:1348–53.

3. Canavan RJ, Unwin NC, Kelly WF, Connolly VM. Diabetes- and nondiabetes-related lower extremity amputation incidence before and after the introduction of better organized diabetes foot care: continuous longitudinal monitoring using a standard method. *Diabet Care* 2008;**31**:459–63.

4. Mayfield JA, Reiber GE, Maynard C, *et al.* Survival following lower-limb amputation in a veteran population. *J Rehabil Res Dev* 2001;**38**:341–5.

5. Horlocker TT, Wedel DJ. Neurologic complications of neuraxial blockade. In: Cousins MJCD, Horlocker TT, Bridenbough BD, eds., *Cousins and Bridenbaugh's Neural Blockade in Clinical Anesthesia and Pain Medicine*, 4th edn. Philadelphia, PA: Lippincott Williams & Wilkins; 2008, 296–315.

6. Subramaniam B, Pomposelli F, Talmor D, Park KW. Perioperative and long-term morbidity and mortality after above-knee and below-knee amputations in diabetics and nondiabetics. *Anesth Analg* 2005;**100**:1241–7.

7. Schofield CJ, Libby G, Brennan GM, *et al.* Mortality and hospitalization in patients after amputation: a comparison between patients with and without diabetes. *Diabet Care* 2006; **29**:2252–6.

8. Kehlet H, Jensen TS, Woolf CJ. Persistent postsurgical pain: risk factors and prevention. *Lancet* 2006;**367**:1618–25.

9. Nikolajsen L, Jensen TS. Phantom limb pain. *Br J Anaesth* 2001;**87**:107–16.

10. Jensen TS, Krebs B, Nielsen J, Rasmussen P. Non-painful phantom limb phenomena in amputees: incidence, clinical characteristics and temporal course. *Acta Neurol Scand* 1984;**70**:407–14.

11. Jensen TS, Krebs B, Nielsen J, Rasmussen P. Phantom limb, phantom pain and stump pain in amputees during the first 6 months following limb amputation. *Pain* 1983;**17**:243–56.

12. Ephraim PL, Wegener ST, MacKenzie EJ, Dillingham TR, Pezzin LE. Phantom pain, residual limb pain, and back pain in amputees: results of a national survey. *Arch Phys Med Rehabil* 2005;**86**:1910–19.

13. Sherman RA, Sherman CJ, Bruno GM. Psychological factors influencing chronic phantom limb pain: an analysis of the literature. *Pain* 1987;**28**:285–95.

14. Wall PD, Gutnick M. Ongoing activity in peripheral nerves: the physiology and pharmacology of impulses originating from a neuroma. *Exp Neurol* 1974;**43**:580–93.

15. Wall PD, Devor M. Sensory afferent impulses originate from dorsal root ganglia as well as from the periphery in normal and nerve injured rats. *Pain* 1983; **17**:321–39.

16. Matzner O, Devor M. Hyperexcitability at sites of nerve injury depends on voltage-sensitive Na^+ channels. *J Neurophysiol* 1994;**72**:349–59.

17. Woolf CJ. Evidence for a central component of post-injury pain hypersensitivity. *Nature* 1983;**306**:686–8.

18. Woolf CJ, Thompson SW. The induction and maintenance of central sensitization is dependent on *N*-methyl-D-aspartic acid receptor activation; implications for the treatment of post-injury pain hypersensitivity states. *Pain* 1991;**44**:293–9.

19. Flor H. Maladaptive plasticity, memory for pain and phantom limb pain: review and suggestions for new therapies. *Expert Rev Neurother* 2008;**8**:809–18.

20. Ypsilantis E, Tang TY. Pre-emptive analgesia for chronic limb pain after amputation for peripheral vascular disease: a systematic review. *Ann Vasc Surg* 2010;**24**:1139–46.

21. Hayes C, Armstrong-Brown A, Burstal R. Perioperative intravenous ketamine infusion for the prevention of persistent post-amputation pain: a

randomized, controlled trial. *Anaesth Intens Care* 2004; **32**:330–8.

22. Wilson JA, Nimmo AF, Fleetwood-Walker SM, Colvin LA. A randomised double blind trial of the effect of pre-emptive epidural ketamine on persistent pain after lower limb amputation. *Pain* 2008;**135**:108–18.

23. Nikolajsen L, Finnerup NB, Kramp S, *et al.* A randomized study of the effects of gabapentin on postamputation pain. *Anesthesiology* 2006;**105**:1008–15.

24. Sherman RA, Sherman CJ, Gall NG. A survey of current phantom limb pain treatment in the United States. *Pain* 1980;**8**:85–99.

25. Baron R, Binder A, Wasner G. Neuropathic pain: diagnosis, pathophysiological mechanisms, and treatment. *Lancet Neurol* 2010;**9**:807–19.

26. Dworkin RH, O'Connor AB, Backonja M, *et al.* Pharmacologic management of neuropathic pain: evidence-based recommendations. *Pain* 2007;**132**:237–51.

27. Finnerup NB, Otto M, McQuay HJ, Jensen TS, Sindrup SH. Algorithm for neuropathic pain treatment: an evidence-based proposal. *Pain* 2005;**118**:289–305.

28. Cook RJ, Sackett DL. The number needed to treat: a clinically useful measure of treatment effect. *BMJ* 1995 **310**:452–4.

29. Robinson LR, Czerniecki JM, Ehde DM, *et al.* Trial of amitriptyline for relief of pain in amputees: results of a randomized controlled study. *Arch Phys Med Rehabil* 2004;**85**:1–6.

30. Bone M, Critchley P, Buggy DJ. Gabapentin in postamputation phantom limb pain: a randomized, double-blind, placebo-controlled, cross-over study. *Reg Anesth Pain Med* 2002;**27**:481–6.

Anaesthesia for carotid artery disease

Mark D. Stoneham

Carotid artery atheromatous disease

Atheroma [Greek *athēra*, gruel] is the furring-up process of arteries which is associated with Western-type diet and lifestyles. Atheroma commonly forms at the bifurcation of major arteries (where blood flow becomes turbulent) such as the aorta in the abdomen and in the neck where the common carotid artery divides into the external carotid artery (supplying the face and neck) and the internal carotid artery (supplying the eye and brain).

Several pathophysiological events may subsequently occur involving the atheromatous plaques which form at the carotid bifurcation. Firstly, blood flow is gradually reduced in the carotid artery as the plaque enlarges which may promote collateral flow through the contralateral internal carotid or the vertebral arteries (although they may obviously have atheromatous plaques developing too). Secondly, small platelet microemboli may be released from the surface of the plaque into the internal carotid artery – these usually cause transient ischaemic attacks (TIA) as the neurological symptoms of hemiplegia or temporary blindness (amaurosis fugax) resolve within 24 hours. Thirdly, a larger embolus of plaque material can cause a more permanent cerebrovascular accident (CVA). Fourthly and finally, acute haemorrhage within the plaque can cause acute complete occlusion of the internal carotid and a devastating stroke.

Surgical techniques

The first reported carotid endarterectomy (CEA) was carried out at St Mary's Hospital, London in 1954 [1], although DeBakey may have performed the first operation in the United States the previous year. The description from the original *Lancet* article is revealing:

In 1954 Pickering, Professor of Medicine at St Mary's Hospital, London, had a 66-year-old female suffering intermittent attacks of right hemiplegia and left monocular blindness. A carotid arteriogram showed a significant stenosis of the left internal carotid artery. He suggested to the Professor of Surgery, Charles Robb, that the lesion might be corrected by surgery. Felix Eastcott, his Assistant Director, performed the operation with oversight by Robb. Before prepping and draping, the patient was covered with a rubber sheet and ice bags until the body temperature reached 28°C, in an attempt to protect the brain during the period of cross-clamping.

Thus these pioneers of vascular surgery clearly understood the principal problem of CEA – namely protection of the brain during carotid cross-clamping.

The standard surgical approach for CEA involves a longitudinal incision from the common carotid artery extended into the internal carotid artery. The carotid plaque is then removed piecemeal by opening an artificial 'plane' within the media of the arterial wall. Tacking sutures may be required at the distal (internal carotid) end of the incision to prevent the intima 'lifting' when blood flow is restored within the artery. If the arterial diameter is sufficient, the artery may be sutured closed directly. However, in smaller arteries, to avoid the development of postoperative stenosis, a patch angioplasty may be performed using a Goretex or Dacron patch.

An alternate surgical approach is eversion endarterectomy. This involves a transverse arterial incision cutting the internal carotid artery off the common carotid artery. The internal carotid artery is everted to remove the plaque from within. A circumferential anastomosis of the internal stump onto the common carotid artery is then performed. Eversion endarterectomy is usually faster than the standard approach as there are fewer sutures required and no patch needed. However, it has been

Core Topics in Vascular Anaesthesia, ed. Carl Moores and Alastair F. Nimmo. Published by Cambridge University Press. © Cambridge University Press 2012.

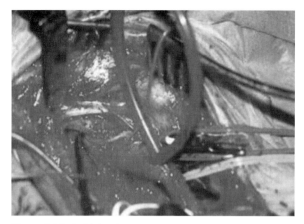

Figure 16.1 Javid shunt.

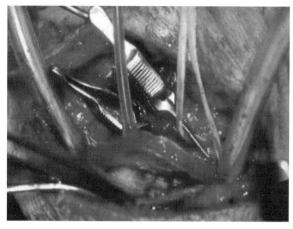

Figure 16.2 Pruitt–Inihara shunt.

shown to be associated with greater haemodynamic instability as, by definition, the carotid sinus nerve is cut during the procedure [2]. In addition, some surgeons find it more difficult to use a shunt with eversion endarterectomy (see below), so, in the author's institution, when using regional anaesthesia, a 'trial cross-clamp' period of 2 minutes is performed and if there is no neurological deterioration, the surgeon proceeds to eversion endarterectomy, whereas if a shunt is required a traditional longitudinal endarterectomy is performed.

Carotid artery shunting

An internal carotid artery shunt may be inserted by the surgeon in order to bypass the clamped portion of the artery and restore blood flow to the brain. The incidence of shunting varies widely, with some surgeons routinely shunting all patients and others never using shunts, instead relying on speed to prevent neurological complications during carotid cross-clamping. However, the majority of vascular surgeons use one or more cerebral monitoring techniques (see below) to identify which patients have inadequate collateral flow around the circle of Willis and to therefore use a shunt on these patients.

Two different types of shunt are available: the Javid shunt (Figure 16.1) which is a simple loop of plastic tubing and the Pruitt–Inihara shunt (Figure 16.2) which has saline-filled balloons used to seal the shunt within the artery and a side tubing allowing aspiration of blood. Insertion of either type of shunt has implications for surgery and anaesthesia including:

- A finite risk of embolic stroke due to plaque material being dislodged by the shunt insertion [3]
- Delay in cross-clamp time due to insertion and removal
- A period of several minutes when the brain can become hypoxic whilst the shunt is inserted and removed
- The possibility of significant haemorrhage due to accidental dislodgement of the shunt
- Some evidence that shunt insertion may be an independent risk factor for the development of postoperative stenosis and postoperative subclinical neurocognitive dysfunction [4,5].

Risks and benefits of carotid artery surgery

There is good evidence from several large, multicentre, randomised controlled trials that CEA improves survival and reduces the incidence of disabling stroke in patients with embolic or ischaemic symptoms (for example TIA, CVA or amaurosis fugax) with an internal carotid artery stenosis greater than 70% [6,7]. Some asymptomatic patients with carotid stenosis are also suitable for surgery [8,9].

The fundamental problem during the operation is maintenance of cerebral oxygenation during carotid cross-clamping. Despite strenuous attempts to make the procedure safer, the perioperative mortality rate from stroke and myocardial infarction (MI) still approaches 5% [10]; thus there is considerable interest in improving surgical and anaesthetic techniques for CEA to minimise this risk. This has led to controversies in surgical technique, anaesthetic technique, haemodynamic management and many other aspects of care.

In addition, the operation does not abolish the risk of stroke, but, like the treatment of hypertension with antihypertensive drugs, makes the patient less likely to suffer disabling stroke. However, the relatively high 30-day morbidity and mortality mean that, on average, the benefits of the operation are not realised unless the patient survives for 12–18 months postoperatively [9]. Thus patients with terminal diseases are not usually considered for carotid surgery.

Complications of carotid endarterectomy

Stroke is a devastating complication of CEA and may have multiple causes including embolus, thrombosis, haemorrhage, hypoperfusion (so-called 'watershed' stroke), and, perhaps, cerebral hyperperfusion syndrome [11]. The latter occurs postoperatively in a small percentage (1–2%) of patients undergoing CEA and may be due to ipsilateral cerebral cortex which was previously protected from extremes of blood pressure, being 'exposed' to high systolic blood pressures following the removal of the stenosis and restoration of blood flow. The features of cerebral hyperperfusion syndrome are headache, cerebral irritability, seizures and, eventually, subarachnoid haemorrhage.

Cardiac complications can also occur as many patients undergoing carotid surgery are arteriopaths who have concomitant ischaemic heart disease. In fact the GALA trial results showed that the incidence of MI is relatively low – only 13 patients out of 3542 (0.37%) of patients suffered MI peroperatively [10].

Cranial nerves may be damaged during the surgery, particularly the hypoglossal nerve and recurrent laryngeal nerve. Other complications of surgery include haemorrhage, which is obviously a possibility but in fact is uncommon, and wound haematoma, which may lead to acute airways obstruction and demands immediate attention and decompression. Airway oedema actually occurs in 100% of patients undergoing CEA – so superadded wound haematoma may be enough to cause airways obstruction [12].

Complications of regional anaesthesia

There are more complications associated with deep block than superficial block [13], although it is more

reliable and gives better postoperative analgesia. Serious potential complications include:

- Intravascular injection, producing immediate unconsciousness or seizures
- Subarachnoid injection, producing total spinal anaesthesia
- Phrenic nerve palsy which occurs in 60% of deep block recipients but is tolerated well, except in patients with underlying respiratory disease, who should receive superficial block alone.

Other potential side-effects of cervical plexus block include local haematoma, hoarseness, dysphagia, stellate ganglion block and Horner syndrome. Aspiration of blood during placement of cervical plexus blocks is common, occurring in up to 30% of patients [14]. Frequent aspiration is therefore vital to avoid intravascular injection of local anaesthetic, which may cause immediate epileptic seizure. This also applies to injection of local anaesthetic by the surgeon, either for local supplementation or carotid sinus blockade.

Preoperative assessment and risk management

As many of these patients are arteriopaths it is clearly important for them to be formally pre-assessed. A history, clinical examination, routine bloods and ECG are required for all patients. Patients with unstable angina or new cardiac symptoms may require referral to a cardiologist and more invasive cardiac assessment. A significant number of patients are discovered to have a significant carotid stenosis whilst being worked up to undergo coronary revascularisation, so by definition they are at a much higher risk of perioperative MI.

It has been recommended by the National Stroke Guidelines that patients are referred for CEA within 2 weeks of their 'presenting event' (TIA, stroke, etc.) [15]. This may cause problems with timing of pre-assessment as well as initiation of new medications following the presenting event.

Regional versus general anaesthesia

In the 1990s, a meta-analysis of trials looking at anaesthetic choice for CEA was published and revealed that there were only 143 patients who had been in randomised trials comparing general with regional anaesthesia but many thousands who were in non-randomised studies. Many of these were from North American institutions reporting on sequences of patients undergoing CEA where local anaesthesia had been arbitrarily introduced at some point and data from several hundred patients were analysed before and after the change to regional anaesthesia. These non-randomised trials suggested a 50% reduction in mortality and stroke from the use of regional as opposed to general anaesthesia [16], whereas from the randomised trial results, the only significant difference was a lower incidence of wound haematoma in the patients receiving regional anaesthesia.

Thus was born the GALA trial [10], a multicentre controlled comparison of anaesthetic techniques for CEA, which between 2000 and 2008 randomised 3526 patients with symptomatic or asymptomatic carotid stenosis from 95 centres in 24 countries randomly assigned to general anaesthesia (GA) ($n = 1753$) or local anaesthesia (LA) ($n = 1773$). The primary outcomes were the percentage of patients with stroke (including retinal infarction), MI and 30-day mortality.

The results were non-conclusive. A primary outcome occurred in 84 (4·8%) patients assigned to surgery under GA and 80 (4·5%) of those under LA; three events per 1000 treated were prevented with LA (95% confidence interval (CI) −11 to 17; relative risk ratio (RRR) 0·94 (95% CI 0·70 to 1·27).

Despite this being the largest published randomised trial of any anaesthetic technique, it was still underpowered to detect a difference in mortality or stroke. Although no differences between the two techniques were found in terms of major morbidity or mortality, any techniques for regional or general anaesthesia was permitted, which could therefore have 'diluted' potential differences between the groups (i.e. introduced a type B statistical error). In addition, there were suggestions that there had been 'entry bias' with some patients deemed unfit to undergo GA and therefore not randomised in the trial and who subsequently received LA as this was perceived to be 'safer' by some. Finally, a significant number of patients randomised to LA actually received GA but under 'intention to treat' were analysed with the other group.

The GALA trial results were therefore disappointing and have not prevented surgeons and anaesthetists continuing their dogmatic views concerning the advantages of one technique over the other.

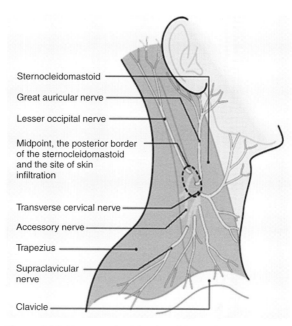

Figure 16.3 Nerve supply of the skin of the neck.

Regional techniques

The neck is supplied via the cervical plexus by cutaneous nerves from C2, 3 and 4 (Figure 16.3). The anterior divisions of the upper four cervical nerves unite to form the cervical plexus, which consists of three loops lying anterior to the cervical transverse processes. The cervical plexus gives rise to deep and superficial branches. Superficial branches, including lesser occipital, great auricular, anterior cutaneous and supraclavicular nerves, supply the neck from above the clavicle up to the angle of the mandible, usually including the earlobe. The deep plexus includes branches to the phrenic, the vagus and the hypoglossal nerves and to the cervical musculature.

Cervical epidural anaesthesia

Cervical epidural anaesthesia is used infrequently in the UK and USA, although there are large case series reporting its simplicity and success, particularly in France and Canada. Typically, 10 ml of bupivacaine 0.5% is injected at the C6–7 level to facilitate surgery. However, as all cervical and upper thoracic nerve roots bilaterally are affected, there is a relatively high incidence of side-effects, including hypotension and bradycardia, respiratory failure (requiring endotracheal intubation in 1–2%), dural puncture and bloody tap.

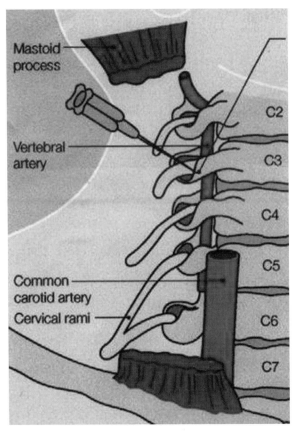

Figure 16.4 Deep cervical plexus block.

Cervical plexus block

Cervical plexus block is easier to perform, affects unilateral nerve roots only and has fewer side-effects than cervical epidural anaesthesia. Deep and/or superficial cervical plexus block may be employed. Deep block may be performed at a single level (usually C3) or at several levels (usually C2, C3 and C4) (Figure 16.4). The patient lies supine, slightly sitting up, with the head turned contralaterally. After skin disinfection, the cervical transverse processes may be palpated, usually 1 cm behind the posterior border of sternocleidomastoid. The third cervical transverse process is located by counting up from the sixth (Chassaignac's tubercle) at the level of the cricoid cartilage. After intradermal infiltration of 1% lidocaine, a 40 mm 25 gauge needle is introduced at C3 perpendicular to the skin, but aiming slightly caudad to avoid intrathecal injection. The transverse process is located 1–2 cm under the skin. Alternatively, it is possible to locate the transverse process and/or cervical plexus using ultrasound.

The patient may report paraesthesia in the distribution of the cervical plexus – typically down to the shoulder or round the front of the neck. Bupivacaine 0.375%, up to 20 ml, is then injected after careful aspiration by a second operator, using an immobile-needle technique.

True superficial block is a simpler technique with fewer reported complications. With the patient similarly positioned, an intradermal 'bleb' of lidocaine 1% is raised at the midpoint of the posterior border of the sternocleidomastoid. Then 10–20 ml bupivacaine 0.375% is injected in the subcutaneous plane along the posterior border of the sternocleidomastoid in cranial and caudal directions from this point. The external jugular vein commonly lies at the exact point where the superficial block is performed so great care needs to be taken to avoid intravascular injection.

Many practitioners of superficial block are, in fact, performing the block deep to the investing layer of deep cervical fascia – which may help to explain why the two blocks may be equally effective for cervical surgery. This has been termed 'intermediate block'.

Whichever regional technique is chosen for CEA, it rarely provides perfect anaesthesia. In some patients, the carotid disease extends so high that the incision needs to be extended into tissues innervated by cranial nerves. Additionally, despite apparently having good surgical anaesthesia, patients commonly complain of pain from the carotid sheath. This may reflect sympathetic afferent carotid innervation. Approximately half the patients will require local anaesthetic supplementation, which should not therefore be looked upon as a failure of the technique. Patients occasionally complain of pain referred to the jaw, molar teeth or the ear, which may be relieved by moving the surgical retractor, by local anaesthetic supplementation or by mandibular nerve block.

Management of the awake patient during carotid endarterectomy

Patient positioning is important to allow smooth progress of awake carotid surgery. Manoeuvres such as use of a 'deck-chair'-type position with a pillow under the knees help this elderly patient population tolerate 2 or more hours of surgery. The patient's bladder should be empty prior to surgery. There are several possible methods of allowing the surgeons adequate access to the neck whilst at the same time avoiding the patient feeling claustrophobic under excessive

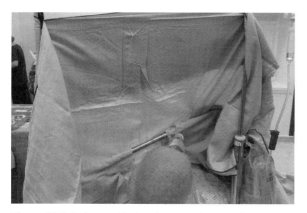

Figure 16.5 Patient positioning during awake carotid surgery.

surgical drapes. The technique in use at the author's hospital is shown in Figure 16.5.

Many patients require a degree of sedation to relax them and allow them to tolerate awake carotid surgery. Several different approaches have been described, including hypnotics such as target-controlled propofol infusion, opioids such as remi-fentanil, and alpha-2 agonists such as clonidine or dexmeditomidine. The author uses a remifentanil infusion, titrated to effect but typically 100–400 μg/hour, to provide reversible, predictable sedo-analgesia during block placement and dissection to enhance patient cooperation. The amount of supplemental local anaesthetic required is significantly reduced using this technique.

During carotid cross-clamping, constant neuro-logical assessment is vital, therefore sedation must be minimal at this stage. A useful cue for the anaes-thetist to know when to turn off the sedation is when the surgeon requests the administration of heparin. If the patient complains of pain during the operation, administering additional sedation is no substitute for augmentation of the block by the surgeon with sup-plemental local anaesthetic.

Oxygen is administered via a standard face mask. Monitoring consists of five-lead ECG, invasive arter-ial pressure measured from the contralateral radial artery, non-invasive blood pressure cuff, pulse oxime-try and capnography, estimated by sampling within the oxygen face-mask. The patient's head must be readily accessible. The anaesthetist must be attentive throughout, particularly during the period of carotid cross-clamping. Verbal communication, cerebral function and grip strength are tested throughout the cross-clamp period. Neurological signs such as slurring of speech, altered grip strength or an alter-ation in conscious level develop in 10–15% of awake patients. The anaesthetist should immediately check that the blood pressure is at, or above, the preopera-tive 'normal' level. Increased oxygen concentrations should be administered by face-mask. Either of these interventions can in itself reverse the developing neurological signs. If this does not work, the surgeon should insert a carotid shunt to maintain ipsilateral carotid flow.

The patient's normal cardiovascular medications are administered on the morning of surgery to help maintain haemodynamic stability. Blood pressure is maintained within 20% of preoperative values, pro-vided absolute systolic values are 120–180 mm Hg. Ephedrine, phenylephrine, metaraminol, labetalol and intravenous nitrates should all be immediately available for close haemodynamic control as appro-priate. Significant blood loss is uncommon; therefore minimal fluids are administered to avoid the problem of a patient needing to void during surgery.

Management of general anaesthesia

The prerequisites for general anaesthetic techniques are maintenance of haemodynamic stability, reduc-tion in cerebral oxygen consumption and rapid emer-gence to allow immediate postoperative neurological assessment.

A conventional technique might include preoxy-genation, intravenous induction with propofol sup-plemented with fentanyl, 2.5 μg/kg, neuromuscular relaxation with a non-depolarizing muscle relaxant such as vecuronium or atracurium to facilitate trach-eal intubation and subsequent ventilation with an air/oxygen/volatile mixture. Alternatively, an ultra-short-acting opioid such as remifentanil may be used, which allows more rapid emergence.

There is evidence from the literature that nitrous oxide should be avoided in patients undergoing CEA as it is associated with raised concentrations of plasma homocysteine and increased incidence of postopera-tive MI [17].

Monitoring should include five-lead ECG, inva-sive and non-invasive arterial pressure, pulse oxime-try, capnography, and the usual oxygen and ventilator pressure alarms. Central venous access is unnecessary – and indeed, inadvertent contralateral carotid punc-ture could lead to cancellation of the surgery because the patient may rely on contralateral carotid blood flow during ipsilateral internal carotid cross-clamping. Accidental carotid arterial puncture may also dislodge carotid plaque material, leading to embolic stroke.

Almost all anaesthetists use intermittent positive pressure ventilation (IPPV) to control arterial carbon dioxide tension tightly, because spontaneous ventilation may lead to hypercapnoea (or hypocapnoea) and undesirable cerebral steal effects. The drawback of IPPV is the need for intubation and extubation, which can precipitate hypertensive crises. Indeed there is evidence from some studies comparing general with regional anaesthesia for CEA that there is a difference in the rate of re-operation due to postoperative haematoma between the two. This is hypothesised to be due to venous hypertension on extubation.

At extubation, the ipsilateral brain is no longer protected by the tight carotid stenosis against sudden increases in perfusion pressure. Rapid-acting drugs such as remifentanil may be used to prevent such hypertensive crises, permitting intubation and ventilation without muscle relaxation and, when used in conjunction with superficial cervical block, allow rapid recovery with excellent postoperative analgesia. Another technique to reduce this risk is to replace the tracheal tube with a laryngeal mask airway (LMA) before emergence. The LMA has also been used as the sole airway during CEA, but cerebral blood flow has been shown to be decreased by the LMA cuff. The significance of this in patients with carotid stenosis is unknown. There could also be a risk of cuff puncture during surgery because the laryngeal mask cuff is situated close to the surgical field.

The use of general anaesthesia does not, of course, preclude the use of local anaesthetic infiltration or superficial cervical plexus blockade in order to provide excellent postoperative analgesia.

Monitoring cerebral perfusion

The ipsilateral cerebral cortex is at risk of hypoperfusion during carotid cross-clamping. There are several methods of monitoring cerebral function during this period. The real value of such monitoring is to identify patients with inadequate cerebral perfusion who may therefore benefit from interventions such as blood pressure augmentation, supplemental oxygenation or internal carotid artery shunting.

The 'gold standard' for cerebral monitoring is recognised to be the awake patient – where changes in speech, cerebration or motor power following carotid cross-clamping provide a more direct monitor of cerebral perfusion. The requirement for shunting is thereby reduced to 10–15%.

Alternate techniques used for cerebral perfusion monitoring during general anaesthesia include:

- Carotid artery stump pressure measurement in which the internal carotid artery is clamped and the pressure 'above' the clamp is measured by a needle placed within the lumen of the artery; this measures the pressure due to collateral flow around the circle of Willis – this is now largely of historical interest
- Transcranial Doppler ultrasound of the middle cerebral artery (which additionally gives audible indication of particulate embolisation during dissection around the carotid artery) – this is the most common technique used in the UK currently for GA patients
- EEG processing
- Somatosensory evoked potential monitoring – usually auditory
- Near-infrared spectroscopy techniques including 'cerebral oximetry'.

These techniques may be used to indicate which patients have inadequate collateral circulation. A shunt may then be used to bypass the internal carotid during cross-clamping. However, the relatively poor sensitivity and specificity of these techniques mean that some surgeons use a shunt on all patients. Other surgeons rely on very rapid surgical technique to limit cross-clamp time to 20 minutes or less. Alternatively, blood pressure may be augmented pharmacologically to maintain cerebral perfusion. Shunt insertion itself makes surgery more difficult and carries a small, but finite, risk of embolic stroke. All randomised trials of regional versus general anaesthesia for CEA have shown a lower incidence of shunt insertion using regional anaesthetic techniques.

Cerebral protection during carotid cross-clamping

Cerebral protection is an oft-quoted benefit and indication for the use of general anaesthesia. However, barbiturates are less commonly used in anaesthesia nowadays and the cerebral protective benefits of volatiles agents and propofol are less clear-cut compared to barbiturates.

The dose of barbiturates used for cerebral protection is of the order of 4 mg/kg initially followed by 0.5 mg/kg per minute during the carotid cross-clamping period [18]. This regimen leads typically to doses of thiopentone of 2000 mg or thereabouts preoperatively which therefore has implications for the speed of recovery and neurological assessment of the patient postoperatively.

Perioperative hypertension and hypotension

Carotid surgery is unique in that one of the principal components of the physiological control mechanisms of arterial pressure – baroreceptors in the carotid sinus – are involved in the disease process itself, and may be affected by the surgical procedure, concurrent therapy, administered drugs and the effects of anaesthesia.

Patients presenting for CEA may be undiagnosed hypertensives and often will have been commenced on antihypertensive medication recently. Thus their 'normal limits' for blood pressure may be changing or have recently changed. For this reason it is important for the anaesthetist to get a feel for the normal blood pressure of the patient and use this as a guide for management thereafter.

The most vulnerable period for the patient perioperatively is whilst the internal carotid artery is cross-clamped. Perfusion of the ipsilateral cerebral cortex during this time is dependent on collateral flow around the circle of Willis. The 'driving pressure' for this collateral flow is the systolic pressure – so during this period the patient's blood pressure should be kept at or above normal – provided there are no signs of myocardial ischaemia.

Postoperatively the reverse is true. The tight carotid stenosis protecting the brain from surges in blood pressure has now been removed, so uncontrolled hypertension can cause haemorrhagic stroke and may be associated with the cerebral hyperperfusion syndrome.

It is important, therefore, that protocols are developed for medical and nursing staff looking after these patients postoperatively so that blood pressure can be brought under control in timely fashion. It is equally important that precipitous falls in blood pressure are avoided as this can itself lead to watershed stroke.

Postoperative management

The choice of where the patients are managed postoperatively depends on the availability of critical care facilities. There is evidence that patients who develop neurological dysfunction after cross-clamping are at greater risk of permanent postoperative deficit [14]. These patients may benefit from closer observation on a high dependency unit.

Haemodynamic complications such as hypertension, hypotension, arrhythmias and myocardial ischaemia are common; therefore, invasive arterial pressure and ECG monitoring should be continued for a period (usually 2–4 hours) postoperatively.

Postoperative hypertension is common after CEA. It is usually transient and peaks in the first few hours after surgery, and is related to impaired baroreceptor function. It predisposes to wound haematoma and myocardial ischaemia, and in some cases may be a harbinger of cerebral hyperperfusion. The incidence of severe postoperative hypertension is up to 66%, with 40% or more patients requiring specific therapeutic intervention. Furthermore, intraoperative hypotension and postoperative hypertension put the patient at risk of developing wound haematoma [19]. Routine CEA causes airway narrowing due to oedema in all cases [12], and a wound haematoma can cause severe airway obstruction by a combination of direct compression and oedema. In some cases emergency wound exploration is needed [20], which carries significant risks [21]. In the NASCET trial, this pathophysiological mechanism was responsible for all non-stroke-related fatal surgical complications [22]. The incidence of postoperative wound haematoma is 3–8%; this may be minimised by surgical manoeuvres such as closing the artery at normal arterial pressure, wound drainage and an aggressive approach to control blood pressure during and after surgery. [19,23].

It remains uncertain whether postoperative hypertension is a causative factor in the development of cerebral hyperperfusion after CEA or a response to increased intracranial pressure [24]. However, there is indirect evidence that prompt control of blood pressure in patients who are hypertensive after CEA does improve outcome by reducing neurological complications, wound complications or both [19,25], and most practitioners would consider prompt, although not precipitous, treatment of postoperative hypertension to be important [26]. In the absence of definitive data, target pressures of <160 mm Hg systolic or within 20% of preoperative values are widely used, but a lower threshold may be appropriate in those at high risk for cerebral hyperperfusion or wound haematoma.

There are also few comparative data on the efficacy of different drugs to prevent or treat hypertension in patients undergoing CEA. Practice in the UK amongst vascular anaesthetists varies widely in terms of thresholds for therapy and preferred hypotensive drugs [27]. Important considerations include the availability of a parenteral formulation, duration of onset and mechanism of action, and co-existing therapy or disease. Most patients should be able to take oral medication within 2 hours of uncomplicated CEA whether performed under general or regional anaesthesia, but intravenous medication is usually required in the early postoperative period.

Though they have been used widely, direct-acting vasodilators (e.g. sodium nitroprusside, glyceryl trinitrate, nicardipine, hydralazine) have theoretical disadvantages after CEA as they cause cerebral vasodilatation. This may be deleterious in patients with newly increased cerebral blood flow and impaired autoregulation after CEA, though this may be outweighed by the effects of therapy on systemic arterial pressure, and it is difficult to predict the precise effects of different drugs on cerebral haemodynamics in individual patients.

Nifedipine capsules also cause cerebral vasodilatation and when administered sublingually can cause precipitous decreases in arterial pressure which have been associated with serious adverse events. Sublingual nifedipine is therefore not indicated for the treatment of acute hypertension [28]. Alpha- or beta-adrenergic antagonists are often effective for the prevention or treatment of postoperative hypertension. Available intravenous preparations include labetalol, esmolol, metoprolol, atenolol or clonidine. Labetalol and esmolol have been found effective in neurosurgical patients and both can be titrated to effect [29], but other drugs may be used [30]. Beta-adrenoceptor antagonists are useful to counteract the reflex tachycardia seen with other agents. Alpha-2-adrenoceptor agonists such as clonidine administered before or during surgery decrease myocardial ischaemia, arterial pressure and plasma catecholamine concentrations [31], though there are no data for the use of clonidine in patients undergoing CEA. Whatever drug is used

it should be given in a controlled manner and titrated against effect as precipitous decreases in blood pressure can be associated with watershed cerebral ischaemia [32]. Beat-to-beat blood pressure monitoring is advised if parenteral drugs are required, and response to therapy should be closely monitored in a high dependency unit or intensive care unit environment if necessary for a period of at least 2–4 hours until arterial pressure is stable. Suggestions for postoperative management of blood pressure are given in Table 16.1.

Postoperative analgesia

Analgesia is not usually required following regional anaesthesia for carotid surgery; however, patients recovering from general anaesthesia without regional block may require small doses of opioid analgesia titrated against their pain. If patients are haemodynamically stable after 2 hours, they are discharged to the ward. Compromise of the airway as a result of oedema or haematoma is not uncommon. Wounds are observed carefully for signs of swelling and, if required, opened in recovery and explored immediately in the operating theatre. This may be done without additional local anaesthetic supplementation following a regional technique. Neurological deficit developing postoperatively requires immediate surgical consultation, because it may indicate developing cerebral ischaemia due to haemorrhage, embolus or obstruction to blood flow.

Carotid artery stenting

An alternative treatment for carotid stenosis is carotid artery stenting (CAS).

Carotid artery stenting is a less invasive procedure than open surgical treatment involving placement of a stent across the carotid stenosis by interventional radiological access from the groin. Initial thoughts were that this might be a safer treatment than open surgery. The first carotid balloon angioplasty was done in 1980 and the first stent placed in 1989. This initial enthusiasm was followed by concerns as it was reported that morbidity and mortality was increased compared to CEA [33]. Since then, several large multicentre randomised controlled trials have been performed in order to answer the question as to whether outcome is improved by CAS [34–6]. Some trials have shown increased morbidity and mortality of CAS particularly due to cardiac events. However, a recent

Table 16.1 Postoperative blood pressure management

(1) Postoperative care unit (PACU): systolic pressure >170 mm Hg

General points

Does the patient have urinary retention or is he/she in pain?

Has the patient received his/her normal anti-hypertensive medication today?

First line

Labetalol: 100 mg labetalol in 20 ml of 0.9% NaCl (5 mg/ml). Give 10 mg (2 ml) boluses *slowly* every 2 minutes up to 100 mg (i.e. 20 ml given over 20 minutes)

If BP remains elevated after 20 minutes, move to second-line agent

If BP decreases and does not rebound, continue regular BP observations

If BP decreases initially but increases again, start infusion at 50–100 mg/hour, titrating dose to BP

(2) *Patient remains in postoperative care unit/high depency unit (HDU) while labetalol infusion is running. Following cessation of the infusion, the patient should remain in PACU/HDU for 2 further hours to minimise rebound hypertension.*

Second line

Hydralazine: 10 mg hydralazine in 10 ml 0.9% NaCl (1 mg/ml). Give 2 mg (2 ml) boluses *slowly* every 5 minutes up to 10 mg (i.e. 10 ml given over 25 minutes)

If BP remains elevated after 25 minutes, move to third-line agent

If BP decreases and does not rebound, continue regular BP observations

If BP decreases initially but increases again, move to third-line agent

Patient remains in PACU/HDU while hydralazine therapy is under way. Following cessation of hydralazine therapy, the patient should remain in PACU/HDU for 2 further hours to minimise rebound hypertension.

Third line

Glyceryl trinitrate (GTN): 50 mg GTN in 50 ml 0.9% NaCl (1mg/ml) start infusion at 5 ml/hour (5 mg/hour), increasing rate to 12 ml/hour (12 mg/hour), titrated to BP

Patient remains in PACU/HDU while GTN infusion is under way. Following cessation of GTN infusion, the patient should remain in PACU/HDU for 2 further hours to minimise rebound hypertension.

meta-analysis of all randomised trials has concluded that overall, CAS offers no advantage over CEA and that surgical treatment of carotid stenosis is recommended unless there are relative contraindications to surgery [37].

Carotid body tumours

The carotid body is derived from both mesodermal elements of the third branchial arch and neural elements originating from the neural crest ectoderm. It is a small ovoid or irregular mass bilaterally situated on the bifurcation of the common carotid artery, and functions as a chemoreceptor sensitive to changes in arterial pO_2, pCO_2 and pH, which induces reflex changes in vasomotor activity and respiration.

Carotid body tumour (also called paraganglioma, glomus tumour or chemodectoma) is a rare, highly vascular tumour arising from the paraganglion cells of the carotid body.

Three types of carotid body tumours are described in the literature: familial, sporadic and hyperplastic. The sporadic form is the most common type, representing approximately 85% of carotid body tumours. The familial type (10–15%) is more common in younger patients. The hyperplastic form is common in patients with chronic hypoxia, including patients living at high altitude and patients with chronic respiratory or cyanotic heart disease.

The most frequent presentation is a palpable neck mass located below the angle of the mandible, which is mobile laterally but not vertically because of its adventitial attachments.

Anaesthetic management of carotid body tumours

Anaesthetic choices for the surgical removal of carotid body tumours are similar to those for CEA, except that the surgery is likely to be more prolonged. For this reason, general anaesthesia has been preferred in the sparse published literature, together with cerebral protection from barbiturates and carotid shunting, together with invasive haemodynamic monitoring and cerebral oximetry. However, carotid body tumours are more common in patients with chronic hypoxic states such as Eisenmenger syndrome, in which regional anaesthesia may be safer and preferable [38].

As with CEA, the surgical field involves part of the blood pressure regulatory control mechanism, therefore haemodynamic instability may be common. Invasive arterial pressure monitoring, immediate availability of vasoactive medications and close postoperative monitoring in a high dependency unit are therefore advisable.

References

1. Eastcott HHG, Pickering GW, Robb CG. Reconstruction of internal carotid artery in a patient with intermittent attacks of hemiplegia. *Lancet* 1954;2:994–6.

2. Mehta M, Rahmani O, Dietzek AM, *et al.* Eversion technique increases the risk for post-carotid endarterectomy hypertension. *J Vasc Surg* 2001;34:839–45.

3. Woodworth GF, McGirt MJ, Than KD, *et al.* Selective versus routine interoperative shunting during carotid endarterectomy: a multivariate outcome analysis. *Neurosurgery* 2007;61:1170–6.

4. Hudorovic N, Lovricevic I, Hajnic H, Ahel Z. Postoperative internal carotid artery restenosis after local anesthesia: presence of risk factors versus intraoperative shunt. *Interact Cardiovasc Thorac Surg* 2010;11:182–4.

5. Mazul-Sunko B, Hromatko I, Tadinac M, *et al.* Subclinical neurocognitive dysfunction after carotid endarterectomy: the impact of shunting. *J Neurosurg Anesthesiol* 2010;22:195–201.

6. North American Symptomatic Carotid Endarterectomy Trial Collaborators. Beneficial effect of carotid endarterectomy in symptomatic patients with high-grade carotid stenosis. *N Engl J Med* 1991;325:445–53.

7. European Carotid Surgery Triallist's Collaborative Group. MRC European Carotid Surgery Trial: interim results for symptomatic patients with severe (70–99%) or with mild (0–29%) carotid stenosis. *Lancet* 1991;337:1235–43.

8. Toole JF. ACAS recommendations for carotid endarterectomy. ACAS Executive Committee. *Lancet* 1996;347:121.

9. Rothwell PM, Slattery J, Warlow CP. A systematic comparison of the risks of stroke and death due to carotid endarterectomy for symptomatic and asymptomatic stenosis. *Stroke* 1996;27:266–9.

10. Lewis SC, Warlow CP, Bodenham AR, *et al.* General anaesthesia versus local anaesthesia for carotid surgery (GALA): a multicentre, randomised controlled trial. *Lancet* 2008;372:2132–42.

11. Moulakakis KG, Mylonas SN, Sfyroeras GS, Andrikopoulos V. Hyperperfusion syndrome after carotid revascularization. *J Vasc Surg* 2009;49:1060–8.

12. Carmichael FJ, McGuire GP, Wong DT, *et al.* Computed tomographic analysis of airway dimensions after carotid endarterectomy. *Anesth Analg* 1996;83:12–17.

13. Pandit JJ, Satya-Krishna R, Gration P. Superficial or deep cervical plexus block for carotid endarterectomy: a systematic review of complications. *Br J Anaesth* 2007;99:159–69.

14. Davies MJ, Silbert BS, Scott DA, Cook RJ, Mooney PH. Superficial and deep cervical plexus block for carotid artery surgery: A prospective study of 1000 blocks. *Reg Anesth* 1997;22:442–6.

15. Royal College of Physicians Intercollegiate Stroke Working Party. *National Clinical Guidelines for Stroke*, 3rd edn. London: RCP, 2008.

16. Tangkanakul C, Counsell CE, Warlow CP. Local versus general anaesthesia in carotid endarterectomy: a systematic review of the evidence. *Eur J Vasc Endovasc Surg* 1997;13: 491–9.

17. Badner NH, Beattie WS, Freeman D, Spence JD. Nitrous oxide-induced increased homocysteine concentrations are associated with increased postoperative myocardial ischemia in patients undergoing carotid endarterectomy. *Anesth Analg* 2000;91:1073–9.

18. McMeniman WJ, Fletcher JP, Little JM. Experience with barbiturate therapy for cerebral protection during carotid endarterectomy. *Ann R Coll Surg Engl* 1984;66:361–4.

19. Beard JD, Mountney J, Wilkinson JM, *et al.* Prevention of postoperative wound haematomas and hyperperfusion following carotid endarterectomy. *Eur J Vasc Endovasc Surg* 2001;21:490–3.

20. Munro FJ, Makin AP, Reid J. Airway problems after carotid endarterectomy. *Br J Anaesth* 1996;76:156–9.

21. Self DD, Bryson GL, Sullivan PJ. Risk factors for post-carotid endarterectomy hematoma formation. *Can J Anaesth* 1999;**46**:635–40.

22. Ferguson GG, Eliasziw M, Barr HW, *et al.* The North American Symptomatic Carotid Endarterectomy Trial: surgical results in 1415 patients. *Stroke* 1999;**30**:1751–8.

23. Hans SS, Glover JL. The relationship of cardiac and neurological complications to blood pressure changes following carotid endarterectomy. *Am Surg* 1995;**61**:356–9.

24. Russell DA, Gough MJ. Intracerebral haemorrhage following carotid endarterectomy. *Eur J Vasc Endovasc Surg* 2004;**28**:115–23.

25. Nielsen TG, Sillesen H, Schroeder TV. Seizures following carotid endarterectomy in patients with severely compromised cerebral circulation. *Eur J Vasc Endovasc Surg* 1995;**9**:53–7.

26. Stoneham MD, Thompson JP. Arterial pressure management and carotid endarterectomy. *Br J Anaesth* 2009;**102**: 442–52.

27. Ahmed I, Thompson JP. Survey of perioperative blood pressure management for carotid endarterectomy. *Anaesthesia* 2008;**63**:214.

28. Grossman E, Messerli FH, Grodzicki T, Kowey P. Should a moratorium be placed on sublingual nifedipine capsules given for hypertensive emergencies and pseudoemergencies? *JAMA* 1996;**276**:1328–31.

29. Goldberg ME, Seltzer JL, Azad SS, *et al.* Intravenous labetalol for the treatment of hypertension after carotid endarterectomy. *J Cardiothorac Anesth* 1989; **3**:411–17.

30. Haas AR, Marik PE. Current diagnosis and management of hypertensive emergency. *Semin Dial* 2006;**19**:502–12.

31. Wallace AW. Clonidine and modification of perioperative outcome. *Curr Opin Anaesthesiol* 2006;**19**:411–17.

32. Krul JM. [Brain infarct as a possible side effect of blood pressure-lowering treatment.] *Ned Tijdschr Geneeskd* 1987;**131**:1778.

33. Hobson RW, Howard VJ, Roubin GS, *et al.* Carotid artery stenting is associated with increased complications in octogenarians: 30-day stroke and death rates in the CREST lead-in phase. *J Vasc Surg* 2004;**40**:1106–11.

34. Gurm HS, Yadav JS, Fayad P, *et al.* Long-term results of carotid stenting versus endarterectomy in high-risk patients. *N Engl J Med* 2008;**358**:1572–9.

35. Mas JL, Chatellier G, Beyssen B, *et al.* Endarterectomy versus stenting in patients with symptomatic severe carotid stenosis. *N Engl J Med* 2006;**355**:1660–71.

36. Ederle J, Dobson J, Featherstone RL, *et al.* Carotid artery stenting compared with endarterectomy in patients with symptomatic carotid stenosis (International Carotid Stenting Study): an interim analysis of a randomised controlled trial. *Lancet* 2010;**375**:985–97.

37. Ederle J, Featherstone RL, Brown MM. Randomized controlled trials comparing endarterectomy and endovascular treatment for carotid artery stenosis: a Cochrane systematic review. *Stroke* 2009;**40**:1373–80.

38. Jones HG, Stoneham MD. Continuous cervical plexus block for carotid body tumour excision in a patient with Eisenmenger's syndrome. *Anaesthesia* 2006;**61**:1214–18.

Anaesthesia for vascular surgery to the upper limb

Carl Moores

Introduction

Vascular surgeons spend a lot of their working life treating patients with ischaemia to the lower limbs. Conversely, upper limb ischaemia is a much more unusual complaint. Compared with the lower limb, degenerative arterial disease is much less common in the upper limb, and it is less likely to lead to critical ischaemia because of a good collateral circulation around the shoulder. However, acute thromboembolism in an upper limb vessel leading to profound ischaemia is a surgical emergency as the ischaemic tolerance of the upper limb is much less than that of the lower limb and tissue loss can occur rapidly [1].

In this chapter upper limb ischaemia, both acute and chronic, is discussed together with its surgical and anaesthetic management. Also discussed is thoracic outlet syndrome, which may be vascular (affecting the subclavian vessels) or neurogenic (affecting nerves of the brachial plexus). Vascular thoracic outlet syndrome can lead to upper limb ischaemia, but neurogenic thoracic outlet syndrome is also often treated by vascular surgeons, even though there are no blood vessels that are directly affected. Finally, thoracoscopic sympathectomy is discussed. Vascular surgeons often carry out this procedure, even though it is not usually done to treat upper limb ischaemia.

Acute upper limb ischaemia

Acute upper limb ischaemia manifests as a painful, white, pulseless arm which may be accompanied by pain, paraesthesia or weakness. The cause of an acutely ischaemic upper limb is usually an embolus. In many cases the embolus originates in the heart as a consequence of atrial fibrillation. The left ventricle may also be the site of thrombus formation, particularly if a segment of ventricular myocardium is

dyskinetic following a myocardial infarction. Rarely, emboli may originate in the venous circulation and pass through an atrial septal defect. Emboli can arise from the aorta, sometimes secondary to a dissection. The subclavian arteries can also be a source of emboli: thrombus can form in a subclavian aneurysm and emboli can be the result of subclavian artery compression by, for example, a cervical rib (see arterial thoracic outlet syndrome below). Iatrogenic damage to the subclavian artery following wire or catheter insertion can also result in embolisation to the upper limb.

Surgical treatment

If the upper limb is acutely threatened, then emergency brachial embolectomy is indicated to restore blood flow. This operation is usually carried out under local anaesthesia. Nevertheless, monitoring and care by an anaesthetist is recommended as these patients often have significant comorbidity and may be restless and in pain.

The surgeon makes an arteriotomy in the brachial artery at the level of the elbow. Balloon embolectomy catheters are passed proximally up the brachial artery and distally down the radial and ulnar arteries to retrieve as much clot as possible. The vessels are then flushed with a heparinised solution and the arteriotomy is closed. Usually, the patient will require anticoagulation postoperatively.

Although the operation is usually well tolerated under local anaesthesia, general anaesthesia may be required if the patient is uncooperative, particularly if the upper limb has been ischaemic for some time and is very painful. In a small number of cases, a compartment syndrome of the forearm muscles can develop, and fasciotomies are then required. Further investigation may reveal a source of the embolus, for example a cervical rib.

Core Topics in Vascular Anaesthesia, ed. Carl Moores and Alastain F. Nimmo. Published by Cambridge University Press.
© Cambridge University Press 2012.

Chronic upper limb ischaemia

Atherosclerotic disease

Because of the good collateral circulation around the shoulder, atherosclerosis of the subclavian artery often does not give rise to symptoms of overt ischaemia and may simply present as a noticeable difference in blood pressure recorded in the two arms. Only in more advanced disease does exercise-induced claudication of the upper limb become apparent. In addition, embolisation from atherosclerotic plaques may lead to acute upper limb ischaemia or areas of digital ischaemia or gangrene.

Subclavian steal syndrome

Stenosis in the proximal subclavian artery can give rise to subclavian steal syndrome. Reduced pressure and flow in the subclavian artery distal to the stenosis may lead to retrograde blood flow in the ipsilateral vertebral artery, often in response to upper limb exercise. This reduces cerebral perfusion which may in turn lead to symptoms including dizziness, light-headedness and, in more severe cases, drop attacks. Coronary–subclavian steal syndrome may occur in patients who have undergone coronary artery bypass graft surgery using the internal mammary artery as a graft. Subclavian artery stenosis can lead to retrograde blood flow in the internal mammary artery graft which can cause cardiac symptoms, including not only angina but also heart failure, ischaemic cardiomyopathy and sudden cardiac death [2].

Radiation disease

Damage to the subclavian artery is sometimes the result of radiation administered for the treatment of breast cancer. Initially, radiation arteritis can lead to stenosis of the artery or may give rise to distal emboli. Later, atherosclerosis may supervene leading to chronic ischaemic symptoms.

Other causes of chronic upper limb ischaemia

Congenital abnormalities of the subclavian artery or its origin from the aortic arch may predispose to chronic upper limb ischaemia, as may trauma to the vessel. Cervical ribs and other structures are discussed below in the section on thoracic outlet syndrome.

Surgical treatment

Where symptoms are due to thoracic outlet syndrome, this should be treated, as described below.

Isolated stenosis of the subclavian artery is usually treated using endovascular techniques. Angioplasty and stenting of the subclavian artery is generally successful, although restenosis rates of between 6% and 20% have been reported [3].

If the subclavian artery is occluded, or if endovascular techniques are not successful, a bypass technique is generally indicated. A carotid subclavian bypass may be carried out, whereby an artificial graft is interposed between the ipsilateral carotid artery and the subclavian artery. An alternative is the subclavian–carotid transposition. In this procedure, the subclavian artery is transected and transposed onto the carotid artery. Prior to either of these procedures, duplex assessment of the carotid artery is required to ensure that it is suitable. Other bypass options include subclavian–subclavian or axillo–axillary bypass techniques, whereby blood is directed through artificial grafts from the contralateral vessels.

Thoracic outlet syndrome

Thoracic outlet syndrome is characterised by symptoms attributable to compression of or injury to the brachial plexus, subclavian artery or subclavian vein as they pass though the thoracic outlet [2,3]. The syndrome can be divided into three distinct forms: arterial, venous and neurogenic, depending on the anatomical structure that is predominantly affected. The neurogenic form of the syndrome is by far the commonest, accounting for over 98% of all cases. Although only a small minority of cases of thoracic outlet syndrome are vascular in aetiology, it is common for vascular surgeons to carry out operative procedures to relieve symptoms in all forms of thoracic outlet syndrome, given the presence of major vessels in the operative field.

Anatomy of the thoracic outlet

The subclavian artery and brachial plexus arch over the first rib in the interscalene triangle which lies between the anterior scalene muscle anteriorly, the middle scalene muscle posteriorly and the first rib inferiorly. The subclavian vein passes over the first rib anterior to the anterior scalene muscle (see Figure 17.1) [4]. Arching over all these structures

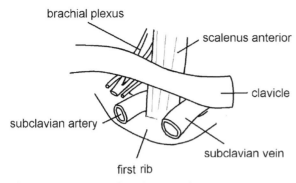

Figure 17.1 Anatomy of the thoracic outlet.

is the clavicle, forming the costoclavicular space between itself and the first rib.

Compression of the neurovascular structures in the thoracic outlet can be the result of congenital variations in the surrounding structures or a consequence of trauma.

Cervical ribs are among the commonest causes of neurogenic and arterial thoracic outlet syndrome. They are present in about 0.5% of individuals and are twice as common in females as in males. If they are present, they are usually bilateral. However, it is thought that only 10–20% of them cause symptoms [4]. A fully developed cervical rib extends forward from the lateral process of the C7 vertebra and articulates with the first rib, often in close proximity to the neurovascular structures of the thoracic outlet. However, smaller less fully developed ribs may also be symptomatic. The tip of the cervical rib may compress adjacent structures, or may 'lift' the subclavian artery off the first rib. In addition, it is common for tight fibrous bands to extend from the tip of the cervical rib to the upper surface of the first rib. These fibrous bands may compress the subclavian artery or the brachial plexus.

Thoracic outlet syndrome may arise as a result of an unusually narrow gap between the anterior and middle scalene muscles. Often the result of overlapping insertions of these muscles on the first rib, this can lead to compression of the subclavian artery or brachial plexus. In some individuals, symptoms may be due to a scalenus minimus muscle, the fibres of which insert into the first rib between the subclavian artery and the T1 nerve root.

Thoracic outlet syndrome may also be the result of anatomical abnormalities of the first rib or overlying clavicle. These may be congenital or as a result of fractures or excessive callus formation in these bones.

Neurogenic thoracic outlet syndrome

Neurogenic thoracic outlet syndrome is characterised by pain, paraesthesia or weakness in the neck, upper trunk or arm. In its most severe form, it is accompanied by muscle wasting. Typically, the pain can be brought on or worsened by the patient adopting a particular neck or head position. It is thought that neurogenic thoracic outlet syndrome is usually precipitated by injury in patients who have a predisposition to the condition. The predisposition may be, for example, a narrow interscalene triangle or a cervical rib. The injury is usually a neck injury, commonly a hyperextension injury, perhaps as a result of a motor accident. Additionally, repetitive strain to the arm and neck (for example in keyboard workers) can trigger the syndrome. Histological studies have demonstrated fibrosis, scarring and other histological abnormalities in scalene muscles that have been excised at operation from sufferers of neurogenic thoracic outlet syndrome [5]. This scarring may be responsible for compression of the trunks of the brachial plexus as they pass through the interscalene triangle. Neurogenic thoracic outlet syndrome can be further divided into true neurogenic thoracic outlet syndrome and disputed thoracic outlet syndrome. The true form is characterised by radiological or other evidence of an abnormality of the thoracic outlet, or by electrophysiological evidence of nerve damage; the 'disputed' form is where there is no such evidence.

Venous thoracic outlet syndrome

Venous thoracic outlet syndrome is caused by compression or occlusion of the subclavian vein as it passes through the thoracic outlet and can be either thrombotic or non-thrombotic [6]. It is characterised by swelling of the affected arm, forearm and hand. This may be associated with distal cyanosis, arm pain, or in more severe cases paraesthesia. The diagnosis is confirmed by duplex ultrasound scanning or venography.

Venous thoracic outlet syndrome may be either primary or secondary. The primary form of the syndrome is presumed to be due to narrowing of the space in the thoracic outlet through which the subclavian vein passes. Secondary venous thoracic outlet syndrome can result from catheters or wires in the subclavian vein, extrinsic compression from tumours or may be as a result of a thrombotic tendency.

Arterial thoracic outlet syndrome

This is the rarest form of thoracic outlet syndrome. It is the result of an anatomical structure compressing the subclavian or axillary artery. This structure may be a cervical rib, an elongated transverse process of C7 or a fibrous band extending from C7 to the first rib. The arterial compression can lead to a reduction in upper limb blood flow, which in turn can lead to upper limb claudication. This is characterised by pain, pallor and early fatigue of the arm on exertion, particularly if the limb is elevated. Distal to the stenosis, turbulent blood flow can lead to post-stenotic dilatation of the artery or even aneurysm formation. This in turn may predispose to thrombus formation which can lead to distal embolisation and acute ischaemia of the arm or hands. In the worse cases, digital gangrene can result.

Surgical treatment of thoracic outlet syndrome

The choice of surgical procedure for treatment of thoracic outlet syndrome depends on the source of the symptoms and the surgeon's preference. For symptoms relating to a cervical rib or for symptoms affecting the upper roots (C5, C6 or C7) of the brachial plexus, a transcervical scalenectomy is carried out. An incision is made above the clavicle and the anterior and middle scalene muscles are exposed. If a cervical rib is present, it is resected. The scalene muscles are resected, with care being taken not to injure the phrenic nerve which lies on the anterior scalene muscle. In resecting the scalene muscles, the interscalene triangle is released, which will hopefully lead to the resolution of symptoms.

For symptoms affecting the lower roots of the brachial plexus (C8 and T1), a first rib resection may be carried out, although there is some dispute among surgeons as to whether this is any more effective than simply carrying out anterior and middle scalenectomies.

First rib resection can be carried out via a supraclavicular incision [7]. Anterior and middle scalenectomies are carried out as described above. The subclavian vessels and brachial plexus are mobilised and the first rib is separated from its posterior periosteum before being divided anteriorly and posteriorly and then removed.

Some surgeons prefer to perform a transaxillary first rib resection. The patient is placed in the lateral position and the arm is extended to approximately right angles to the torso (the upper arm is therefore held in a vertical position). The surgeon makes an incision at the base of the axilla against the chest wall, and dissects upwards towards the apex of the axilla until the lower border of the first rib is reached. The subclavian vessels and brachial plexus are carefully dissected off the rib. The scalene muscles are divided at their attachments to the rib and the subclavius tendon and the costocoracoid ligaments are divided anteriorly. The rib is then free from all its attachments. The rib is carefully dissected away from its posterior periosteum and is divided anteriorly and posteriorly before being removed completely [8]. Recently, endoscopically assisted transaxillary first rib resection has been described [9].

Anaesthetic management

General anaesthesia is required for thoracic outlet surgery and care must be taken in patient positioning, particularly for transaxillary first rib resection, given the risk of brachial plexus injury. Intubation and ventilation are required for these procedures, given the risk of pneumothorax. If a pneumothorax does occur, it can be treated with a chest drain at the end of the procedure.

Haemorrhage can be heavy if the subclavian artery or vein is injured, and bleeding can be difficult to control because of the limited surgical access. For this reason, good venous access and the ready availability of blood products are essential.

Complications

Neurological symptoms, including altered sensation in the arm, are often reported following transaxillary first rib resection, and are presumably related to traction on the brachial plexus during the procedure. These symptoms are generally self-limiting and more serious injuries to the brachial plexus are rare.

Supraclavicular thoracic outlet surgery may be complicated by damage to the phrenic nerve which may result in dyspnoea, although this is usually temporary. It may also be complicated by lymph collections, particularly on the left-hand side in relation to the thoracic duct. Occasionally, a Horner syndrome may result.

Thoracoscopic sympathectomy

Thoracoscopic sympathectomy is the division of the thoracic sympathetic chain as it passes over the necks of the upper thoracic ribs. It is a procedure that is often carried out by vascular surgeons as it remains an option for the relief of symptoms of upper limb ischaemia. However, this is rarely the indication for which it is performed these days.

Indications

Thoracoscopic sympathectomy has been performed for a number of conditions related to sympathetic nerve function [10]. These include reflex sympathetic dystrophy, Raynaud disease, hypertension, long QT syndrome [11], ventricular dysrhythmias [12,13], abdominal visceral pain, facial flushing and upper limb ischaemia. However, the condition for which the procedure is most commonly employed is upper limb hyperhidrosis. Thoracoscopic sympathectomy can be used for palmar or axillary hyperhidrosis, although medical treatments of axillary hyperhidrosis, such as aluminium salts or botulinum toxin injections, are generally tried first [14].

Surgical technique

The surgeon inserts a thoracoscope into the chest through an incision made between two ribs. The patient may have a simple endotracheal tube in situ and the lung collapses passively, or many anaesthetists use a double-lumen tube to aid lung deflation. The sympathetic chain is identified alongside the vertebral column and is divided as it passes over the neck of one or more of the ribs. The level at which the chain is divided depends upon the symptoms for which the procedure is being carried out [15].

The chain is divided at the level of the second rib for facial flushing. For the treatment of reflex sympathetic dystrophy and palmar hyperhidrosis, the chain is divided at the level of both the second and third ribs. For axillary hyperhidrosis, the chain is divided at the level of the third rib and possibly also the fourth rib. Either simple division of the chain is carried out, or a small segment is resected. Figure 17.2 shows a sympathetic chain after surgical division.

Anaesthetic management

General anaesthesia is required for this procedure. One-lung ventilation can be achieved using a double-lumen endobronchial tube, or a bronchial blocker. If the patient is in a semi-recumbent position, the lung can deflate passively with the aid of

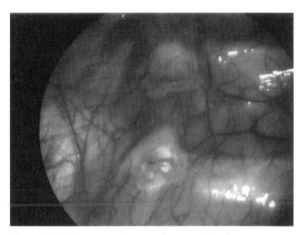

Figure 17.2 Thoracoscopic sympathectomy. The thoracoscope is looking at the posterior wall of the thorax. The second and third ribs are the whitish structures on the right. The thoracic sympathetic chain has been divided as it passes over the ribs. See plate section for colour version.

gravity. Some surgeons use carbon dioxide insufflation into the chest cavity in order to cause the lung to collapse; if this is the case, it is possible to perform the procedure using a single-lumen endotracheal tube.

Division of the sympathetic chain is usually achieved using an electrocautery device. This is often inserted into the chest through a second port, although it is possible to carry out the procedure through a single thoracoscopy port using a dedicated channel for electrocautery [16]. Once the chain has been divided, the two cut nerve ends are cauterised. Often, the surgeon will extend the electrocautery incision on the second rib laterally for a centimetre or so. This is to divide any putative direct sympathetic nerve connections between the second thoracic ganglion and the brachial plexus (so-called nerves of Kuntz), although there is some doubt as to whether such pathways actually exist [17].

Once the nerve chain is divided, haemostasis is secured and the lung is reinflated as the thoracoscope is removed from the chest. A chest drain is not usually required if care is taken to make sure that the lung is completely reinflated as the thoracoscope is withdrawn from the chest.

Postoperative analgesia can be provided by leaving a narrow catheter (for example an epidural catheter) in the pleural cavity as the thoracoscope is withdrawn, with the tip of the catheter positioned in the area of surgery The catheter exits the patient's chest through the surgical incision, and local anaesthetic can be injected into the intrapleural space through the catheter [18].

Complications

The more common complications of thoracoscopic sympathectomy include compensatory sweating which often occurs over the trunk. This can occur in 20–80% of cases, although it is rarely disabling [10]. Less common is Horner syndrome, which can affect up to 5% of patients. Rarer complications include large pneumothorax, chylothorax and oesophageal or lung injury.

References

1. Thompson JF, Kinsella DC. Vascular disorders of the upper limb. In Beard JD, Gaines PA, eds., *Vascular and Endovascular Surgery: A Companion to Specialist Surgical Practice*. Amsterdam: Elsevier, 2009.

2. Takach TJ, Reul GJ, Cooley DA, *et al*. Myocardial thievery: the coronary–subclavian steal syndrome. *Ann Thorac Surg* 2006;**81**:386–92.

3. Rogers JH, Calhoun RF 2nd. Diagnosis and management of subclavian artery stenosis prior to coronary artery bypass grafting in the current era. *J Card Surg* 2007;**22**:20–5.

4. Atasoy E. Thoracic outlet syndrome: anatomy. *Hand Clin* 2004;**20**:7–14.

5. Sanders RJ, Hammond SL, Rao NM. Thoracic outlet syndrome: a review. *Neurologist* 2008;**14**:365–73.

6. Sanders RJ, Hammond SL. Venous thoracic outlet syndrome. *Hand Clin* 2004;**20**:113–18.

7. Sanders RJ, Hammond SL. Supraclavicular first rib resection and total scalenectomy: technique and results. *Hand Clin* 2004; **20**:61–70.

8. Atasoy E. Combined surgical treatment of thoracic outlet syndrome: transaxillary first rib resection and transcervical scalenectomy. *Hand Clin* 2004;**20**:71–82.

9. Abdellaoui A, Atwan M, Reid F, Wilson P. Endoscopic assisted transaxillary first rib resection. *Interact Cardiovasc Thorac Surg* 2007;**6**:644–6.

10. Krasna MJ. Thoracoscopic sympathectomy. *Thorac Surg Clin* 2010;**20**:323–30.

11. Li J, Wang L, Wang J. Video-assisted thoracoscopic sympathectomy for congenital long QT syndromes. *Pacing Clin Electrophysiol* 2003;**26**: 870–3.

12. Gutierrez O, Garita E, Salazar C. Thoracoscopic sympathectomy for incessant polymorphic ventricular tachycardia in chronic chagasic myocarditis: a case report. *Int J Cardiol* 2007; **119**:255–7.

13. Scott PA, Sandilands AJ, Morris GE, Morgan JM. Successful treatment of catecholaminergic polymorphic ventricular tachycardia with bilateral thoracoscopic sympathectomy. *Heart Rhythm* 2008;**5**:1461–3.

14. Moffat CE, Hayes WG, Nyamekye IK. Durability of botulinum toxin treatment for axillary hyperhidrosis. *Eur J Vasc Endovasc Surg* 2009;**38**:188–91.

15. Weksler B, Luketich JD, Shende MR. Endoscopic thoracic sympathectomy: at what level should you perform surgery? *Thorac Surg Clin* 2008; **18**:183–91.

16. Weight CS, Raitt D, Barrie WW. Thoracoscopic sympathectomy: a one-port technique. *Aust N Z J Surg* 2000;**70**:800.

17. Ramsaroop L, Partab P, Singh B, Satyapal KS. Thoracic origin of a sympathetic supply to the upper limb: the 'nerve of Kuntz' revisited. *J Anat* 2001; **199**:675–82.

18. Assalia A, Kopelman D, Markovitz R, Hashmonai M. Intrapleural analgesia following thoracoscopic sympathectomy for palmar hyperhidrosis: a prospective, randomized trial. *Surg Endosc* 2003;**17**:921–2.

Chapter 18

Surgery for vascular access in renal dialysis

Carl Moores

Procedures establishing vascular access in patients requiring haemodialysis are among the commonest operations carried out by vascular surgeons. Partly, this is because the number of patients with end-stage renal disease has been steadily rising over the past few years. For example, in 2008 in the United Kingdom, over 47 000 patients were receiving renal replacement therapy and in the same year 6 600 patients started renal replacement therapy. Of these, some 70% were undergoing haemodialysis at 3 months [1]. Furthermore, there is a relatively high reintervention rate to keep arteriovenous grafts and fistulas functioning, and a relatively high long-term failure rate means that many patients will require multiple grafts or fistulas during their time on dialysis.

For successful haemodialysis it is necessary to have vascular access that can provide an extracorporeal blood flow rate of at least 300 ml/minute and can be used up to three times per week. There are three main forms of vascular access:

- indwelling dialysis catheters
- arteriovenous fistulas
- arteriovenous grafts.

Indwelling dialysis catheters

In some patients, vascular access is obtained via an indwelling dialysis catheter sited in a central vein. Indwelling catheters have the advantage that they can be used for dialysis immediately after they have been inserted without the 'maturation' time required for arteriovenous fistulas and grafts. However, they have the disadvantage of a relatively high incidence of catheter infection and thrombosis. In particular, central vein thrombosis is a serious complication of these catheters and they are often only used when a patient is waiting for surgery to create an arteriovenous

fistula or graft, while waiting for a graft to mature, or following the failure of a fistula or graft. Where long-term use is anticipated, a dialysis catheter is usually tunnelled to reduce the risk of infection.

Arteriovenous fistulas

An arteriovenous fistula is a direct surgical anastomosis made between an artery and vein. After a period of maturation, dialysis needles can be inserted into the dilated vein [2–5]. There are three sites in the upper limb where arteriovenous fistulas are routinely created (see Figure 18.1):

- between the radial artery and the cephalic vein at the wrist
- between the brachial artery and the cephalic vein in the upper arm
- between the brachial artery and the basilic vein in the upper arm.

The site of the fistula is usually dictated by the size and condition of the arteries and veins. Duplex ultrasound can be used preoperatively to assess the diameter of vessels and to estimate the blood flow through them. This information allows the surgeon to choose a suitable site to create the fistula. Best practice is to site the fistula as distally as possible, which reduces the risk of distal limb ischaemia postoperatively.

The most distal fistula is the radiocephalic fistula, or Brescia–Cimino fistula, first described in 1966. It is created at the wrist by anastomosing the radial artery to the cephalic vein at the level of the distal radius, or alternatively by anastomosing the thenar branch of the radial artery to the cephalic vein in the anatomical snuffbox.

A radiocephalic fistula must support an adequate initial blood flow to allow it to mature to the stage

Core Topics in Vascular Anaesthesia, ed. Carl Moores and Alastair F. Nimmo. Published by Cambridge University Press.
© Cambridge University Press 2012.

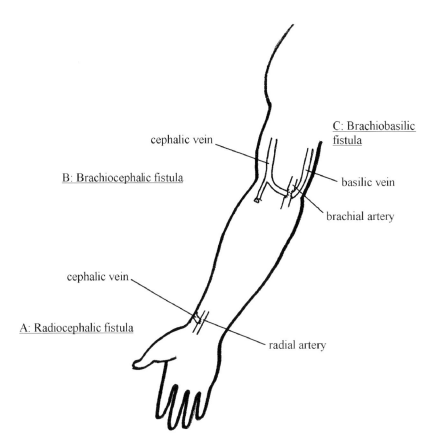

cephalic vein

C: Brachiobasilic
fistula

B: Brachiocephalic fistula

basilic vein

brachial artery

cephalic vein

A: Radiocephalic fistula

radial artery

Figure 18.1 Three common sites of arteriovenous fistula formation in the arm. (A) Radiocephalic (Brescia–Cimino) fistula. (B) Brachiocephalic fistula. (C) Brachiobasilic fistula. The basilic vein is situated deep in the arm, and so needs to be transposed to a more superficial position.

where it can be used for haemodialysis. If the radial artery is narrow and calcified or the cephalic vein is small in diameter, as assessed by ultrasound examination, this is unlikely to happen and a more proximal site is selected.

Either a brachiocephalic or a brachiobasilic fistula may be formed in the upper arm just above the elbow. The cephalic vein is quite superficial and therefore well placed for haemodialysis; however the basilic artery lies deep in the arm and requires to be transposed to a more accessible position before it can be used for dialysis. This transposition may be done at the time of the fistula formation, or later after the fistula has matured.

An arteriovenous fistula matures over a period of several weeks in response to the increased blood flow. Typically, the artery increases in diameter by 50% and, in the majority of cases, there is retrograde blood flow in the artery distal to the anastomosis: in other words, blood flows back from distal limb towards the fistula. The flow through the vein increases from a few millilitres per minute to over 500 ml/minute. The

vein dilates in response to the increase in blood pressure and to increased shear-stress in the vein wall caused by the higher blood flow. The vein diameter increases by about 150% until, after maturation, blood flow is sufficient to support haemodialysis and the vein wall is sufficiently thickened not to tear during needle insertion.

Maturation takes 4–6 weeks for upper arm fistulas and up to 8 weeks for radiocephalic fistulas. Furthermore, 20–50% of newly created fistulas never reach the stage where they can be used for haemodialysis (primary failure), either because of thrombosis or a failure to mature, and therefore additional surgical intervention and a further period of maturation may be required. For these reasons, fistulas are usually created some time before dialysis is anticipated. The Renal Association in the United Kingdom recommends that fistulas should be created shortly after a patient reaches chronic kidney disease stage 4 [6]. This generally means creating a fistula between 3 months and 1 year prior to dialysis being required. This allows adequate time for a fistula to mature while reducing the risk of fistulas being created which turn out not to be required.

Arteriovenous grafts

An arteriovenous graft is formed by interposing a length of graft material between an artery and a vein. The graft is usually artificial (e.g. polytetrafluoroethylene, PTFE) although cadaveric human or animal veins can also be used. The dialysis needles are inserted directly into the graft. There are a number of sites where an arteriovenous graft can be sited (Figure 18.2): in the forearm between the radial artery and a vein in the antecubital fossa, and in the upper arm between the brachial artery and the axillary vein. The grafts may be straight or formed into a loop. It is also possible to place grafts in sites outwith the upper limb, although this is usually only done where it is not possible to site an upper limb graft. For example, a loop of graft may be placed between the femoral artery and the femoral vein (looped thigh graft) or across the upper chest between the axially artery and the contralateral axillary vein ('necklace' graft).

Arteriovenous grafts can be used after only 2–3 weeks, compared to the longer period of maturation that is required for arteriovenous fistulas; indeed synthetic polyurethane grafts can be used after only 24 hours. Furthermore, the primary failure rate for arteriovenous grafts, 15–20%, is lower than for arteriovenous fistulas. Nevertheless, the long-term patency rate for arteriovenous grafts is lower than for arteriovenous fistulas and they carry a significant risk of infection. For these reasons, the UK Renal Association recommends that an arteriovenous fistula is formed in the first instance where possible.

Anaesthetic management

Radiocephalic and brachiocephalic fistulas are often formed under local infiltrative anaesthesia, although regional or general anaesthesia can be used. The formation of a brachiobasilic fistula may also be done under local anaesthesia, but the transposition of the basilic vein requires general or regional anaesthesia.

General anaesthesia

Patients presenting for surgery for vascular access for haemodialysis are often quite elderly (the median age

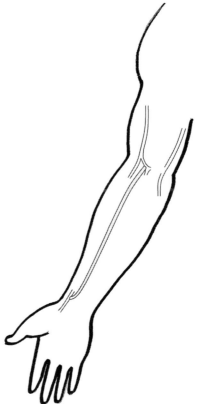

Figure 18.2 Example of a forearm arteriovenous graft, between the radial artery and an antecubital fossa vein. Dialysis needles are inserted into the graft itself.

of patients starting haemodialysis in the United Kingdom is 64) and renal failure is associated with a number of comorbidites. In the United Kingdom, 25% patients starting renal replacement therapy have diabetes, which in itself increases perioperative risk. Furthermore, renal disease is an independent predictor of cardiovascular disease; about 25% of patients starting renal replacement therapy have established ischaemic heart disease, 10% have cerebrovascular disease and 12% have peripheral vascular disease [7].

Some patients undergoing vascular access surgery will be in end-stage renal failure, but many will have surgery before they reach this stage in order to allow time for arteriovenous fistulas or grafts to mature. In these patients, it is therefore important that everything possible is done to preserve what renal function they have left, and nephrotoxic drugs, hypotension and dehydration should be avoided at all costs.

Renal patients are very often chronically anaemic. However, for the formation of a fistula or graft this rarely requires treatment. Renal failure has a complex effect on coagulation. Although uraemia may influence platelet function (uraemic thrombocytopathy), it has nevertheless been shown in studies using thromboelastography that these patients are often hypercoagulable. Overall, studies support the use of intravenous heparin during the formation of arteriovenous fistulas in order to reduce the risk of early thrombosis leading to primary fistula failure.

Patients who are already undergoing haemodialysis are usually dialysed the evening before surgery. This can lead then to be relatively fluid depleted, which is further complicated by the fact that they are generally fluid restricted.

Pharmacology in renal failure

Renal failure can have multiple effects on the pharmacokinetics of drugs. Albumin concentration is low although the concentration of other proteins to which drugs bind may be elevated. Furthermore, the protein binding of drugs can be affected by acidaemia and also the accumulation of organic acids. Some drugs, or active metabolites, undergo predominantly renal excretion, and these will accumulate in renal failure.

The pharmacokinetics of propofol is unchanged in renal failure and total intravenous anaesthesia can be used. Morphine should be used with caution in renal patients, as morphine-6-glucuronide, an active metabolite of morphine, is excreted by the kidneys and can therefore accumulate. The clearance of fentanyl is reduced in renal failure, but it undergoes hepatic metabolism with no active metabolites. The elimination of alfentanil is not altered by renal failure, although reduced protein binding means that a smaller dose may be required. Atracurium is the neuromuscular blocking drug of choice in renal failure, as it undergoes Hoffman degeneration and hepatic metabolism and so its duration of action is not altered. Despite initial concerns about sevoflurane being associated with raised plasma fluoride levels, its use is not associated with changes in sensitive indices of renal tubular function and it would therefore appear that it is a safe agent for use in patients with chronic renal failure.

Regional anaesthesia

Surgery with a brachial plexus block offers an alternative to general anaesthesia in what is a relatively high-risk group of patients.

Initiating a brachial plexus block with lidocaine provides a block of rapid onset and sufficiently long duration to complete an arteriovenous fistula or graft. The duration of brachial plexus blocks does not appear to be different in patients in renal failure compared to other patients. The choice of brachial plexus block depends upon the site of surgery and the preference of the anaesthetist. In general, axillary blocks or supraclavicular blocks are suitable for forearm anastomoses. Using a regional technique for basilic vein transposition may well require anaesthesia of the upper inner aspect of the arm. The intercostobrachial nerve supplies this area of skin and may need to be blocked separately.

There may be advantages to creating arteriovenous fistulas or grafts under regional anaesthesia. In one study of patients undergoing vascular access surgery under axillary brachial plexus blocks, both the basilic and cephalic veins underwent a mean dilatation of 1.5 mm, to the extent that either the site of operation or the type of procedure (fistula as opposed to graft) was changed in a third of cases [8].

Other studies in patients undergoing surgery with a brachial plexus block have shown an increased blood flow through fistulas that persisted into the immediate postoperative period. A similarly increased blood flow through newly created arteriovenous fistulas has also been shown to follow stellate ganglion blocks [9]. There is, however, no evidence to suggest that regional anaesthesia confers any long-term benefit in terms of the longevity of either fistulas or grafts.

Complications of arteriovenous fistulas and grafts

Failure

Unfortunately, both arteriovenous fistulas and grafts have a relatively high failure rate. In terms of longevity, arteriovenous fistulas can be expected to last for about 5 years, with a failure rate of about 30% in the first year. Arteriovenous grafts last about 2–3 years.

In the first instance, fistulas may fail to mature sufficiently to support dialysis. One reason for this is that tributaries of the vein can divert blood out of the fistula. These tributaries can be located using ultrasound and ligated, increasing the blood flow through the fistula and promoting maturation. A fistula may fail to mature simply because there is insufficient blood flow through the arteriovenous anastomosis. The anastomosis may therefore require revision, or the fistula may need to be resited. Factors associated with primary failure of fistulas include: female sex, diabetes, obesity and peripheral vascular disease.

The commonest reasons for late failure of an arteriovenous fistula or graft are stenosis and/or thrombosis. In both grafts and fistulas, stenosis is most likely to occur on the venous side. Neointimal hyperplasia of the vein or venous anastomosis is the most common cause of stenosis, and is caused by the proliferation of smooth muscle cells in response to vascular injury. Treatments include thrombolysis, angioplasty, embolectomy, surgical thrombectomy and surgical revision. Fistulas are generally more amenable to treatment than grafts, but often it is necessary to create a new anastomosis.

Aneurysm formation

Aneurysmal dilatation of an arteriovenous fistula can, if severe enough, lead to necrosis of the overlying skin. If the skin appears threatened, a surgical repair may be needed. The aneurysmal segment can either be shortened, or excised and bypassed.

Infection

Arteriovenous grafts are prone to infection. This is unsurprising, given that they are made of artificial material and are repeatedly punctured by needles passing through the overlying skin. Furthermore, renal patients usually suffer from a degree of immunosuppression. Antibiotics can be used to treat graft infections, but it may be necessary to remove part or all of the graft.

Claudication

Both arteriovenous fistulas and grafts can lead to steal causing ischaemic symptoms in the distal part of the affected limb. These symptoms are more usually associated with grafts or fistulas formed in the upper arm and are sometimes so severe as to warrant surgical

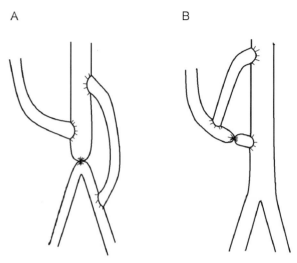

Figure 18.3 Operative approaches to relieve forearm steal. A In a distal revascularisation interval ligation (DRIL) procedure, blood is directed from the proximal brachial artery to a forearm artery. The brachial artery is ligated distal to the original anastomosis with the arteriovenous fistula or graft. B In a proximalisation procedure, blood is directed between the proximal brachial artery and arterial end of the arteriovenous fistula or graft. The original anastomosis with the distal brachial artery is closed.

intervention. In order to reduce the blood flow through the fistula or graft, the anastomosis may be narrowed by surgical revision, or by placing a band around it.

In an alternative approach to relieving steal, blood can be diverted from the proximal part of the brachial artery (where blood flow is high) to either the fistula itself or to a forearm artery (see Figure 18.3). In the distal revascularisation and interval ligation (DRIL) procedure, blood from the proximal brachial artery is taken via a graft past the fistula to the distal artery. The artery is then ligated just distal to the fistula. In a proximalisation of arterial inflow procedure, a bypass is constructed between the proximal artery and the fistula itself. The original anastomosis is then closed.

References

1. Ansell DC.C. *UK Renal Registry 12th Annual Report.* Bristol: UK Renal Registry, 2009. Available from: www.renalreg.com/reports/2009.html.

2. Konner K. A primer on the av fistula – Achilles' heel, but also Cinderella of haemodialysis. *Nephrol Dial Transplant* 1999;**14**:2094–8.

3. Maya ID, Allon M. Vascular access: core curriculum 2008. *Am J Kidney Dis* 2008;**51**:702–8.

4. Singh N, Starnes BW, Andersen C. Successful angioaccess. *Surg Clin North Am* 2007;**87**:1213–28.

5. Vazquez MA. Vascular access for dialysis: recent lessons and new insights. *Curr Opin Nephrol Hypertens* 2009;**18**: 116–21.

6. Fluck RK, Kumwenda M. *Vascular Access for Haemodialysis.* 2011. Petersfield: Renal Association, Available from: www.renal.org/

Clinical/GuidelinesSection/
VascularAccess.aspx.

7. Craig RG, Hunter JM. Recent
    developments in the perioperative
    management of adult patients
    with chronic kidney disease.
    Br J Anaesth 2008;**101**:296–310.

8. Laskowski IA, Verhagen HJ, Gagne
    PJ, *et al.*, Regional nerve block allows
    for optimization of planning in the
    creation of arteriovenous access for
    hemodialysis by improving
    superficial venous dilatation.
    Ann Vasc Surg 2007;**21**:730–3.

9. Yildirim V, Doganci S,
    Yanarates O, *et al.*, Does
    preemptive stellate ganglion
    blockage increase the patency
    of radiocephalic arteriovenous
    fistula? *Scand Cardiovasc J* 2006;
    40:380–4.

Index

abciximab, 35, 76
abdominal aortic aneurysm, 10,
    101–107
  anaesthesia, 103
  emergency procedure, 137–145
  epidemiology, 101
  intraoperative monitoring, 104–105
  postoperative management,
    105–106
  preoperative assessment, 102
  risk factors, 102
  ruptured. *See* aortic aneurysm
    rupture
  screening, 101
  surgical blood loss, 105
  surgical technique, 102
  symptomatic, 144
abdominal compartment syndrome,
    63
ACE inhibitors, 26, 40, 103
acidosis, 79
activated clotting time, 81
activated partial thromboplastin time,
    80
acute aortic syndrome. *See* aortic
    dissection
acute coronary syndromes, 22–23, 34
acute kidney injury, 123
acute limb ischaemia, 148
  treatment, 153
acute normovolaemic haemodilution,
    95
adenosine, 131
ADP receptor inhibitors.
    See clopidogrel and prasugrel
aerobic capacity, 14
aerobic fitness, 14
aldosterone blockers, 26
alpha2-adrenergic agonists, 39
amaurosis fugax, 170–171
amlodipine, 40
amputation. *See* lower limb
    amputation
anaerobic threshold, 15
anaesthesia, 48–51
  epidural. *See* epidural anaesthesia
  general, 48–50
  intravenous, 50
  postoperative care, 50

procedures
  abdominal aortic aneurysm, 103
  carotid body tumours, 180
  carotid endarterectomy, 170–179
  EVAR, 124–127
  lower limb amputation, 163
  renal dialysis, vascular access, 190
  revascularisation, 154–155
  thoracic outlet syndrome, 185
  thoracoabdominal aneurysm, 111
  thoracoscopic sympathectomy,
    186
  regional. *See* regional anaesthesia
  volatile, 50
angina pectoris, 23
angioplasty, 3
angiotensin converting enzyme
    inhibitors. *See* ACE inhibitors
angiotensin receptor blockers, 40, 103
ankle-brachial index, 2, 149
anterior spinal artery syndrome, 113
anticoagulants, 76–78, 95
  See also individual drugs
antifibrinolytics, 78
antihypertensive therapy, 25
antiplatelet therapy, 32–34, 75–76, 95
  and neuraxial blocks, 35
  and stents, 42
  dual, 34–35
  haemorrhage versus thrombosis, 43
  peripheral arterial disease, 150
  preoperative, 103
  response to, 35
  See also individual drugs
antithrombin, 72, 74
aortic aneurysm, 4–7
  abdominal. *See* abdominal aortic
    aneurysm
  clinical presentation, 5
  management, 5–6
  pathology, 4
aortic aneurysm rupture, 8, 137–144
  assessment, 139–140
  endovascular repair, 139, 144
  management, 138–139
  open repair, 140–144
  pre-operative fluid resuscitation,
    140
  presentation and diagnosis, 137–138

aortic cross clamping, 104
aortic dissection, 7–8
aortic occlusion, acute, 144
aortic visceral debranching, 122
aorto-caval fistula, 138
aorto-enteric fistula, 138
aorto-femoral bypass grafts, 152
  anaesthesia, 155
aorto-uni-iliac stent grafts, 120, 139
apheresis, 92
aprotonin, 78
arterial blood pressure, 54
arterial thoracic outlet syndrome, 185
arteriovenous fistula, 188–190
arteriovenous grafts, 190
artery of Adamkiewicz, 126
ASCET, 3
aspirin, 32–33, 75, 103
  haemorrhage risk, 33
  peripheral arterial disease, 150
  thrombosis risk, 33
  with clopidogrel, 34
  with dipyridamole, 34
ASTRAL trial, 2
atenolol, 142, 178
atherosclerosis, 1–2
  and upper limb ischaemia, 183
atracurium, 175
autologous transfusion, 95
  acute normovolaemic
    haemodilution, 95
  intraoperative cell salvage, 96
  preoperative autologous blood
    donation, 95
axillo-bifemoral grafts, 153

balanced electrolyte solutions, 63
balloon angioplasty, 3
balloon embolectomy, 153
bare metal stents, 23, 42
BASIL trial, 3
beta-blockers, 26, 37–39
  and heart rate, 38
  chronic blockade, 39
  efficacy of, 38
  patient selection, 39
  preoperative, 103
biomarkers, 20
bleeding, 71

blood component therapy, 92–93
  practical aspects, 99
blood conservation, 94–97
  autologous transfusion, 95
  preoperative management, 95
blood pressure
  arterial, 54
  invasive monitoring, 141
blood transfusion, 92–99
body mass index (BMI), 17
brachial plexus block, 191
brain natriuretic peptide, 20, 60
branched stent grafts, 120

CABG, 23–24, 41
  preoperative, 103, 111
calcium channel blockers, 40
cardiac biomarkers, 60–61
cardiac output, 56–57
cardiac resynchronisation, 27
cardiac risk scoring, 18–19
cardiopulmonary exercise testing.
    See CPET
CardioQ™, 57
carotid angioplasty and stenting, 4
carotid artery disease, 3–4, 170–179
carotid artery shunting, 171
carotid artery stenting, 178
carotid body tumours, 179–180
carotid endarterectomy, 3, 10
  awake patients, 174–175
  complications, 172
  general anaesthesia, 172, 175–176
  perioperative hypertension/
    hypotension, 177
  postoperative management,
    177–178
  preoperative assessment and risk
    management, 172
  regional anaesthesia, 172–174
  risks and benefits, 171
  surgical techniques, 170–171
carotid-subclavian bypass, 6
CARP trial, 41
CASP-19 scale, 12
catheter-directed thrombolysis, 153
central neuraxial blockade, 124–125
  contraindications, 129
central venous pressure, 54, 142
cerebral monitoring, 176
cerebral protection, 176
cerebrospinal fluid. See CSF
cerebrovascular accident. See stroke
cervical epidural anaesthesia, 173
cervical plexus block, 174
cervical ribs, 184
choice of procedure, 11
chronic obstructive pulmonary
    disease. See COPD

chronological age, 13
cilostazol, 150
citrate phosphate dextrose (CPD), 92
clamp and go technique, 6
clevidipine, 125
clonidine, 39, 178
clopidogrel, 23, 33–34, 75, 103
  perioperative, 34
  peripheral arterial disease, 150
  with aspirin, 34
clot strength, 82
clotting time, 83
coagulation, 72
  limitation of, 74
coagulation time analysers, 80
co-existing disease, 22
  management, 28
colloids, 62, 64–67
  dextrans, 65
  effects on coagulation, 67, 79
  effects on renal function, 67–68
  gelatins, 64
  human albumin solution, 66
  hydroxyethyl starches, 65–66
computerised tomographic
    angiography, 3, 151
continuous peripheral nerve blockade,
    167
contrast nephropathy, 124
COPD, 22, 28
coronary artery bypass grafting.
    See CABG
coronary artery disease
  acute coronary syndromes, 22–23
  revascularisation. See coronary
    artery revascularisation
coronary artery revascularisation,
    23–24, 40–43
  future of, 43
  implications for anaesthesia, 42
  See also CABG and stents.
CPET, 14–17, 28, 102
  anaerobic threshold, 15
  peak oxygen consumption, 14
  ventilatory equivalents, 15
C-reactive protein, 20
creatinine kinase, 60
Creutzfeld Jacob disease, variant
    (vCJD), 92–93
critical limb ischaemia, 147
cryoprecipitate, 93, 97–98
crystalloids, 62
CSF drainage, 116
  EVAR, 126–128, 129
  TEVAR, 129
  thoracoabdominal aneurysm,
    114–115
customised probability model
    (CPM), 19

dabigatran, 77
D-dimer, 75
DECREASE-V trial, 41
dexmeditomidine, 39
dextrans, 65
diabetes mellitus, 22, 26, 146, 161
  treatment, 150
diamorphine, 155
digital subtraction angiography, 151
diltiazem, 40
dipyridamole, 33, 76
  with aspirin, 34
dipyridamole thallium scanning, 19
dobutamine stress echocardiography,
    19
drug-eluting stents, 23, 42
duplex ultrasound, 2, 151
Dutch Randomised Endovascular
    Aneurysm Management
    (DREAM) trial, 133
dyslipidaemia, 146

ECG, 52–54
  exercise, 19
echocardiography
  transoesophageal.
    See transoesophageal
    echocardiography
ECST, 3
Edinburgh Artery Study, 2
Edinburgh Ruptured Aneurysm
    (ERA) score, 138
efficacy of vascular surgery, 10
Eisenmenger's syndrome, 180
electrocardiogram. See ECG
electrocautery, 186
EloHaes®, 66
endarterectomy, 153
endoleaks
  classification, 132
  detection, 130
endovascular aortic repair. See EVAR
endovascular repair, 5
endovascular stent grafts. See EVAR
enteral nutrition, 105
epidural anaesthesia, 48
  cardiac complications, 49
  cervical, 173
  EVAR, 125
  mortality, 49
  phantom limb pain, 167
  respiratory complications, 48
epsilon-aminocaproic acid, 78
eptifibatide, 35, 76
erythropoietin, 95
esmolol, 125, 178
etomidate, 141
EVAR, 119–136
  abdominal position (EVAAR), 134

EVAR (cont.)
  anaesthesia, 124–127
    central neuraxial blockade,
      124–125
    general, 125
    local, 124
  complications, 132–133
  evolution of, 119
  haemodynamic manipulation,
    131–132
  hybrid procedures, 121–122
  indications and contraindications,
    122–123
  intraoperative monitoring, 126–131
    CSF drainage, 126–129
    invasive arterial monitoring, 130
    SEPs and MEPs, 128–130
    transoesophageal
      echocardiography, 130–131
  outcome, 133–134
  perioperative renal protection,
    123–124
  preoperative evaluation, 123
  retroperitoneal incision/approach,
    121
  types of, 120
EVAR 1 study, 13, 133
exercise ECG, 19
exercise therapy
  intermittent claudication, 150

factor IX, 72
factor VII, 72
factor VIII, 72
factor X, 72
factor Xa inhibitors, 77
fasciotomy, 153
fatty streak, 1
femoro-distal bypass grafts, 153
femoro-femoral bypass grafts, 3, 153
femoro-popliteal bypass grafts, 153
fenestrated stent grafts, 120
fentanyl, 140–141, 155, 175
FEV$_1$, 16
fibrin, 72
fibrin degradation products, 75
fibrinogen, 72, 97
  concentrate, 87
  concentration, 80
  reduced levels, 78
fibrinolysis, 74
fibrinolytics, 78
fibrous cap, 1
FloTrac/Vigileo, 57
fluid responsiveness, 58–60
fondaparinux, 77
fresh frozen plasma (FFP), 87, 92–93,
  97–98
FTc, 57

functional haemodynamic
  monitoring, 58–60
FVC, 16

gabapentin
  phantom limb pain, 167
gelatins, 64
Gelofusin®, 64
general anaesthesia, 48–50
  carotid endarterectomy, 175–176
global end diastolic volume index, 59
glyceryl trinitrate, 142, 178
glycoprotein IIb/IIIa inhibitors, 35, 76
  See also individual drugs
glycoprotein IIb/IIIa receptor, 74
graft occlusion, 89–90

Haemaccel®, 64
haemorrhage, 43
haemostasis, 71–75
  clot formation, 71
  drugs affecting, 75–78
  impaired, 78–79
    diagnosis, 79–88
    treatment, 87–88
  point of care testing, 80
haemostatic sealants/glues, 96
HAES-Steril®, 66
health objectives of surgery, 10
heart failure, 26–28
Heart Outcomes Prevention
  Evaluation (HOPE) study, 150
heart rate, 38
Hemocue®, 105
Hemohes®, 66
heparin, 76, 157
  and thrombocytopaenia, 76
  low molecular weight, 76
  preoperative, 103
Hespan®, 65–66
Hetastarch, 66
Hexastarch, 66
Hextend®, 66
HMG coenzyme A reductase
  inhibitors. See statins
hospital acquired generalised
  interstitial oedema
  (HAGIE), 63
human albumin solution, 66
hydralazine, 178
hydroxyethyl starches, 65–66
  effects on renal function, 68
hyperchloraemic acidosis, 63
hypercholesterolaemia, 22, 24
hyperfibrinolysis, 79
hyperhomocysteinaemia, 147
hyperkalaemia, 99
hyperlipidaemia
  treatment, 150

hypertension, 22, 25–26, 147
  perioperative, 177
  postoperative, 177
  treatment, 150
hypocalcaemia, 79, 99, 112
hypomagnesaemia, 112
hypotension
  intraoperative, 127
  perioperative, 177
hypotensive resuscitation, 140
hypothermia, 79, 99, 105, 112
  spinal cord protection, 115
hypovolaemia, 142

ilio-femoral bypass grafts, 3
indwelling dialysis catheters, 188
inferior mesenteric artery, 102
infra-inguinal arterial bypass
  grafts, 153
  anaesthesia, 156
infrainguinal disease, 3
innominate artery disease, 4
inspiratory capacity (IC), 16
intermittent claudication, 2, 3, 147
  treatment, 149
intermittent positive-pressure
  ventilation, 176
International Normalised Ratio
  (INR), 78
intraoperative blood pressure
  monitoring, 25
intraoperative cell salvage (ICS),
  96, 105
intrathoracic blood volume index, 59
intravenous fluid therapy, 62
  effects on coagulation, 64
  effects on renal function, 63
  optimisation of volume, 68
  See also individual constituents
ischaemic colitis, 106
ischaemic heart disease, 22
ivabradine, 40

Javid shunt, 171

ketamine, 141, 155
  phantom limb pain, 167

labetalol, 178
laryngeal mask airway, 176
Lee's Revised Cardiac Risk Index, 18
left carotid subclavian bypass, 121
lethal surgery, 11
levobupivacaine, 155
LiDCO, 57, 59, 105
lidocaine, 167
local anaesthesia
  EVAR, 124
low molecular weight heparins, 76

lower limb amputation, 161–169
  diabetes mellitus, 161
  incidence, 161
  intraoperative care, 162–164
  level of, 162
  mortality, 164
  phantom sensation, 165
  post-amputation pain
    pathophysiology, 165–166
    phantom limb pain, 165–167
    stump pain, 165
  postoperative care, 164–165
  preoperative assessment, 162
  vascular disease, 161
lower limb ischaemia, 2–3
lower limb revascularisation.
    See revascularisation

magnetic resonance angiography, 2, 151
Marfan's syndrome, 5, 108
maximum voluntary ventilation
    (MVV), 16
MEPs, 113, 128–130
mesenteric artery disease, 4
mesenteric ischaemia, 2
metoprolol, 178
mivazerol, 39
modular bifurcated stent grafts, 120
monitoring, 52–61
  integrated, 61
  See also individual modalities
morphine, 141
  in renal failure, 191
motor evoked potentials. *See* MEPs
myocardial infarction, 32
  perioperative, 106
  postoperative, 37
  post-revascularisation, 158
  ST elevation. *See* STEMI
myocardial ischaemia, 37, 157
  ECG changes, 53

naftidrofuryl, 150
naloxone, 115
neuraxial blocks, 35
neurogenic thoracic outlet syndrome, 184
NHS Abdominal Aortic Aneurysm
    Screening Programme
    (NAAASP), 101
nicardipine, 178
nifedipine, 40, 178
nitrates, 40
non-steroidal anti-inflammatory
    drugs. *See* NSAIDs
NSAIDs, 106

oesophageal Doppler monitoring, 57,
    104
overweight, 17

papaverine, 115
paracetamol, 106
paraplegia, 113
patient controlled analgesia, 107
peak oxygen consumption, 14
Penfield homunculus, 166
Pentaspan®, 66
Pentastarch, 66
pentoxifylline, 151
percutaneous coronary interventions,
    23, 41
  preoperative, 103
  See also stents.
percutaneous transluminal
    angioplasty, 152
perioperative risk reduction,
    32–38
peripheral arterial disease, 2–3, 146
  assessment, 148–149
    ankle-brachial index, 149
  classification, 148
  clinical presentation, 2, 147–148
  epidemiology, 2, 146
  investigations, 2, 151
  natural history, 147
  pathophysiology, 146
  risk factors, 146–147
  treatment, 149–151
    interventional, 151
    revascularisation.
      See revascularisation
peripheral revascularisation, 49
permissive hypotension, 140, 144
phantom limb pain, 165
  prevention, 166–167
  treatment, 167
phantom sensation, 165
physical fitness, 26
physiological age, 13
PiCCO, 59, 105
plaque, 1, 146, 170
Plasmalyte A, 63
Plasmalyte B, 63
Plasmasteril®, 66
plasmin, 74
plasminogen, 74
platelet concentrate, 93, 98
platelet count, 80
platelet function analysers, 85
platelet transfusion, 87, 97
platelets, 72
postimplantation syndrome, 132
postoperative care, 50
  See also individual procedures
postoperative survival curves, 11
prasugrel, 76
preoperative autologous blood
    donation, 95
preoperative risk, 10–11

preserved systolic function, 28
propofol, 50, 141–142
  in renal failure, 191
protamine, 77
protein C, 74
  activated, 79
protein S, 74
prothrombin, 72
prothrombin complex concentrate,
    78, 97
prothrombin time, 78, 80
Pruitt-Inihara shunt, 171
pulmonary artery catheterisation,
    55–56
pulmonary artery flotation catheter
    (PAFC), 104
pulmonary artery occlusion pressure,
    55
pulse contour analysis, 56, 105
pulse pressure variation, 59

quality of life, 12

radiation arteritis, 183
randomised controlled trials
    (RCTs), 10
rapid ventricular pacing, 132
REACH registry, 2
red cell concentrate (RCC), 92–94
  age of blood, 94
  risks, 93
  transfusion threshold, 94
regional anaesthesia, 48–50
  and peripheral revascularisation, 49
  carotid endarterectomy, 172–174
  complications, 172
  lower limb amputation, 164
  renal dialysis, vascular access, 191
remifentanil, 175
renal dialysis, vascular access,
    188–193
  anaesthesia, 190–191
  arteriovenous fistula, 188–190
  arteriovenous grafts, 190
  complications, 191–192
  indwelling dialysis catheters, 188
renal failure
  dialysis vascular access, 188–193
  pharmacology, 191
renal impairment, 28
renal protection, 115, 123, 124
reperfusion hypotension, 126
resting metabolic rate (RMR), 17
revascularisation
  anaesthesia, 154–155
  complications, 158–159
  intraoperative considerations,
    156–158
  postoperative care, 158

revascularisation (cont.)
  preoperative assessment and risk
    management, 153
  See also individual procedures
Revised Cardiac Risk Index, 18
right atrial inflow occlusion, 132
right ventricular end diastolic
    volume, 55
Ringer's lactate, 63
risk stratification, 11–12
rivaroxaban, 77
ROTEM® analyser.
      See thromboelastography/
      thromboelastometry
ruptured aortic aneurysm. See aortic
    aneurysm rupture

SEPs, 113, 128–130
Serious Hazards of Transfusion (SHOT)
    haemovigilance scheme, 93
serotonergic noradrenergic reuptake
    inhibitors (SNRIs), 167
smoking, 26, 146
smoking cessation, 149
sodium nitroprusside, 178
somatosensory evoked potentials.
      See SEPs
spinal cord ischaemia, 106
spinal cord protection
  CSF drainage. See CSF drainage
  drugs for
    naloxone, 115
    papaverine, 115
  hypothermia, 115
  intraoperative management, 113
  procedures
    EVAR, 126–129
    TEVAR, 129
    thoracoabdominal aneurysm,
      113–116
  surgical strategies, 113
statins, 3, 26, 35–37, 103, 150
  efficacy, 35–37
  safety, 37
STEMI, 22
stents, 3, 41–42
  and antiplatelet therapy, 42
  bare metal, 23, 42
  carotid artery, 178
  drug-eluting, 23, 42
  endovascular stent grafts. See EVAR
  implications for anaesthesia, 42
streptokinase, 78
stroke, 170–172
  watershed, 172
stroke volume, 59
subclavian artery disease, 4
subclavian steal syndrome, 183

supra-renal aneurysm repair, 6
surgery. See individual procedures
survival, 11
  and aerobic fitness, 14
survival age, 13
survival hazard ratios, 16
survival variables, 13
suxamethonium, 141
systolic blood pressure, 25
systolic pressure variation, 59

TAAA. See thoracoabdominal
    aneurysm
TEG® analyser.
      See thromboelastography/
      thromboelastometry
tenase (FVIIIa/IXa) complex, 72
Tetraspan®, 66
Tetrastarch, 66
TEVAR, 6
  complications, 132
  CSF drainage, 129
  outcome, 134
  paraplegia after, 129
  preoperative revascularisation, 122
  See also EVAR
thermodilution, 56
thiopentone, 141
thoracic endovascular aneurysm
    repair. See TEVAR
thoracic outlet syndrome, 183–185
thoracoabdominal aneurysm,
      6, 108–112
  anaesthesia, 111
  classification, 108
  distal aortic perfusion, 109
  extent I, II, III and V repair, 110–111
  intraoperative management, 112–113
  intraoperative monitoring, 112
  postoperative management, 116–117
  preoperative assessment, 111
  renal injury protection, 115
  spinal cord protection, 113–116
thoraco-laparotomy, 116
thoracoscopic sympathectomy, 185–187
thrombin, 72
thrombin burst, 72
thrombin inhibitors, 77
thromboelastography/
      thromboelastometry, 81–85
  value and limitations, 85
thromboembolism, 71
thrombomodulin, 74
thromboplastin, 80
thrombosis, 43, 71, 88–90
  graft occlusion, 89–90
  venous thromboembolism, 88–89
thromboxane A2, 72

tirofiban, 35, 76
tissue factor pathway inhibitor, 74
tissue factor protease inhibitor, 72
tissue plasminogen activator,
    recombinant, 78
total intravenous anaesthesia (TIVA),
    50
tramadol, 167
tranexamic acid, 78
transfusion associated lung injury
    (TRALI), 98
Transfusion Requirements in Critical
    Care (TRICC) trial, 94
transient ischaemic attacks, 171
transoesophageal echocardiography,
    57–58
  avoidance of high contrast dye load
    exposure, 130
  cardiac assessment, 131
  diagnosis of aortic pathology, 130
  endoleak detection, 130
  EVAR, 130–131
  guidewire, sheath and endograft
    location, 130
  TAAA, 112
transversus abdominis plane blocks, 107
tricyclic antidepressants, 167
troponins, 60
tube grafts, 120

underweight, 17
upper limb ischaemia, 182–187
  acute, 182–183
  chronic, 183
  thoracic outlet syndrome, 183–185
  thoracoscopic sympathectomy,
    185–187
urokinase, 78

vasodilators, 104
vasopressors, 104
vecuronium, 175
Venofundin®, 65–66
venous thoracic outlet syndrome,
    184
venous thromboembolism, 88–89
ventilatory equivalents, 15
verapamil, 40
Virchow's triad, 89
visceral ischaemia, 112
vitamin K antagonists, 77
VO_2, 16
Volulyte®, 66
Voluven®, 65–66
von Willebrand factor, 72

warfarin, 77
windsock effect, 131